AF846802

Studies in Big Data

Volume 80

Series Editor

Janusz Kacprzyk, Polish Academy of Sciences, Warsaw, Poland

The series "Studies in Big Data" (SBD) publishes new developments and advances in the various areas of Big Data- quickly and with a high quality. The intent is to cover the theory, research, development, and applications of Big Data, as embedded in the fields of engineering, computer science, physics, economics and life sciences. The books of the series refer to the analysis and understanding of large, complex, and/or distributed data sets generated from recent digital sources coming from sensors or other physical instruments as well as simulations, crowd sourcing, social networks or other internet transactions, such as emails or video click streams and other. The series contains monographs, lecture notes and edited volumes in Big Data spanning the areas of computational intelligence including neural networks, evolutionary computation, soft computing, fuzzy systems, as well as artificial intelligence, data mining, modern statistics and Operations research, as well as self-organizing systems. Of particular value to both the contributors and the readership are the short publication timeframe and the world-wide distribution, which enable both wide and rapid dissemination of research output.

** Indexing: The books of this series are submitted to ISI Web of Science, DBLP, Ulrichs, MathSciNet, Current Mathematical Publications, Mathematical Reviews, Zentralblatt Math: MetaPress and Springerlink.

More information about this series at http://www.springer.com/series/11970

Chinmay Chakraborty · Amit Banerjee ·
Lalit Garg · Joel J. P. C. Rodrigues
Editors

Internet of Medical Things for Smart Healthcare

Covid-19 Pandemic

Springer

Editors
Chinmay Chakraborty
Department of Electronics
and Communication Engineering
Birla Institute of Technology
Ranchi, Jharkhand, India

Amit Banerjee
Department of Physics
Bidhan Chandra College
(Kazi Nazrul University)
Asansol, West Bengal, India

Lalit Garg
Department of Information
and Communication Technology
University of Malta
Msida, Malta

Joel J. P. C. Rodrigues
Federal University of Piauí
Teresina, PI, Brazil

Instituto de Telecomunicações
Covilhã, Portugal

ISSN 2197-6503 ISSN 2197-6511 (electronic)
Studies in Big Data
ISBN 978-981-15-8096-3 ISBN 978-981-15-8097-0 (eBook)
https://doi.org/10.1007/978-981-15-8097-0

© The Editor(s) (if applicable) and The Author(s), under exclusive license to Springer Nature Singapore Pte Ltd. 2020
This work is subject to copyright. All rights are solely and exclusively licensed by the Publisher, whether the whole or part of the material is concerned, specifically the rights of translation, reprinting, reuse of illustrations, recitation, broadcasting, reproduction on microfilms or in any other physical way, and transmission or information storage and retrieval, electronic adaptation, computer software, or by similar or dissimilar methodology now known or hereafter developed.
The use of general descriptive names, registered names, trademarks, service marks, etc. in this publication does not imply, even in the absence of a specific statement, that such names are exempt from the relevant protective laws and regulations and therefore free for general use.
The publisher, the authors and the editors are safe to assume that the advice and information in this book are believed to be true and accurate at the date of publication. Neither the publisher nor the authors or the editors give a warranty, expressed or implied, with respect to the material contained herein or for any errors or omissions that may have been made. The publisher remains neutral with regard to jurisdictional claims in published maps and institutional affiliations.

This Springer imprint is published by the registered company Springer Nature Singapore Pte Ltd.
The registered company address is: 152 Beach Road, #21-01/04 Gateway East, Singapore 189721, Singapore

Preface

The general interest in the Internet of medical things for smart healthcare has been growing significantly because of its enormous and promising application prospects in the advancement of human civilization. Among literally thousands of different technologies related to the Internet of things for smart healthcare, there are some definite trends that have a high impact in the future healthcare and are focused in the current title. This title focuses on the recent advances and different research issues in smart healthcare by seeking out for theoretical, methodological, well-established and validated empirical work dealing with these different topics and covers the interests of a very vast audience from basic science to engineering and technology experts and learners. This hence deserves to be recommended as textbook for engineering and biomedical students, science masters programs and for researchers. The prominent biomedical advances highlighted here may transform the way we look at healthcare, particularly the innovative health technologies and eHealth solutions which address global health concerns on COVID-19 this moment and the importance of these technologies toward improved health system for current and any future pandemic. Some of these technologies offer a solution to many COVID-19 medical needs, focusing on under-resourced regions, developing framework for assessment, management, regulation, by scientific and commercial perspective. The exciting topics included in the current volume : COVID-19 analysis by using machine and deep learning, transmission dynamics and estimation of basic reproduction number (R0) from early outbreak of novel coronavirus (COVID-19) in India, MML classification techniques for the pathogen based on pnuemonia-nCOVID-19 and the detection of closely related lung diseases using efficacious learning algorithms, diagnosing COVID-19 lung inflammation using machine learning algorithms: A comparative study, factors affecting the success of Internet of things for enhancing quality and efficiency implementation in hospitals sector in Jordan during the crises of COVID-19, IoMT-based smart diagnostic/therapeutic kit for pandemic patients, the prediction analysis of COVID-19 cases using ARIMA and Kalman filter models: A case of comparative study, exploration of cough recognition technologies grounded on sensors and artificial intelligence, clinical deep dive and role of Ai/ml techniques in tackling

COVID-19, a review on use of data science for visualization and prediction of the COVID-19 pandemic and early diagnosis of COVID-19 using machine learning models and finally fuzzy cellular automata model for discrete dynamical system representing spread of MERS and COVID-19 virus. We sincerely hope this book title will be extremely useful in providing valuable knowledge and insight related to the application of Internet of medical things for smart healthcare in managing current pandemic and averting many future health crises.

Ranchi, India — Chinmay Chakraborty
Asansol, India — Amit Banerjee
Msida, Malta — Lalit Garg
Teresina, Brazil — Joel J. P. C. Rodrigues

Contents

Editors and Contributors

About the Editors

Dr. Chinmay Chakraborty is an Assistant Professor (Sr.) in the Department of Electronics and Communication Engineering, BIT Mesra, India. His primary areas of research include Wireless body area network, Internet of Medical Things, point-of-care diagnosis, Wireless Networks, Telemedicine, m-Health/e-health, and Medical imaging. Dr. Chakraborty is co-editing Eight books on Smart IoMT, Healthcare Technology, and Sensor Data Analytics with CRC Press, IET, Pan Stanford, and Springer. He received a Young Research Excellence Award, Global Peer Review Award, Young Faculty Award, and Outstanding Researcher Award.

Dr. Amit Banerjee joined the Advanced Device Research Division, Research Institute of Electronics, Shizuoka University, National University Corporation, Japan as a Scientific Researcher in 2016 and was also part of the Innovative Photonics Evolution Research Center at Hamamatsu, Japan. He later joined the Microelectronic Technologies & Devices, Department of Electrical and Computer Engineering of the prestigious National University of Singapore, as Scientist in 2017. Currently Amit is member of 30+ international advisory boards, including Ocuro Science and Technology (biomed-startup); Ominar Innovations (biomed-startup); EDGE196, EntrepreneursFace, Digivalley Innovations; ULVAC Technologies Inc, ISF Analytica & Informatica; Asentrex Global, Arohan Educan Ltd. London, UK; Ambassador, Bentham Science Publishers, among others. Amit holds Ph.D. degree in Semiconductor Technology and has co-authored several scientific papers, presented in several international conferences as plenary and keynote speakers, received several national/international awards, edited seven books. His current work is on THz detectors, compatible with the state-of-the-art medium-scale semiconductor device fabrication processes, with commercial viability as on-chip integrable detector arrays for terahertz imaging.

Dr. Lalit Garg is a Senior Lecturer in Computer Information Systems at the University of Malta, Malta. He is also an Honorary Lecturer at the University of Liverpool, UK. His research interests are missing data handling, machine learning, data mining, mathematical and stochastic modeling, operational research, and their applications, especially in the healthcare domain. He has published over 80 technical papers in refereed high impact journals, conferences, and books and has more than 500 citation count to his publications. He has organized many conferences and also delivered keynotes in many other conferences.

Prof. Joel J. P. C. Rodrigues [S'01, M'06, SM'06, F'20] is a professor at the Federal University of Piauí, Brazil; senior researcher at the *Instituto de Telecomunicações*, Portugal; and collaborator of the Post-Graduation Program on Teleinformatics Engineering at the Federal University of Ceará (UFC), Brazil. He is the leader of the Next Generation Networks and Applications (NetGNA) research group (CNPq), an IEEE Distinguished Lecturer, Member Representative of the IEEE Communications Society on the IEEE Biometrics Council. He was Director for Conference Development—IEEE ComSoc Board of Governors, a Past-Chair of the IEEE ComSoc TCs on eHealth and on Communications Software. He is the editor-in-chief of the International Journal of E-Health and Medical Communications. He has authored or coauthored over 900 papers in refereed international journals and conferences, 3 books, 2 patents, and 1 ITU-T Recommendation. Senior member of ACM and Fellow of IEEE.

Contributors

Abbas M. Ali Department of Software Engineering, Salahaddin University-Erbil, Erbil, Iraq

Sharf Alzubi Jordan University of Science and Technologym, Irbid, Jordan

Sumita Basu Bethune College, Kolkata, India;
Guest Faculty, Department of Mathematics, The Heritage College, Kolkata, India

Umesh Chandra Department of Computer Science, Banda University of Agriculture and Technology, Banda, UP, India

Shiv Kumar Choubey Department of Electronics and Communication Engineering, Birla Institute of Technology Mesra, Patna Campus, India

Kayhan Zrar Ghafoor Department of Software Engineering, Salahaddin University-Erbil, Erbil, Iraq;
School of Mathematics and Computer Science, University of Wolverhampton, Wolverhampton, UK

D. Ghosh Industrial Service and Research Group, CSIR-Central Mechanical Engineering Research Institute, Durgapur, West Bengal, India

Debasmita Ghosh Indian Institute of Science Education and Research(IISER), Bhopal, India

Sreeya Ghosh Department of Applied Mathematics, University of Calcutta, Kolkata, India

V. Gowrishankar Department of Electronics and Communication Engineering, Velalar College of Engineering and Technlology, Erode, Tamil Nadu, India

Murali Krishna Iyyanki Defence Research Development Organization, Hyderabad, India

Vidya Kameshwari St.Peter's Institute of Higher Education and Research, Avadi, Chennai, Tamil Nadu, India

M. Kannan PhD Research Scholar, Department of Computer Science, Vels Institute of Science, Technology and Advanced Studies (VISTAS), Chennai, India

S. K. Laha Industrial Service and Research Group, CSIR-Central Mechanical Engineering Research Institute, Durgapur, West Bengal, India

Halgurd S. Maghdid Department of Software Engineering, Faculty of Engineering, Koya University, Koysinjaq, Kurdistan Region, Iraq

Himani Maheshwari Department of Computer Science and Engineering, Uttarakhand Technical University, Dehradun, Uttarakhand, India

Aos Mulahuwaish Department of Computer Science and Information Systems Saginaw, Valley State University, Itta Bena, MI, United States

M. Murugan Department of Electronics and Communication Engineering, SRM Valliammai Engineering College, Kattankulathur, Chengalpatu, Tamil Nadu, India

Malik Mustafa Gulf College, Seeb, Oman

Harshit Naman Department of Electronics and Communication Engineering, Birla Institute of Technology Mesra, Patna Campus, India

M. Parimala Devi Department of Electronics and Communication Engineering, Velalar College of Engineering and Technlology, Erode, Tamil Nadu, India

S. R. Preethi Department of Electronics and Communication Engineering, SRM Valliammai Engineering College, Kattankulathur, Chengalpatu, Tamil Nadu, India

Jayanthi Prisilla Technical Support Engineering, The Airports Authority of India Ltd, Hyderabad, India

C. Priya Associate Professor, Department of Information Technology, Vels Institute of Science, Technology and Advanced Studies (VISTAS), Chennai, India

G. Boopathi Raja Department of Electronics and Communication Engineering, Velalar College of Engineering and Technlology, Erode, Tamil Nadu, India

A. R. Revathi Department of Information Technology, SRM Valliammai Engineering College, Kattankulathur, Chengalpatu, Tamil Nadu, India

T. Sathya Department of Electronics and Communication Engineering, Velalar College of Engineering and Technlology, Erode, Tamil Nadu, India

Selva Kumar Selvaraj St.Peter's Institute of Higher Education and Research, Avadi, Chennai, Tamil Nadu, India

Avinash Sharma Maharishi Markandeshwar Deemed to be University Mullana, Ambala, Haryana, India

Sangeetha Sundaramoorthy St.Peter's Institute of Higher Education and Research, Avadi, Chennai, Tamil Nadu, India

B. Swarnakar Industrial Service and Research Group, CSIR-Central Mechanical Engineering Research Institute, Durgapur, West Bengal, India

Dharminder Yadav Department of Computer Science and Technology, Glocal University, Saharanpur, UP, India

Transmission Dynamics and Estimation of Basic Reproduction Number (R_0) from Early Outbreak of Novel Coronavirus (COVID-19) in India

S. K. Laha, Debasmita Ghosh, D. Ghosh, and B. Swarnakar

Abstract Novel coronavirus (COVID-19) caused by severe acute respiratory syndrome coronavirus 2 (SARS-CoV-2) is an epidemic declared by the World Health Organization (WHO). Till now in June 13, 2020, the total COVID-19 cases in different countries around the world are 77,56,905 with 4,28,576 deaths and 3,974,422 recovered. The virus has taken spread in India as well, whereas of June 13, 2020, 3,09,603 cases are confirmed with 8,890 deaths and 1,54,330 recovery. It this situation, it is vital to know the potential danger posed by the pandemic and the epidemic trajectory. In this paper, the basic reproduction number (R_0) of COVID-19 from the early epidemic data in India is estimated. The course of the pandemic in India as well as the worst affected seven states in India, namely Maharashtra, Tamil Nadu, Delhi, Gujarat, Uttar Pradesh, Rajasthan and West Bengal is also analyzed. The early outbreak data from the Ministry of Health and Family Welfare (MoHFW), Government of India, are collected for the analysis. The two R packages 'R0' and 'earlyR' to estimate the basic reproduction number are used. An attempt is also made to forecast near-future incidence cases based on statistical methods. The results show that R_0 varies from 1.53 to 3.25 accounting to different methodologies and serial intervals adopted, whereas WHO estimations are from 2 to 2.5. Due to effect of lockdown, the time-dependent reproduction number has reduced to near about 1.22. It is predicted that by July 15, cumulative number of COVID-19 cases may reach around 1.2 million if the current effective reproduction number remains same over the next one month. Finally, it can be concluded that in the coming months, the novel

S. K. Laha (✉) · D. Ghosh · B. Swarnakar
Industrial Service and Research Group, CSIR-Central Mechanical Engineering Research Institute, M.G. Avenue, Durgapur 713209, West Bengal, India
e-mail: sk_laha@cmeri.res.in

D. Ghosh
e-mail: dghosh@cmeri.res.in

B. Swarnakar
e-mail: b.swarnakar@cmeri.res.in

D. Ghosh
Indian Institute of Science Education and Research(IISER), Bhopal, India
e-mail: debasmita18@iiserb.ac.in

© The Editor(s) (if applicable) and The Author(s), under exclusive license to Springer Nature Singapore Pte Ltd. 2020

C. Chakraborty et al. (eds.), *Internet of Medical Things for Smart Healthcare*, Studies in Big Data 80, https://doi.org/10.1007/978-981-15-8097-0_1

coronavirus will pose a severe challenge to the Indian healthcare system. Thus, it is necessary to predict how the virus may spread so that the healthcare system may be prepared in advance. The time-dependent reproduction number shows the positive effect of lockdown, as this number has gone down.

Keywords Basic reproduction number · Novel coronavirus · Transmission dynamics

1 Introduction

Coronavirus in the form of COVID-19 poses a pandemic threat in most of the countries all over the world in 2020. The COVID-19 is spreading at alarming rate in almost all countries over the globe. It has first originated in Wuhan, Hubei province, Republic of China [1] at the end of December 2019. The 41 cases existing as 'pneumonia of unknown reasons' are reported by the Wuhan Municipal Health Committee [2]. On January 01, 2020, the seafood wholesale market in Wuhan is announced as the epicenter of the outbreak of COVID-19 and is decided to be closed. After few days, human-to-human transmission is reported in Wuhan [3]. In first week of February 2020, the virus outbreak causes more than 24,000 total confirmed cases and 494 deaths and spreads in 25 countries around the world. The outbreak is a major concern in Italy, Spain, Iran followed by England, USA, Russia, UAE, Australia, Canada, Singapore, India and many other countries. The outbreak is increasing day by day and poses a major threat to healthcare system in different countries. Till now in June 13, the total cases in different countries around the world are 7,756,905 with 4,28,576 deaths and 3,974,422 recovery [4]. The most affected states and union territories in India are Maharashtra, Tamil Nadu, Delhi, Gujarat, Uttar Pradesh, Rajasthan and West Bengal. 98% of the patients are having mild symptoms or asymptomatic, and rest 2% are in critical and serious condition of acute respiratory problems. The problem of rapid outbreak in India is also very alarming and spread to almost every states in May 2020. The total no of cases in India up to June 13, 2020 are 3,09,603 with 8,890 deaths and 1,54,330 recovery [5].

The first case of COVID-19 in India is reported in 30 January 2020 in Kerala. There has been a gradual increase in the number of infections (1,251 on March 30, among which 32 deaths and 102 recovered cases). In response, Indian government has implemented international travel bans, Janata curfew and strict lockdown throughout the country from 25th March onward. The major event in connection with COVID-19 outbreak is listed in Table 1.

India is having second highest population after China around the world with very large population density, limited infrastructure and healthcare systems to cater to very large demands of COVID-19 patients. On the other hand, factors like warmer climate as well as humidity [6–9], a large proportion of the young population, and possible immunity due to BCG vaccinations [8], may favor India. Most of the infected patients in India are asymptomatic or mild symptoms, which is quite unusual as compared

Table 1 Key events and decisions taken by Indian government

Dates	Key events
January 30, 2020	First confirmed positive case
March 6, 2020	International passenger screenings at airports
March 12, 2020	First confirmed death
March 13, 2020	Suspension of non-essential traveler visas
March 15, 2020	100 confirmed positive cases
March 22, 2020	One-day Janata curfew Passenger air travel suspended till further notice
March 25, 2020	First national lockdown imposed till April 14
March 28, 2020	1000 confirmed positive cases
March 30, 2020	100 confirmed recoveries
April 2, 2020	Government announces plans to convert trains and stadiums into isolation wards
April 14, 2020	10,000 confirmed Covid-19 cases National lockdown extended till May 3
May 01, 2020	Nationwide lockdown further extended till May 17
May 17, 2020	Nationwide lockdown further extended till May 31
May 29, 2020	Highest number of recovered cases recorded
June 01, 2020 till date	Lockdown to continue in containment zone

to Europeans and North American countries. India is experiencing early lockdown followed by China in view of favorable effect in controlling the final epidemic size. However, considering the huge population (almost 1.35 billion), with high population density, poses significant challenges to mitigate the pandemic situation due to COVID-19 spreading, without affecting economic and social issues. In this context, it is very important to consider the huge demand of healthcare systems (like ICU beds, PPE, ventilator, oxygenerator, etc.) and also enforce social distancing and avoid spreading in a larger scale through community transmission. So the prediction of possible COVID-19 outbreak is very important for formulation of policy-making decision regarding healthcare system lockdown and social distancing. The trend of spread in India is confined in some specific hotspot areas, especially in highly population dense area, where the timely decision of lockdown, social distancing and rapid diagnosis of infected cases play a major role to prevent pandemic situation.

Mathematical modeling is frequently used to predict the outbreaks of different diseases in epidemiology [10, 11]. Infectious disease models under epidemiology aim at understanding the mechanisms that influence the spread of diseases and predicting disease transmission. Mathematical models are popular to evaluate the potential impact of different control measures of pandemic diseases and to guide public health policy decisions of certain union government. Different models used earlier to predict the nature of the out breaks of Ebola pandemic diseases at African countries are reported in different literatures [12–14]. The different models used to predict the pandemic disease outbreak mainly consist of two types of models such as statistical models [15] and mechanistic models [16]. The forecasting of different diseases by mathematical modeling in case of dengue, influenza and chikungunya is reported in different literature [17–19]. In all models, a balance must be shown between obtaining precise forecasts, considering for all uncertainties, both in the data and in the dynamics of transmission.

Mathematical modeling is used to understand the dynamics of the pandemic in its early stages and to predict the rate of spreading from the infector to receiver. The basic reproduction number (R_0) measures the average number of secondary infections generated by primary cases in a fully susceptible population. A schematic diagram of basic reproduction number with a value of 2.0 is shown in Fig. 1

Liu et al. [20] reviewed and listed reproduction numbers reported in literatures in PubMed, bioRxiv and Google Scholar. Twelve studies in the period between January 1, 2020–February 7, 2020, were covered in their paper. It was shown that the estimates of reproduction number range from 1.49 to 6.49, with a mean of 3.28, a median of 2.79 and interquartile range (IQR) of 1.16. They attribute that such a large deviation to the estimation method adopted such as stochastic method, mathematical methods and exponential growth method. Zhang et al. [21] estimated the value of R_0 and probable outbreak dynamics in the Diamond Princess cruise ship.

In this study, data is obtained from Govt. of India, the Ministry of Health and Family Welfare (MoHFW) for the period from 2 March to 1 April to estimate the R_0 of COVID-19 by applying different statistical models. No new cases of COVID-19 have been detected in India from January 31 to 1 March 1, 2020; therefore in the modeling, the number of the samples has been taken from March 2, 2020 onward.

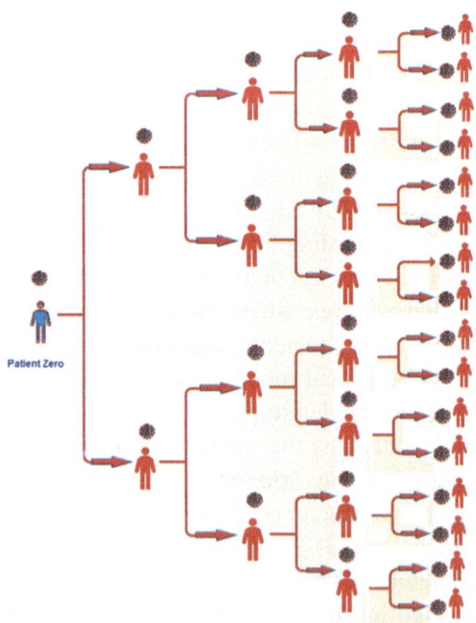

Fig. 1 A schematic diagram of basic reproduction number

The gradual increase of infected cases is observed on March 2, 2020 onward. The 'projections' package in R is used to get an idea about the possible epidemic trend in India.

2 Materials and Methods

The incidence data is taken from the Ministry of Health and Family Welfare (MoHFW) of the Government of India and COVID 10 tracker in India [5], which tracks the country-wise COVID-19 cases in India. To estimate the reproduction number, three serial interval (SI) distributions reported in the literature: (1) by Li et al. [22]; (2) by Nishihura et al.; [23] and (3) by Du et al. [24].

Two R packages 'earlyR' [25] and 'R0' [26, 27] are used to estimate the basic reproduction number (R_0). The 'earlyR' package estimates this number using the maximum likelihood (ML) method as illustrated by Cori et al. [28]. The 'R0' package uses five different methods to estimate the number: (1) from attack rate, (2) maximum likelihood, (3) exponential growth rate, (4) Bayesian approach and (5) time-dependent reproduction number. In this paper, three methods from the 'R0' package: (1) exponential growth rate (EG), (2) maximum likelihood (ML) and (3) time-dependent (TD) reproduction number are used. The maximum likelihood (ML) method of estimation in 'R0' package follows the algorithm proposed by White and Pagano [29], whereas the exponential growth rate method follows the paper by Wallinga and Lipsitch [30], and the time-dependent method is proposed by Wallinga and Teunis [31]. Nouvellet et al. [32] presented a simple approach to forecast near-future incidence cases based on a statistical method. In their model, the daily incidence I_t can be approximated by the renewal equation which is assumed to be a Poisson's process as given by $I_t \sim \text{Pois}\left(R_t \sum_{s=0}^{t} I_{t-s}\omega_s\right)$ where ω is the serial interval and R_t is the instantaneous reproduction rate. Their method is implemented in the R package named 'projections' [33].

2.1 *Serial Interval*

To estimate the reproduction number, it is necessary to know about generation time, which is the time lag between infection in primary cases (infectors) and secondary cases (infectee). It is generally obtained from the serial interval (SI) which is defined as the time lag between the onset of symptoms in primary cases and secondary cases. It is assumed the serial interval has gamma distribution. In the analysis of the early outbreak of novel coronavirus in the form of COVID-19 in the city of Wuhan, China, Li et al. [22] estimated that the SI has a mean of 7.5 days and an SD of 3.4 days. However, Nishiura et al. [23] estimated that the mean and standard deviation of SI are 4.7 days (95% CI: [3.7, 6.0]) and 2.9 days, respectively. They have estimated the parameters based on the dataset of 28 infector/infectee pairs. Du et al. [24] also obtained similar SI distribution, where mean is 3.96 days (95% CI: [3.53, 4.39]) and SD is 4.75 days (95% CI: [4.46, 5.07]). Their dataset consists of 468 COVID-19 transmission events.

3 Results

3.1 Analysis of COVID-19 in India

3.1.1 Epidemic Curve and Preliminary Analysis

The epidemic curve of incidence cases in India from March 2, 2020 to April 1, 2020, is shown in Fig. 2. An exponential model is also fitted to the epidemic curve and is shown in Fig. 2. The fitted curve shows that daily cases are doubling in approximately four days.

3.1.2 Estimation of R_0

Table 2 shows our estimation of R_0 along with the 95% confidence interval for three reported SI data and the R package used in the analysis. The range of estimated values of R_0 is from 1.53 to 3.25 with a mean of 2.18. It seems that the 'R0' package tends to overestimate the reproduction number slightly. Also, the R_0 value estimated with SI mean = 7.5 and 3.4 is higher than that obtained with other SI data. The mean value obtained (i.e., 2.18) in this analysis falls within the WHO recommended value.

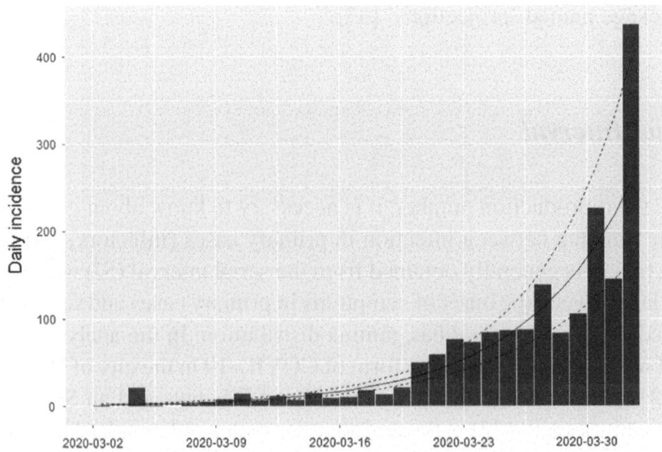

Fig. 2 Epidemic curve of COVID-19 in India (March 02, 2020–April 01, 2020)

Table 2 Estimation of R_0 with confidence interval

Serial interval (SI) (days)	R_0 [95% confidence interval (CI)]	
SI mean = 4.7, SD = 2.9	ML method, 'R0' package	2.05 [1.92, 2.19]
	EG method, 'R0' package	2.15 [2.08, 2.22]
	ML method, 'earlyR' package	1.53 [1.47, 1.60]
SI mean = 3.96, SD = 4.75	ML method, 'R0' package	1.94 [1.82, 2.07]
	EG method, 'R0' package	1.98 [1.93, 2.04]
	ML method, 'earlyR' package	1.68 [1.60, 1.75]
SI mean = 7.5, SD = 3.4	ML method, 'R0' package	2.99 [2.80, 3.19]
	EG method, 'R0' package	3.25 [3.03, 3.43]
	ML method, 'earlyR' package	2.08 [1.99, 2.18]

Figure 3 shows the daily observed incidence and model predicted incidence using ML and EG methods. This fitted incidence is then used to estimate R_0. It can be seen from Fig. 3 that the predicted model fits quite well to the observed incidence data.

The likely values of the basic reproduction number implemented with the 'earlyR' package are shown in Fig. 4.

As deviations are observed concerning serial interval distribution, a sensitivity analysis of SI on the R_0 value is also carried out. The serial interval is assumed to have gamma distribution. The mean and standard deviation of the SI are varied over a range of 1–7 days and 2–5 days, respectively, and then R_0 numbers are estimated using the ML method. Figure 5a shows three different serial distributions considered

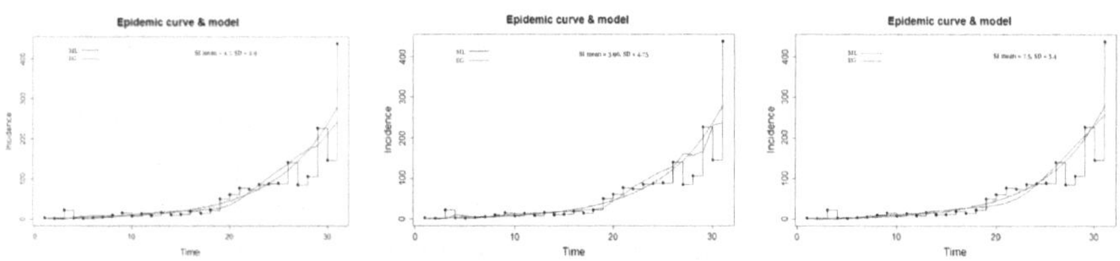

SI mean = 4.7, SD = 2.9 SI mean = 3.96, SD = 4.75 SI mean = 7.5, SD = 3.4

Fig. 3 Observed incidence and model predicted incidence using ML and EG

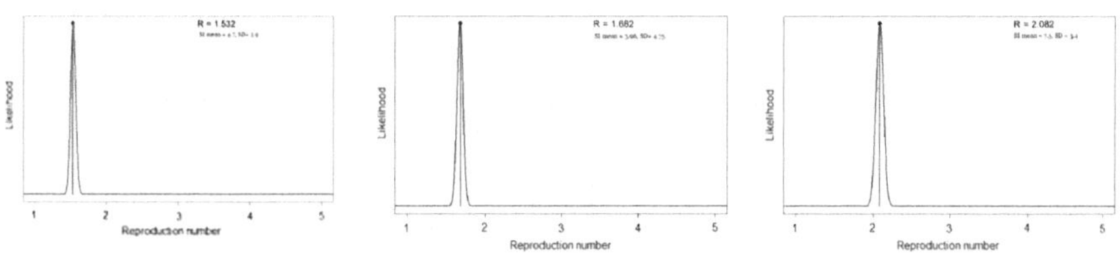

SI mean = 4.7, SD = 2.9 SI mean = 3.96, SD = 4.75 SI mean = 7.5, SD = 3.4

Fig. 4 Estimation of basic reproduction number (R_0), 'earlyR' package

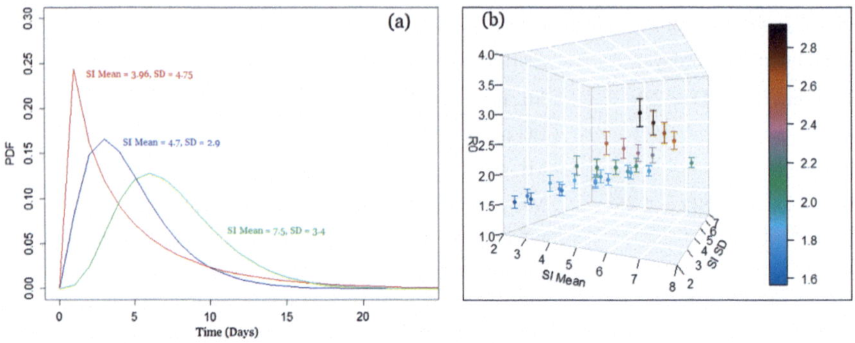

Fig. 5 **a** Serial interval distribution, **b** sensitivity of serial interval distribution to R_0

in the present study. Figure 5b depicts the sensitivity of R_0 to SI mean and standard deviation. From the sensitivity analysis, it can be seen that R_0 has a maximum value of 2.9 when SI mean and SD are seven days and two days, respectively.

Figure 6 shows the time-dependent reproduction number ($R(t)$) over the period from March 14, 2020 to June 10, 2020. The epidemic curve is also shown for this period. The SI mean and the SD are assumed to be 7.5 days and 3.4 days, respectively. The start of lockdown, i.e., March 25, 2020, is also marked on the figure. It can be seen that there is a reduction in reproduction number from April 15 onward, mainly due to the imposition of travel restriction, closure of public places and the imposition

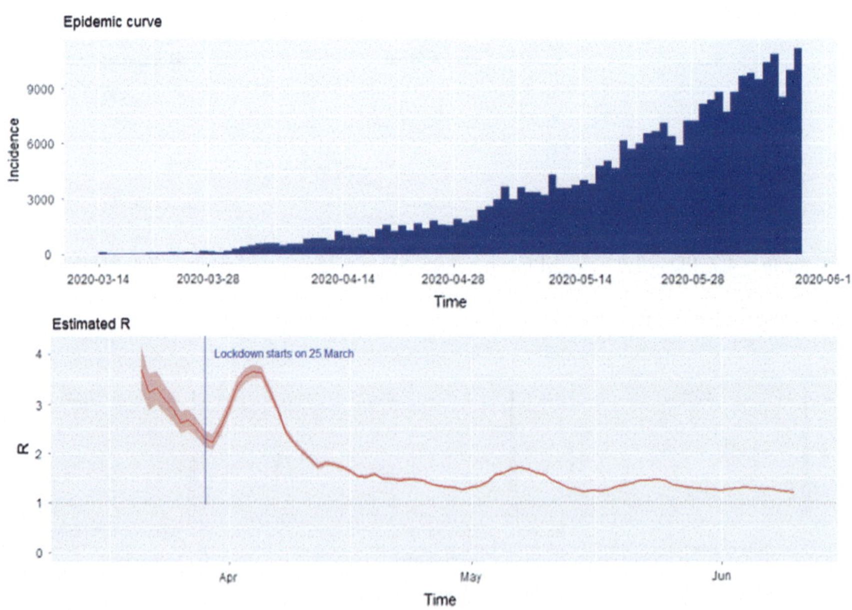

Fig. 6 Epidemic curve and the time-dependent reproduction number in India

of lockdown. For the last twenty days or so, the effective reproduction number has reduced to nearly 1.22 as an effect of the lockdown. However, for containing the spread of the virus, it is necessary to reduce the value of reproduction number below one.

3.2 *Forecasting Near-Future Incidences in India*

An attempt has been made to forecast near-future incidences up to August 12 using the R package 'projections' developed by Thibaut et al. [33]. The first forty-five days' data starting from March 14 is used for learning the model. Further, during the projection, the reproduction number as given in the renewal equation is assumed to be constant during the projection. This reproduction number is obtained from the average of last seven days of the time-dependent reproduction number, while the serial interval has a mean and standard deviation of 7.5 and 3.4 days, respectively. Figure 7a shows the predicted daily incidences in India from April 28 to August 12. The actual daily incidences from April 28 to June 10 are also shown in Fig. 7a. It can be seen that predicted cases by the present methodology fit quite well with the observed cases. Figure 7b shows the predicted cumulative daily incidences up to August 12. With the present epidemic trajectory, it is estimated that predictions are as follows: On 15 June, cumulative incidences are 305,477 (range: 291,402–319,738); on 25 June, cumulative incidences are 492,903 (range: 469,785–517,156); on 05 July, cumulative incidences are 781,432 (range: 741,211–821,212); on 15 July, cumulative incidences are 1,225,636 (range: 1,159,404–1,289,513); on 25 July, cumulative incidences are 1,909,548 (range: 1,802,053–2,011,688); on 01 August, cumulative incidences are 2,597,702 (range: 2,447,797–2,738,595). It may be noted that these are conservative estimates, assuming the present rate of infection persists. However, if the restrictions of lockdown are eased up, then it is expected that R_0 will increase which will result in more number of COVID-19 cases in India.

3.3 *Analysis of COVID-19 in States and UT of India*

Analysis of the COVID-19 cases is also carried out for seven worst affected Indian states, namely Maharashtra, Tamil Nadu, Delhi, Gujarat, Uttar Pradesh, Rajasthan and West Bengal. A map of Indian states and the distribution of active COVID-19 cases are shown in Fig. 8. A probable projection of COVID-19 cases in those states is given in Table 3. It may be noted that the predictions are based on the assumption that reproduction number remains same in the prediction horizon which may not be correct particularly for long-term projection.

It may be noted that first 45 days staring from March 14, 2020, is used for future prediction of COVID-19 cases.

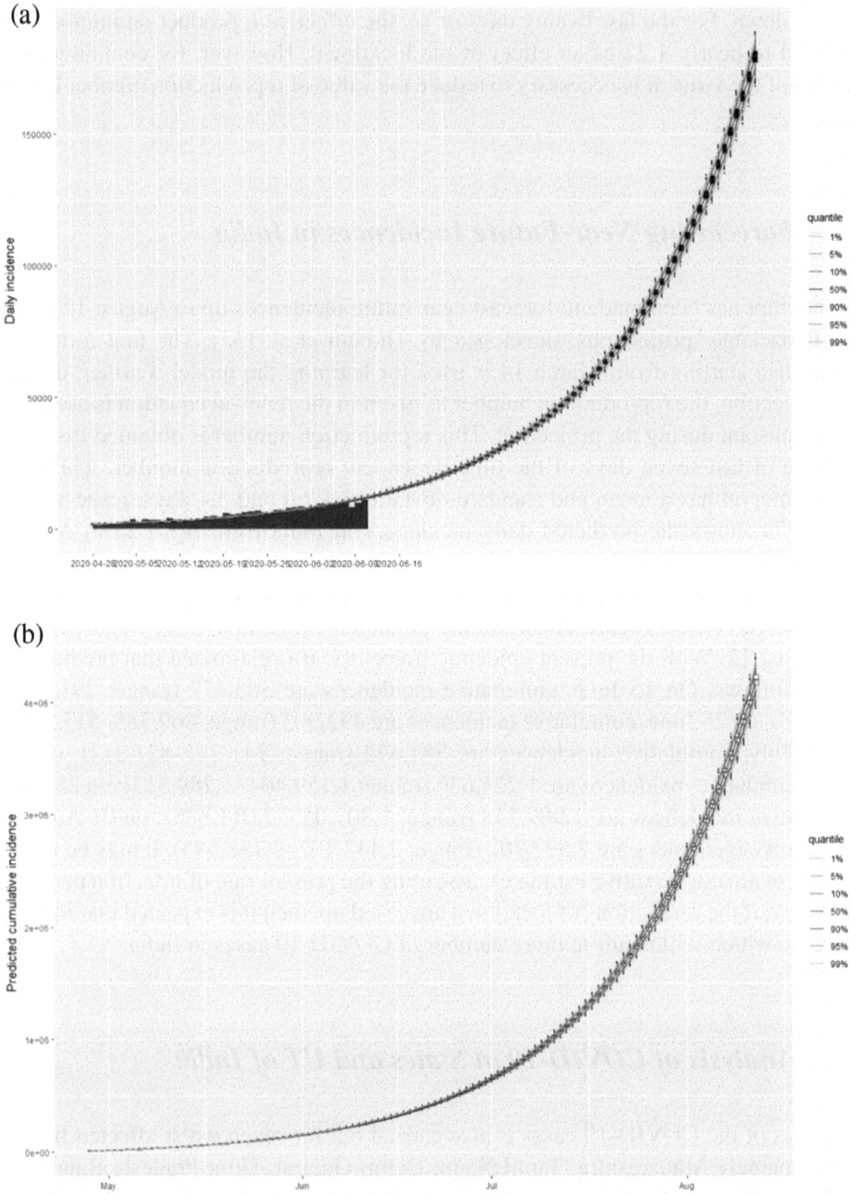

Fig. 7 **a** Predicted daily incidence and actually observed incidence in India, **b** predicted cumulative daily incidence in India

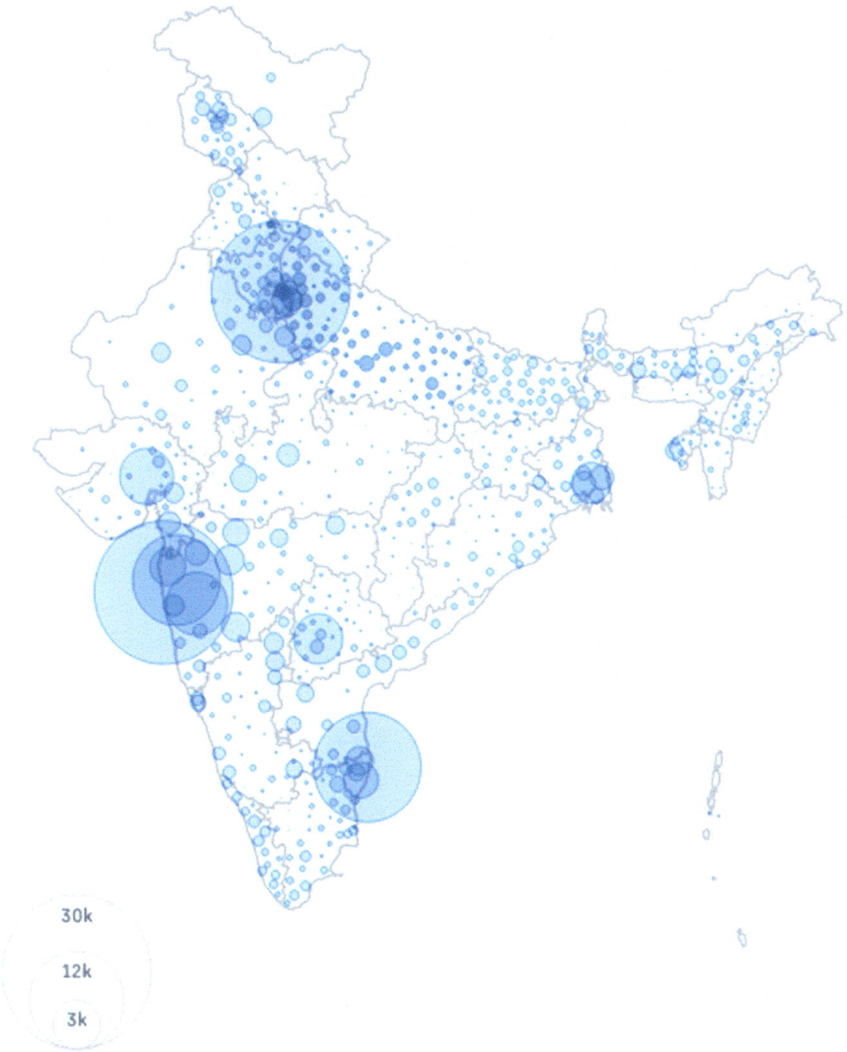

Fig. 8 COVID-19 active cases in India as on June 10, 2020 [5]

Maharashtra

Maharashtra has the highest number of COVID-19 cases in India. As of June 10, total confirmed cases in Maharashtra is 1,04,568 with 51,379 active cases, 49,346 recovered and 3,830 death cases. The epidemic curve and the time-dependent reproduction number in Maharashtra are shown in Fig. 9. However, on a positive note, it can be observed that the effective reproductive number in Maharashtra has reduced to 1.08 on June 10, 2020.

Table 3 Prediction of COVID-19 cases in India and Indian states

Date	India			Maharashtra			Tamil Nadu		
	Mean	Lower	Upper	Mean	Lower	Upper	Mean	Lower	Upper
2020-04-28	1896	1740	2053						
2020-05-03	12,495	12,050	12,952	4258	3986	4493			
2020-05-08	25,570	24,759	26,545	8620	8137	9077	1397	1174	1646
2020-05-13	41,792	40,320	43,395	13,933	13,144	14,658	2497	2044	2985
2020-05-18	61,923	59,630	64,488	20,406	19,236	21,692	4085	3374	4937
2020-05-23	86,897	83,426	90,801	28,290	26,654	30,243	6374	5301	7846
2020-05-28	117,893	113,158	123,070	37,897	35,700	40,623	9677	8035	12,028
2020-06-02	156,355	149,728	162,426	49,602	46,641	53,253	14,442	11,924	18,033
2020-06-07	204,083	195,379	212,843	63,862	59,643	68,735	21,317	17,658	26,902
2020-06-12	263,301	251,309	275,276	81,234	75,701	87,650	31,231	25,795	39,725
2020-06-17	336,792	321,074	352,712	102,404	95,329	110,658	45,538	37,414	57,858
2020-06-22	47,961	407,835	448,972	128,186	118,970	138,726	66,167	54,046	84,404
2020-06-27	541,096	515,459	567,873	159,598	148,018	172,972	95,928	78,153	122,683
2020-07-02	681,469	647,452	715,597	197,861	183,073	214,722	138,852	113,061	178,137
2020-07-07	855,630	811,174	899,752	244,469	225,496	265,685	200,758	163,385	258,080
2020-07-12	1,071,730	1,014,653	1,127,095	301,247	277,250	327,715	290,058	235,918	373,564
2020-07-17	1,339,864	1,267,169	1,409,990	370,415	340,230	402,883	418,865	341,404	539,923
2020-07-22	1,672,591	1,579,711	1,761,329	454,689	417,365	494,771	604,680	492,070	780,292
2020-07-27	2,085,442	1,967,294	2,197,288	557,358	511,271	606,560	872,704	709,482	1,127,071
2020-08-01	2,597,702	2,447,797	2,738,595	682,426	626,142	743,292	1,259,305	1,024,474	1,628,398
2020-08-06	3,233,306	3,043,299	3,409,553	834,789	766,260	910,949	1,816,953	1,477,593	2,352,016

(continued)

Table 3 (continued)

Date	India			Maharashtra			Tamil Nadu		
	Mean	Lower	Upper	Mean	Lower	Upper	Mean	Lower	Upper
2020-08-11	4,021,977	3,781,000	4,241,460	1,020,407	937,085	1,115,301	2,621,322	2,132,404	3,396,833
Date	Delhi			Gujarat			Uttar Pradesh		
	Mean	Lower	Upper	Mean	Lower	Upper	Mean	Lower	Upper
2020-04-28									
2020-05-03	1208	1055	1358						
2020-05-08	2578	2268	2854	1810	1638	1988	1436	1206	1676
2020-05-13	4333	3766	4802	3475	3159	3768	2255	1863	2659
2020-05-18	6586	5676	7420	5254	4780	5691	3209	2631	3764
2020-05-23	9475	8142	10,708	7159	6461	7865	4316	3536	5148
2020-05-28	13,185	11,201	14,990	9198	8255	10,150	5604	4590	6742
2020-06-02	17,947	15,128	20,567	11,382	10,207	12,529	7104	5804	8572
2020-06-07	24,058	20,048	27,567	13,721	12,182	15,241	8847	7252	10,681
2020-06-12	31,900	26,376	36,667	16,226	14,424	18,215	10,874	8799	13,140
2020-06-17	41,968	34,583	48,416	18,906	16,810	21,379	13,233	10,653	16,083
2020-06-22	54,882	45,062	63,611	21,780	19,404	24,860	15,973	12,786	19,355
2020-06-27	71,460	58,536	82,877	24,852	22,005	28,433	19,162	15,268	23,389
2020-07-02	92,731	75,907	107,574	28,145	24,831	32,345	22,869	17,974	27,882
2020-07-07	120,024	98,052	139,199	31,669	27,811	36,474	27,177	21,207	33,085
2020-07-12	155,049	126,217	180,156	35,439	30,834	40,776	32,188	24,930	39,432
2020-07-17	199,996	162,565	232,298	39,477	34,092	45,472	38,016	29,259	46,846

(continued)

Table 3 (continued)

Date	Delhi			Gujarat			Uttar Pradesh		
	Mean	Lower	Upper	Mean	Lower	Upper	Mean	Lower	Upper
2020-07-22	257,687	209,109	299,430	43,801	37,588	50,617	44,795	34,336	55,474
2020-07-27	331,725	268,959	385,103	48,432	41,296	56,085	52,677	40,268	65,502
2020-08-01	426,735	345,574	495,017	53,391	45,393	62,137	61,844	47,260	77,359
2020-08-06	548,664	444,309	636,888	58,700	49,611	68,362	72,507	55,244	91,039
2020-08-10	705,140	570,643	819,369	64,386	54,190	75,218	84,906	64,669	107,040

Date	Rajasthan			West Bengal		
	Mean	Lower	Upper	Mean	Lower	Upper
2020-04-28						
2020-05-03	713	598	837	174	127	222
2020-05-08	1368	1096	1582	499	400	602
2020-05-13	2113	1729	2522	917	726	1159
2020-05-18	2968	2371	3586	1453	1122	1824
2020-05-23	3942	3108	4763	2140	1616	2744
2020-05-28	5057	3976	6168	3023	2188	3882
2020-06-02	6334	4953	7805	4156	2912	5361
2020-06-07	7792	6070	9602	5610	3901	7312
2020-06-12	9458	7309	11,870	7477	5173	9758
2020-06-17	11,365	8666	14,417	9870	6783	12,880
2020-06-22	13,544	10,177	17,422	12,943	8927	16,904
2020-06-27	16,037	12,015	20,843	16,888	11,641	22,140
2020-07-02	18,891	14,146	24,786	21,949	15,110	28,968
2020-07-07	22,149	16,537	29,351	28,443	19,608	37,778

(continued)

Table 3 (continued)

Date	Rajasthan			West Bengal		
	Mean	Lower	Upper	Mean	Lower	Upper
2020-07-12	25,868	19,271	34,615	36,772	25,223	49,052
2020-07-17	30,127	22,248	40,612	47,466	32,734	63,530
2020-07-22	35,015	25,702	47,427	61,185	42,281	81,992
2020-07-27	40,631	29,558	55,631	78,800	54,633	105,528
2020-08-01	47,081	34,078	64,936	101,403	70,349	135,786
2020-08-06	54,500	39,104	75,391	130,410	90,494	174,158
2020-08-11	63,018	44,810	87,472	167,644	116,337	223,809

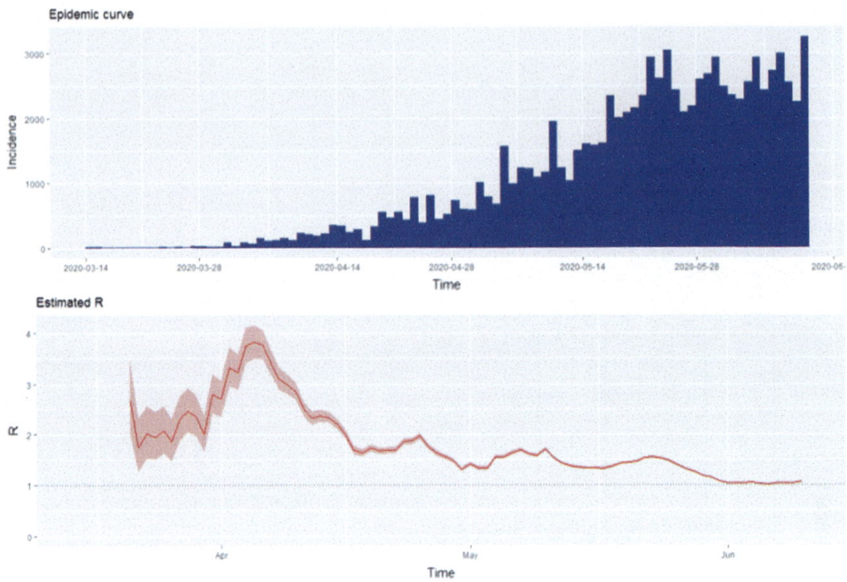

Fig. 9 Epidemic curve and the time-dependent reproduction number in Maharashtra

Figure 10a shows the predicted daily incidences in Maharashtra from April 28 to August 12, whereas Fig. 10b shows the cumulative projection in Maharashtra during that period. The predictions for Maharashtra are as follows: On 30 June, cumulative incidences are 1,81,648 (range: 1,68,149–1,97,195), and on 15 July, cumulative incidences are 3,41,105 (range: 3,13,764–3,70,958).

Tamil Nadu:

Tamil Nadu has second highest number of COVID-19 cases in India. On June 13, Tamil Nadu has observed total 42,687 confirmed cases, 18,881 active cases, 23,490 recovered cases and 397 deaths. Among the worst affected seven states considered in this study, Tamil Nadu has lowest infection death rate. The majority of cases are mainly concentrated in and around of Chennai, which is considered to be the epicenter of Tamil Nadu. However, even after the end of lockdown, the time-dependent reproduction number is still on the higher side. On June 10, 2020, the reproduction number in Tamil Nadu is 1.49 which is higher compared to other Indian states and national average. Also, slight upward trend in the time-dependent reproduction number can be observed (Fig. 11).

Plots indicating future incidences in Tamil Nadu are shown in Figs. 12a and b. It is predicted that cumulative cases may reach 1,19,781 (range: 97,668–1,53,513) on 30 June and 3,61,632 (range: 2,94,560–4,65,707). However, it be noted that such high numbers are predicted for Tamil Nadu can be attributed to higher reproduction number. It is quite possible that actual cases may be much lower, as infection rate may go down due to control measures (Fig. 12).

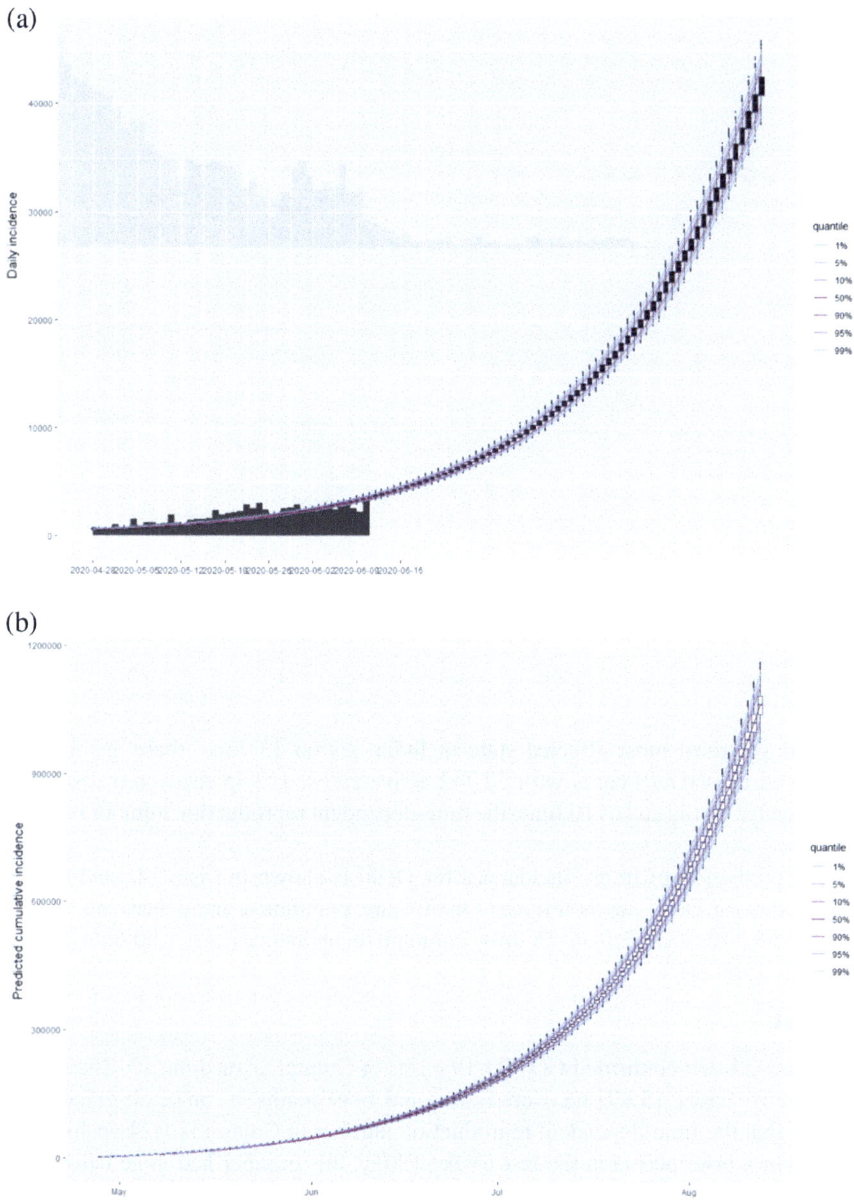

Fig. 10 **a** Predicted daily incidence and actually observed incidence in Maharashtra, **b** predicted cumulative daily incidence in Maharashtra

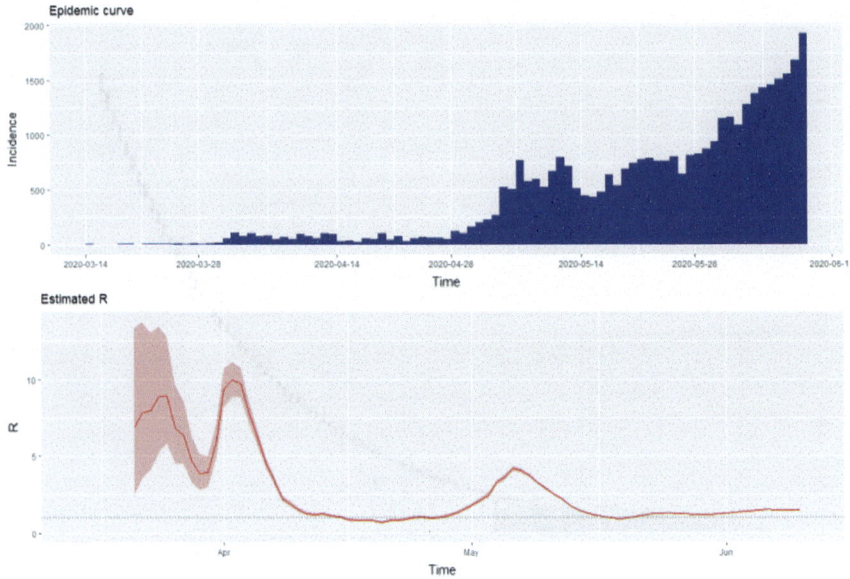

Fig. 11 Epidemic curve and the time-dependent reproduction number in Tamil Nadu

Delhi

Delhi is the third most affected state in India. As on 13 June, there are 3,85,98 confirmed COVID-19 cases with 22,742 active cases, 14,945 recovered cases and 1271 deaths. At the end of 10 June, the time-dependent reproduction number in Delhi is 1.19.

The prediction of future incidences for Delhi is shown in Figs. 14a and b. The predictions for Delhi are as follows: On 30 June, cumulative incidences are 83,585 (range: 68,370–97,017); on 15 July cumulative incidences are 1,80,666 (range: 1,46,961–2,09,867).

Gujarat

There are 23,079 confirmed COVID-19 cases in Gujarat as on June 13, 2020, with 5,739 active cases, 15,891 recovered cases and 1449 deaths. It can be observed from Fig. 15 that the time-dependent reproduction number in Gujarat is 1.24 on June 10, 2020. For a brief period at the last week of May, this number had gone below 1.0, but then again it is increased.

The prediction of future incidences in Gujarat is shown in Figs. 16a and b. From the simulation, it is predicted that cumulative cases in Gujarat may reach 26,802 (range: 23,705–30,779) on 30 June and 37,829 (range: 32,761–43,559) on July 15.

Uttar Pradesh

In Uttar Pradesh, there are 13,118 confirmed cases of COVID-19 resulting in 4,858 active cases, 7,875 recovered and 385 deaths on 13 June. The epidemic curve of

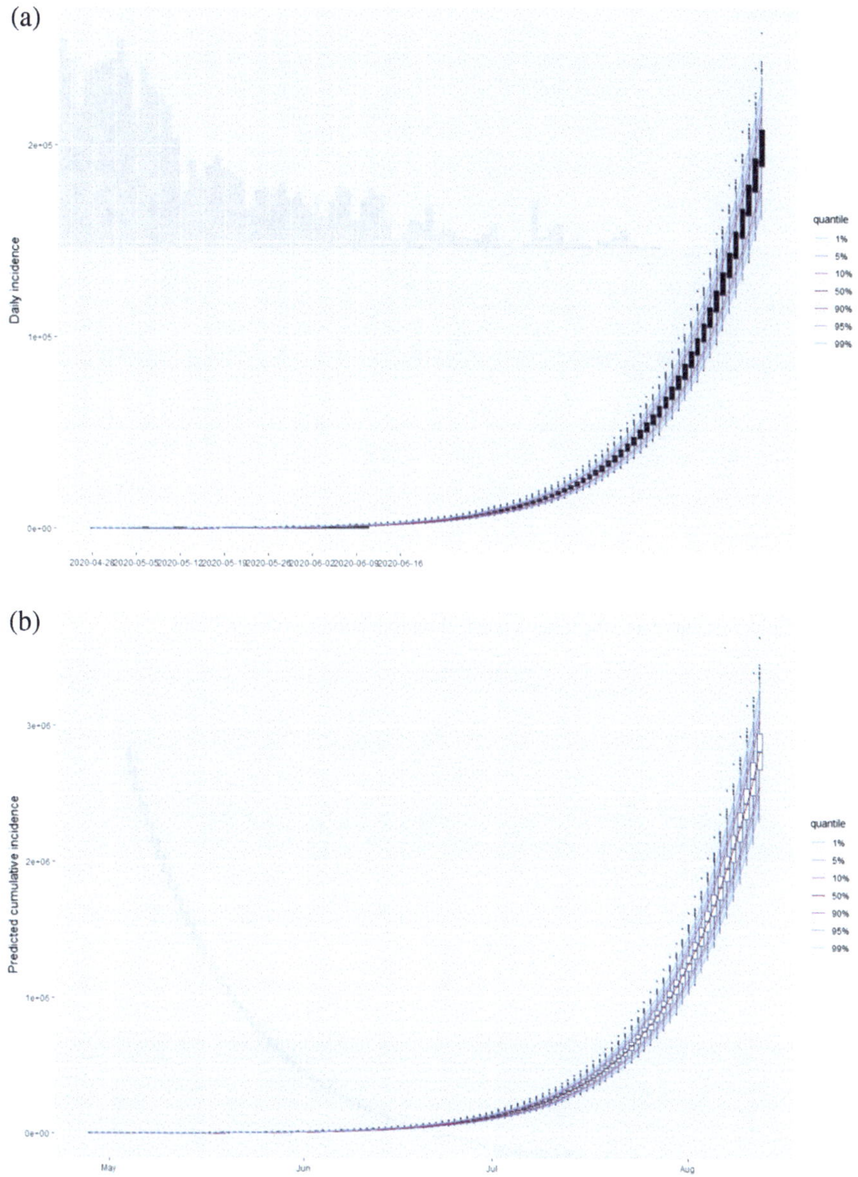

Fig. 12 **a** Predicted daily incidence and actually observed incidence in Tamil Nadu, **b** predicted cumulative daily incidence in Tamil Nadu

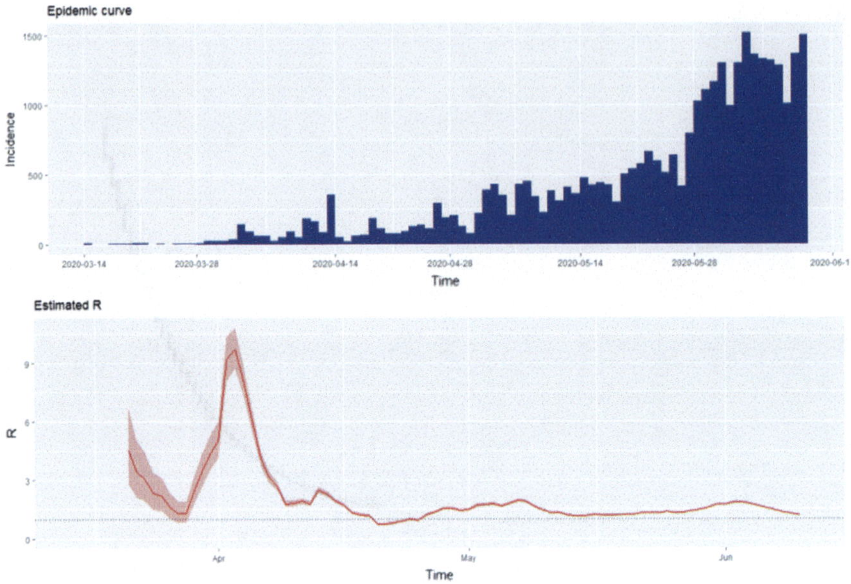

Fig. 13 Epidemic curve and the time-dependent reproduction number in Delhi

(a)

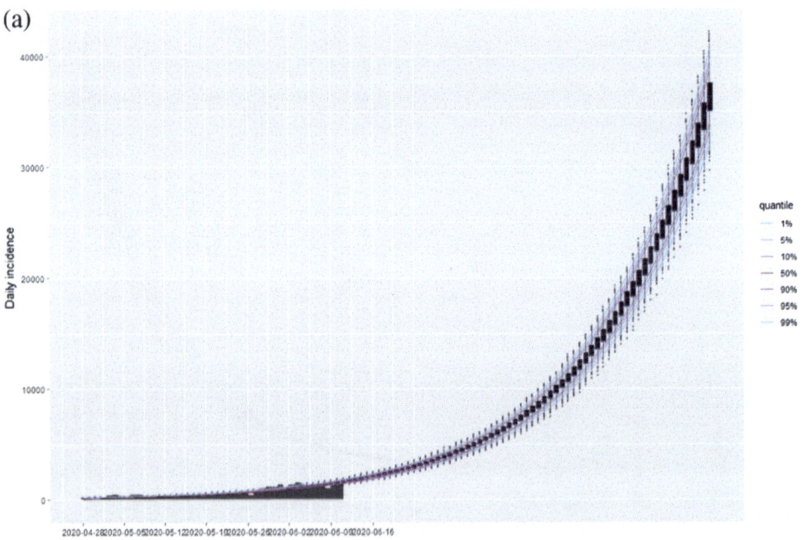

Fig. 14 **a** Predicted daily incidence and actually observed incidence in Delhi, **b** predicted cumulative daily incidence in Delhi

(b)

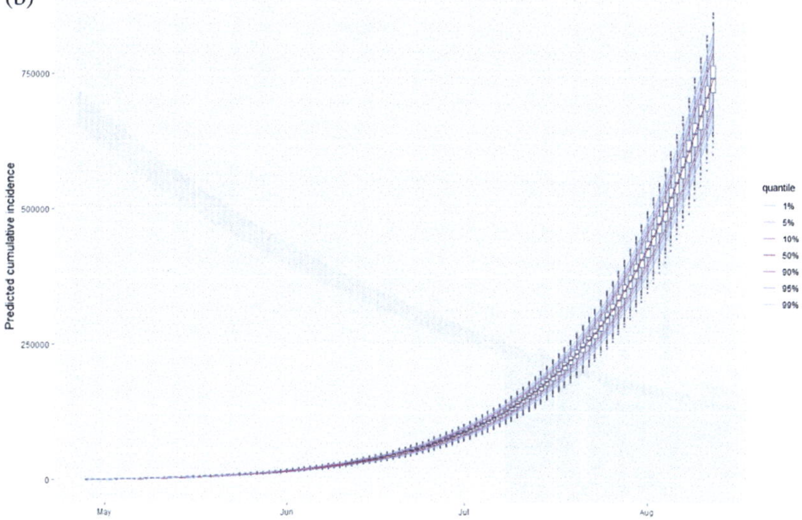

Fig. 14 (continued)

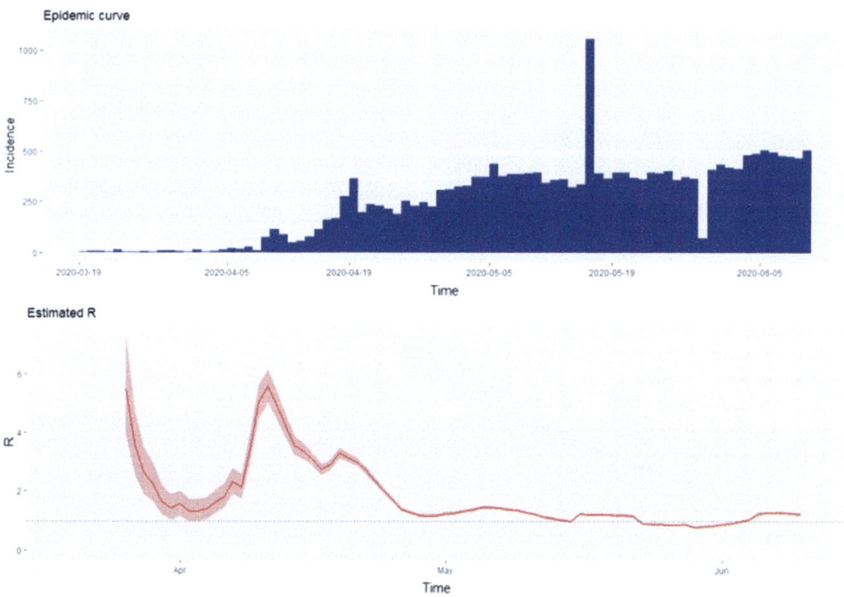

Fig. 15 Epidemic curve and the time-dependent reproduction number in Gujarat

(a)

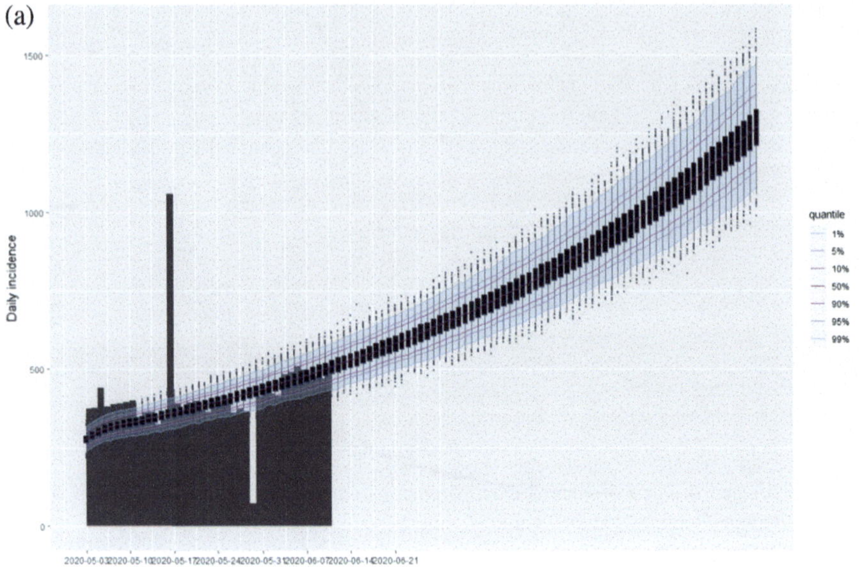

(b)

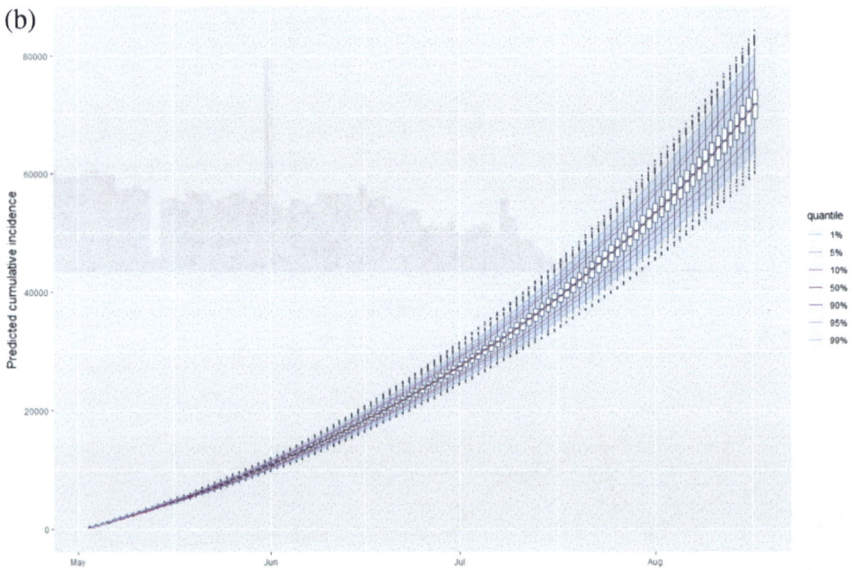

Fig. 16 **a** Predicted daily incidence and actually observed incidence in Gujarat, **b** predicted cumulative daily incidence in Gujarat

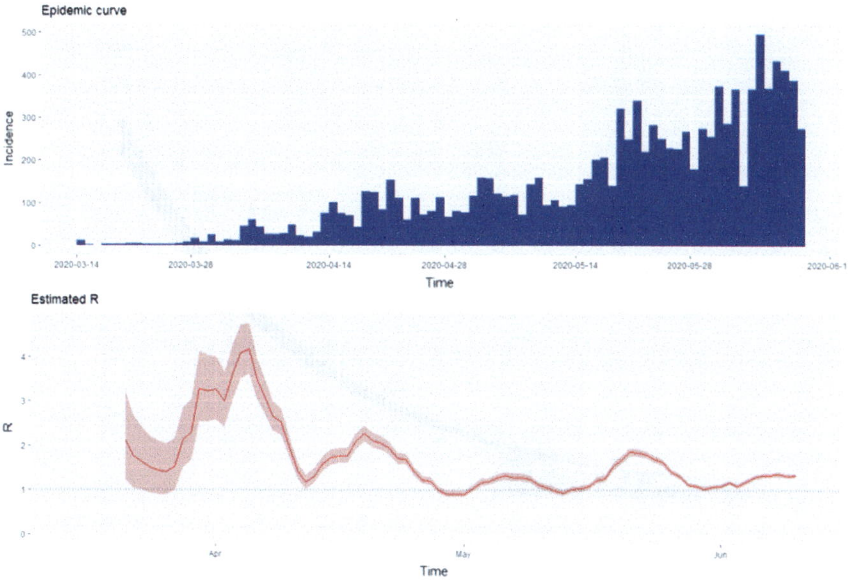

Fig. 17 Epidemic curve and the time-dependent reproduction number in Uttar Pradesh

Uttar Pradesh and the variation of reproduction number with time are shown in Fig. 17. Reproduction number at 10 June is 1.34. Also a slight upward trend in the time-dependent reproduction number can be seen from June 01 onward.

The predicted daily incidence and cumulative incidences in Uttar Pradesh is shown in Fig. 18a and b. It is estimated that is the current rate of infection persists then June 30 and July 15. The predicted value of cumulative cases on July 15 may reach 21,320 [range: 23,705-30,779] and 35,580 [range: 27,453-43,777], respectively.

Rajasthan

For the state of Rajasthan, there are 12,068 confirmed cases of COVID-19 patients along with 2785 active cases, 9011 recovered cases and 272 deaths as on June 13, 2020. The epidemic curve and the time-dependent reproduction number for Rajasthan are shown in Fig. 19. $R(t)$ has downward trend from the week preceding June 01, and on June 10 the value is 1.09.

The predicted daily incidence and cumulative incidences in Rajasthan are shown in Fig. 20a and b, respectively. The predictions for Rajasthan are as follows: On 30 June, cumulative incidences are 17,706 (range: 13,275–23,073); on 15 July, cumulative incidences are 28,354 (range: 20,979–38,153).

West Bengal

West Bengal is one of the highly populous states in India. On June 13, 2020, there are 10698 confirmed cases along with 5693 active cases, 4542 recovered cases and 463 deaths. The epidemic curve and the variation of reproduction number for West

(a)

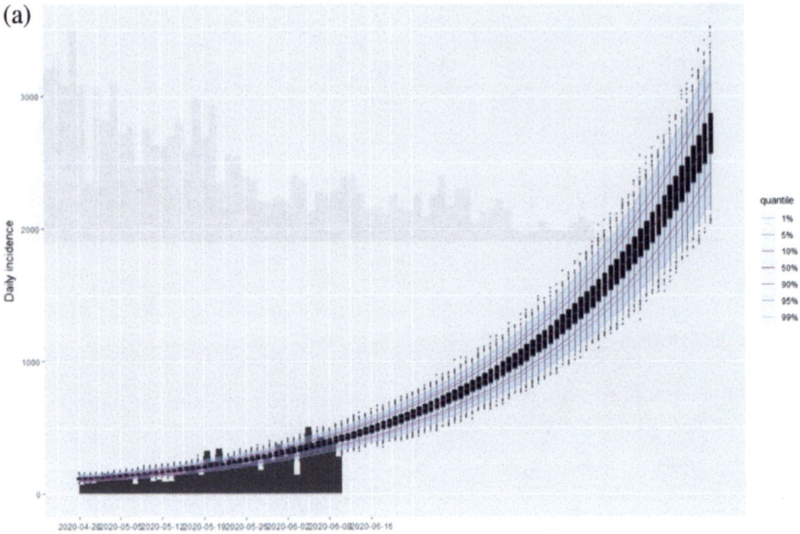

Fig. 18 **a** Predicted daily incidence and actually observed incidence in Uttar Pradesh, **b** predicted cumulative daily incidence in Uttar Pradesh

(b)

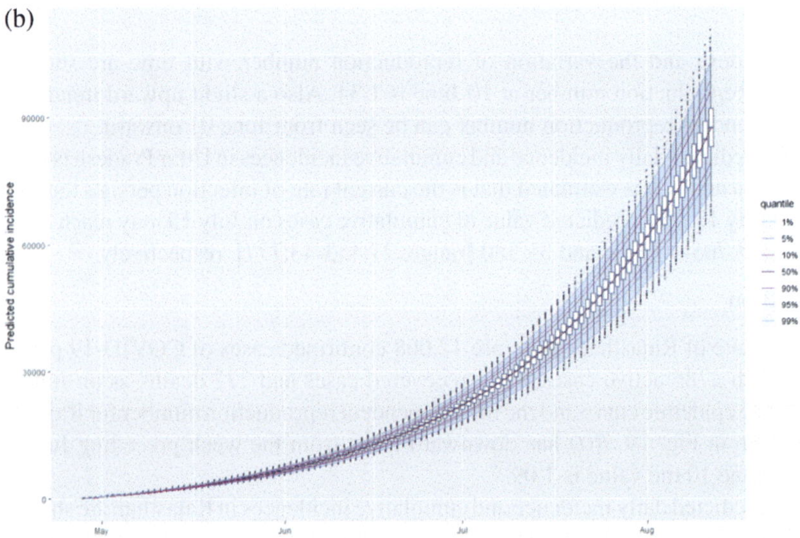

Fig. 18 (continued)

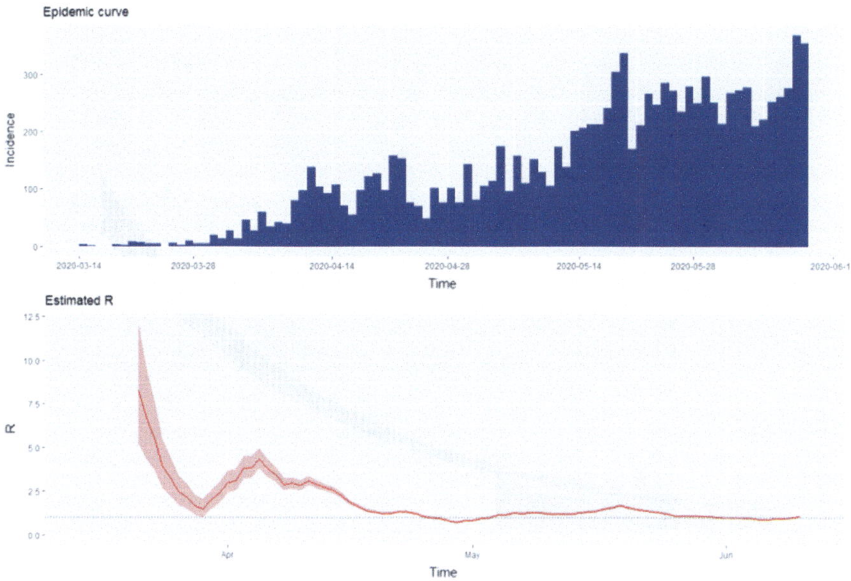

Fig. 19 Epidemic curve and the time-dependent reproduction number in Rajasthan

Bengal are shown in Fig. 21. A downward trend in the reproduction number from 01 June can be observed from the figure. Its value on 10 June is nearly 1.31.

The predicted daily incidence and cumulative incidences in West Bengal are shown in Fig. 22a and b, respectively. The predictions for West Bengal are as follows: On 30 June, cumulative incidences are 19,772 (range: 13,584–26,044); on 15 July, cumulative incidences are 42,864 (range: 29,526–57,359).

4 Discussion

In this study, the basic reproduction number of novel coronavirus (COVID-19) is estimated from the early outbreak of the disease in India. From the results, it is found that the number varies from 1.53 to 3.25 with a mean of 2.18. This variation is due to the method for estimating the number. Also in this study, an attempt is made to predict near-future incidences in India and also in different Indian states. However, it must be noted that these predictions serve as general guidelines rather than absolute certainty. The predictions in India and also in different states help the central and also the state government to formulate the policy for near-future healthcare system in terms of COVID hospitals, doctors, health workers, ICU beds, ventilators, PPE, etc. to fight against COVID-19 pandemic. The predictions also help to take decision regarding further lockdown in hotspot/epicenter area, infrastructure set up for COVID patients, economic and social issues, etc.

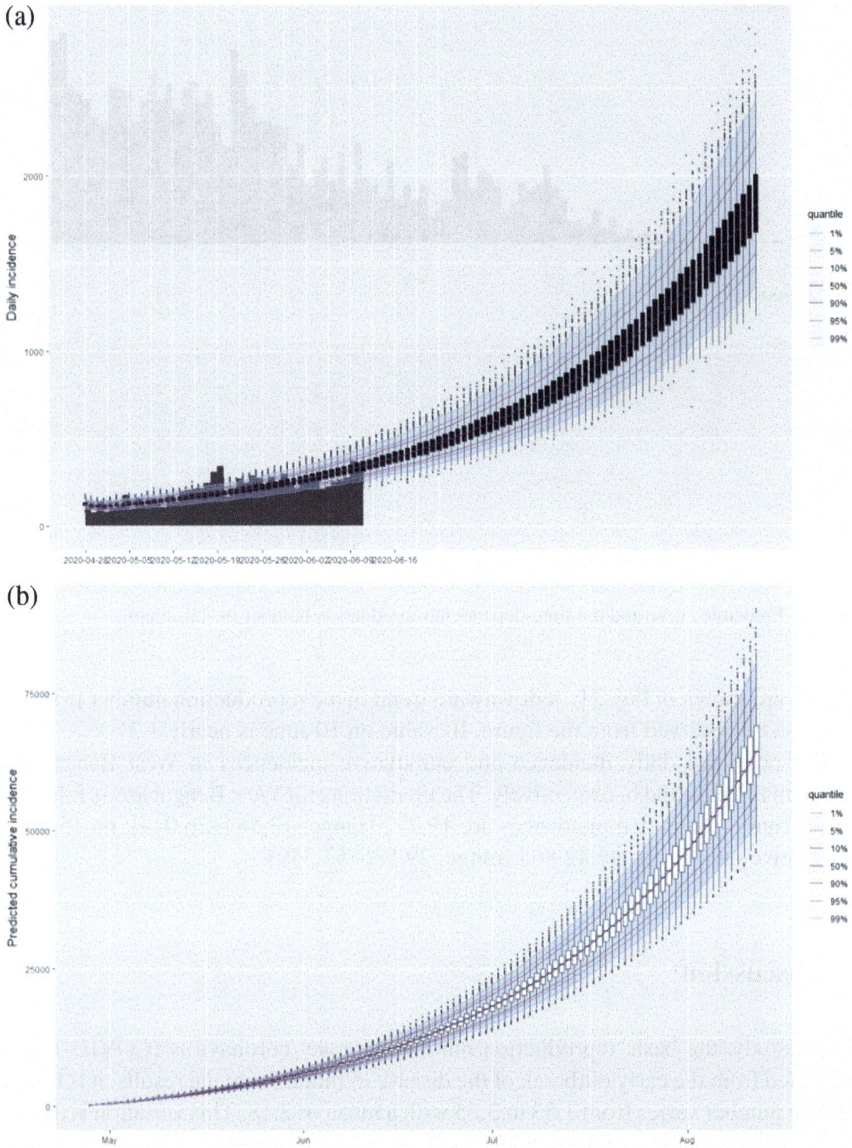

Fig. 20 **a** Predicted daily incidence and actually observed incidence in Rajasthan, **b** predicted cumulative daily incidence in Rajasthan

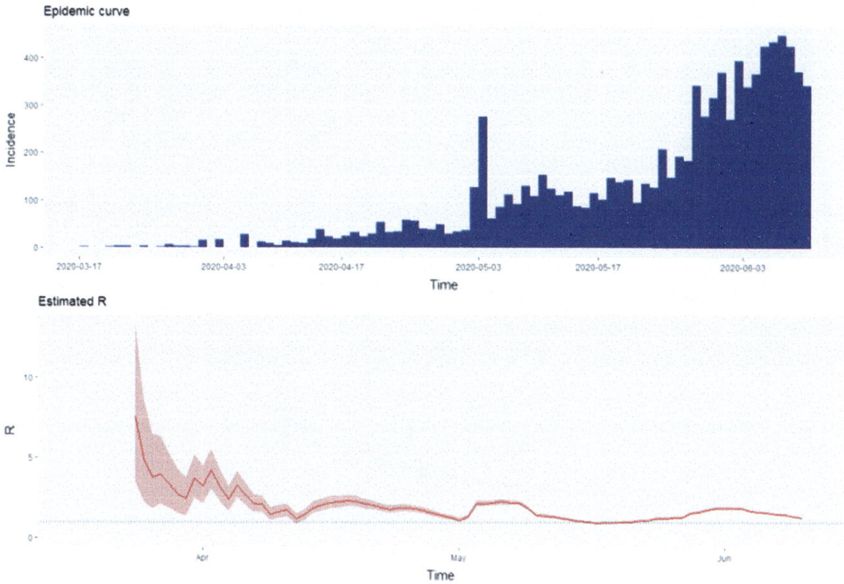

Fig. 21 Epidemic curve and the time-dependent reproduction number in West Bengal

(a)

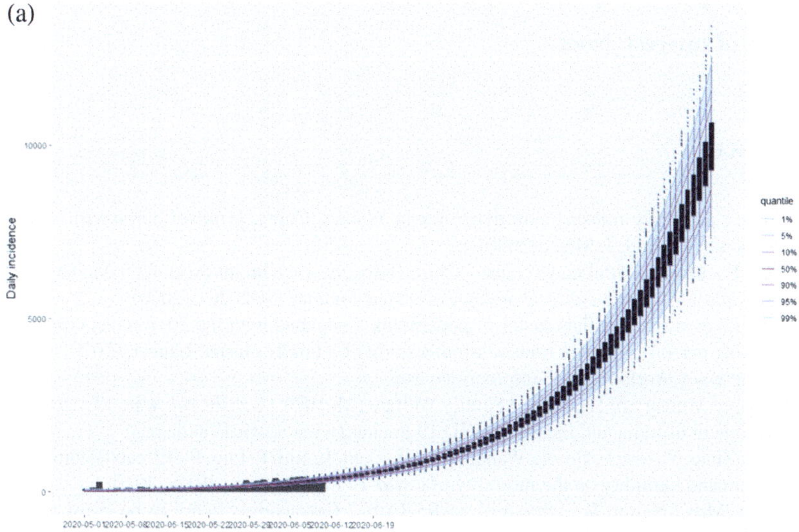

Fig. 22 **a** Predicted daily incidence and actually observed incidence in West Bengal, **b** predicted cumulative daily incidence in West Bengal

(b)

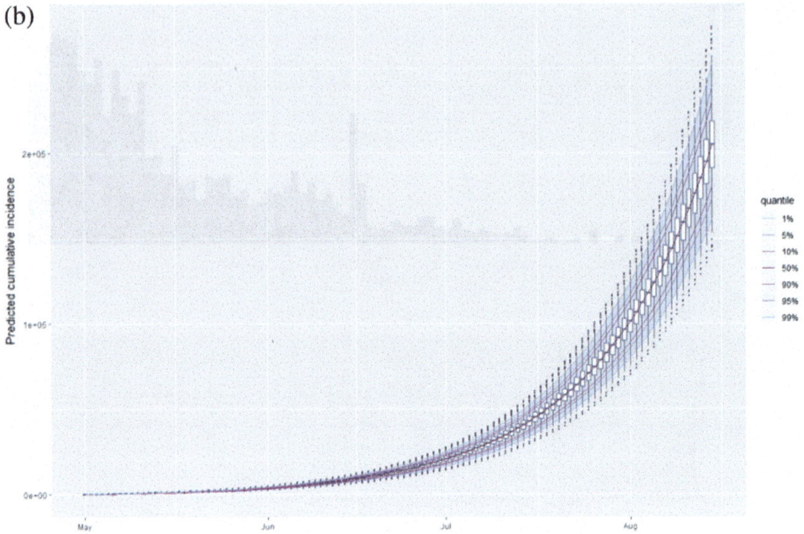

Fig. 22 (continued)

Financial support & sponsorship: None.

Conflicts of Interest: None.

References

1. Li, Q. et al.: Early transmission dynamics in Wuhan, China, of novel coronavirus-infected pneumonia. N. Engl. J. Med., (2020)
2. WHO: Pneumonia of unknown cause—China (https://www.who.int/csr/don/05-January- *2020-pneumonia-of-unkown-cause-china/en/; accessed January 30, 2020)*, (2020)
3. Chan, J.F.et al.: A familial cluster of pneumonia associated with the 2019 novel coronavirus indicating person-to-person transmission: a study of a family cluster. Lancet, (2020)
4. Website:www.Worldometers/ info/coronavirus
5. Data from Ministry of Health and Family Welfare (MoHFW) website(www.mohfw.gov.in) the Government of India and Indian COVID 19 tracker (www. covid19india.org)
6. Ma, Y., Zhao, Y., Liu, J., He, X., Wang, B., Fu, S., Yan, J., Niu, J., Luo, B.: Effects of temperature variation and humidity on the mortality of covid-19 in Wuhan. medRxiv, 2020
7. Araujo, M.B., Naimi, B.: Spread of SARS-CoV-2 Coronavirus likely to be constrained by climate. medRxiv, 2020
8. Salman, S., Salem, M.L.: The mystery behind childhood sparing by COVID-19. Int. J. Cancer Biomed. Res. 10 (3 Apr 2020)
9. Luo, W., Majumder, M., Liu, D., Poirier, C., Mandl, K., Lipsitch, M, Santillana, M.: The role of absolute humidity on transmission rates of the covid-19 outbreak. (2020)
10. Nsoesie, E.O., Brownstein, J.S., Ramakrishnan, N., Marathe, M.V.: A systematicreview of studies on forecasting the dynamics of influenza outbreaks. Influenza. Other. Respir. Viruses. **8**(3), 309–316 (2014)
11. Chretien, J.-P., Riley, S., George, D.B.: Mathematical modeling of the West Africa Ebola epidemic. eLife. **4**, e09186 (2015)

12. WHO Ebola Response Team: Ebola virus disease in West Africa—the first 9 months of the epidemic and forward projections. N. Engl. J. Med. **371**(16), 1481–1495 (2014)
13. WHO Ebola Response Team: West African Ebola epidemic after one year-slowing but not yet under control. N. Engl. J. Med. **372**(6), 584–587 (2015)
14. WHO Ebola Response Team: Ebola virus disease among children in West Africa. New Engl. J. Med. **372**(13), 1274–1277 (2015)
15. Goldstein, E., Cobey, S., Takahashi, S., Miller, J.C., Lipsitch, M.: Predicting the epidemic sizes of influenza A/H1N1, A/H3N2, and B: a statistical method. PLoSMed. **8**(7), e1001051 (2011)
16. Meltzer, M.I., Atkins, C.Y., Santibanez, S., Estimating the future number of cases in the Ebola epidemic—liberia and sierra leone. MMWR Suppl. **63**(3), 1–14 (2014–2015)
17. Influenza Forecasting. http://predict.phiresearchlab.org/flu/index.html (2017)
18. Dengue Forecasting. http://dengueforecasting.noaa.gov/. (2017)
19. Chikungunya Forecasting. http://www.darpa.mil/news-events/ (2017)
20. Liu, Y. et al.: The reproductive number of COVID-19 is higher compared to SARS coronavirus. J. Travel. Med. (2020)
21. Zhang, S. et al.: Estimation of the reproductive number of novel coronavirus (COVID-19) and the probable outbreak size on the Diamond Princess cruise ship: a data-driven analysis. Int. J. Infect. Dis. **93**, 201–204 (2020)
22. Li, Q. et al.: Early transmission dynamics in Wuhan, China, of novel coronavirus-infected pneumonia. New England J. Med. (2020)
23. Nishiura, H., Linton, N.M., Akhmetzhanov, A.R.: Serial interval of novel coronavirus (COVID-19) infections. Int. J. Infect. Dis. (2020)
24. Du, Z. et al.: The serial interval of COVID-19 from publicly reported confirmed cases. medRxiv (2020)
25. Jombart, T. et al.: earlyr: Estimation of transmissibility in the early stages of a disease outbreak. Available from: https://cran.r-project.org/package=earlyR
26. Boelle, P.-Y., Obadia, T.: R0: Estimation of R0 and Real-Time Reproduction Number from Epidemics. Available from: https://cran.r-project.org/package=R0
27. Obadia, T., Haneef, R., Boëlle, P.Y.: The R0 package: a toolbox to estimate reproduction numbers for epidemic outbreaks. *BMC* Med. Inf. Decis. Making. **12**(1), 147 (2012)
28. Cori, et al.: A new framework and software to estimate time-varying reproduction numbers during epidemics. Am. J. Epidemiol. **178**(9), 1505–1512 (2013)
29. Forsberg White, L., Pagano, M.: A likelihood-based method for real-time estimation of the serial interval and reproductive number of an epidemic. Stat. Med. **27**(16), 2999–3016 (2008)
30. Wallinga, J., Lipsitch, M.: How generation intervals shape the relationship between growth rates and reproductive numbers. Proc. Roy. Soc. B: Biol. Sci. **274**(1609), 599 (2007)
31. Wallinga, J., Teunis, P.: Different epidemic curves for severe acute respiratory syndrome reveal similar impacts of control measures. Am. J. Epidemiol. **160**(6), 509–516 (2004)
32. Nouvellet, et al.: A simple approach to measure transmissibility and forecast incidence. Epidemics **22**, 29–35 (2018)
33. Thibaut, et al.: Projections: project future case incidence. Available from: https://cran.r-project.org/package=projections

COVID-19 Analysis by Using Machine and Deep Learning

Dharminder Yadav, Himani Maheshwari, Umesh Chandra, and Avinash Sharma

Abstract Coronavirus is the pandemic in the whole world due to infection spread with community transfer. World Health Organization renames coronavirus to COVID-19, and the full name of coronavirus is severe acute respiratory syndrome coronavirus (SARS-CoV). COVID-19 belongs to the Betacoronavirus family and affects the respiratory system of humans. Machine learning is the part of artificial intelligence which used existing machine learning algorithms and dataset pattern to find an adequate solution for the problem. This chapter used machine learning algorithms supervised and unsupervised to analyze the spreading pattern such as confirmed case, recovered case, and death case of coronavirus worldwide. Analysis of the infection rate and mortality rate of coronavirus in the top 10 countries of the world. Analysis the effect of coronavirus in Asia and Europe visualized the result on the map. Choropleth is a thematic map which divides the world geographical area into different colors on the base of the data variable. This chapter used machine learning algorithms such as support vector machine, navies Bayes theorem, linear regression, decision tree repressors, random forest, and prophet algorithm for future prediction and to test the accuracy of prediction. The analysis of confirmed, recovered, and death cases is visualized by using Matplotlib in Python. Time series analysis of recovered,

D. Yadav (✉)
Department of Computer Science and Technology, Glocal University, Saharanpur, UP, India
e-mail: ydharminder@yahoo.com

H. Maheshwari
Department of Computer Science and Engineering, Uttarakhand Technical University, Dehradun, Uttarakhand, India
e-mail: himani_bahmah@yahoo.com

U. Chandra
Department of Computer Science,
Banda University of Agriculture and Technology, Banda, UP, India
e-mail: uck.iitr@gmail.com

A. Sharma
Maharishi Markandeshwar Deemed to be University Mullana, Ambala, Haryana, India
e-mail: asharma@mmumullana.org

© The Editor(s) (if applicable) and The Author(s), under exclusive license to Springer Nature Singapore Pte Ltd. 2020

C. Chakraborty et al. (eds.), *Internet of Medical Things for Smart Healthcare*, Studies in Big Data 80, https://doi.org/10.1007/978-981-15-8097-0_2

confirmed, and death cases of coronavirus predicted the future infection of the virus on the world. Analysis of the effect of Coronavirus, Country-wise, and State wise on top infected countries. Deep learning algorithm, long short-term memory (LSTM), is a recurrent neural network-type algorithm used to predict the future infection rate of coronavirus in the world. In this study, different machine learning algorithms were implemented and find the algorithm which gives the highest accuracy. Bar graph and pie are used to visualize the result of the experiment by using Python which helps to better understand the result. Analysis of the effect of coronavirus on Russia, Italy, the USA, the UK, Iran, Turkey, Germany, France, and Brazil finds the infection rate, mortality rate, and recovery rate of these countries. Analyze the precision, recall, and f1-score of these algorithms, and plot the graph. Find the recovered and death rates per one thousand patients of confirmed cases.

Keywords Machine learning · SVM · LSTM · ARIMA · Deep learning · COVID-19 · SARS-CoV

1 Introduction of Machine Learning and COVID-19

Coronavirus is not a new virus, but other coronavirus exits in the world such as sever acute respiration syndrome coronavirus (SARS-CoV), human coronavirus NL63 (HCoV-NL63), human coronavirus HKU1 (HCoV-HKU1), and Middle East respiratory syndrome coronavirus (MERS-CoV) identified in years 2003, 2004, 2005, and 2012, respectively [1, 2]. In 1930, first time coronavirus was discovered in chickens caused by infectious bronchitis virus (IBV), which attacks respiration system, kidney, reproductive system [3]. In 1931, new respiration disease was found in chicken with 40–90% mortality rate [4]. Mouse hepatitis virus (MHV) and transmissible gastroenteritis virus, and two other animal coronaviruses were discovered in 1940, but human coronavirus was discovered in 1960 with upper respiratory infection in children [5–7]. New coronavirus B814 was found in an adult in 1965 with symptoms of respiratory tract and common cold [8]. Hamre and Procknow discovered a new coronavirus Hamre's virus in 1965, which later she called 229E [9]. McIntosh et al. discovered a new group of virus named organ culture (OC or OC43), which is searched by using organ culture [10]. The word coronavirus is a combination of two words corona + virus; corona word comes from the Latin root word crown, because it shows crown-like appearance and it is new genus of virus [11–15]. Hoek et al. discovered a new coronavirus name NL63, and Fouchier et al. reported a virus NL in a 8-month boy, 2004 [16, 17]. HCoV new coronavirus was found in children with cough, and rhinorrhea was present in most of the children but this virus is different from the NL63 and 229E. Table 1 shows the virus with their name and discovery year.

Middle East respiratory syndrome coronavirus (MERS-CoV) was first reported in 2012 but till July 2015, confirmed cases were found in the 21 countries [18, 19]. SARS-CoV-2 is the new virus reported in Wuhan, China, at the end of 2019. World Health Organization provides official name of SARS-CoV-2 as COVID-19 on

Table 1 Different types of virus details

Sr. no.	Virus	Location	Group	Year	References
1	HCoV-229E	Chicago	I	1966	[46, 47]
2	HCoV-OC43	USA	II	1967	[48, 49]
3	SARS	China	IV	2003	[50, 51]
4	NL63*	Netherlands	I	2004	[16, 51, 52]
5	NL*	Netherlands	I	2004	[17]
6	HCoV-NH*	New Haven, CT	I	2005	[53]
7	HKU1	Hong Kong	II	2005	[43, 54, 55]
8	MERS-CoV	Saudi Arabia	II	2012	[56]
9	SARS-CoV-2	China	II	2019	[1]

February 11, 2020 [20, 21]. It may be a positive-sense single-stranded RNA infection of the Coronaviridae family [22, 23]. The first case of COVID-19 outside the China was found in Thailand in January 13, 2020, and in March 2020 it is declared as epidemic for world and covers more than 200 countries [24]. Coronavirus' scientific name is Orthocoronavirinae or Coronavirinae, infected to mammal and birds' respiration system [25–27]. There are four genera of coronavirus present such as Alphacoronavirus, Betacoronavirus, Gammacoronavirus, and Deltacoronavirus of the Coronaviridae family; first two are responsible for mammal infection, and last two are responsible for bird infection [27–29]. Seven human coronaviruses were found such as 229E, OC43, HKU1, NL63, SARS-CoV, MERS-CoV, and SARS-CoV-2 [16, 17]. Coronaviruses OC43 and HKU1 are the Betacoronavirus, 229E and NL63 are the Alphacoronavirus with mild symptoms, and SARS-CoV, MERS-CoV, and SARS-CoV-2 are the Betacoronavirus with severe symptoms. Common cold, fever, and sore throat are the symptoms of coronavirus [30]. No vaccine and medicine are developed for treatment of COVID-19; social distancing, lockdown, and precaution are the safety measures [31, 32]. Table 2 shows the genus of coronavirus with their species. Table 2 shows the genus and type of species of coronavirus with their species.

In this study, different supervised machine learning algorithms such as linear regression, Bayes theorem, and SVM are used to find the accuracy of study; time series algorithm long short-term memory (LSTM) and prophet are used to predict the future confirmed cases. LSTM is the deep learning algorithm which is the part of artificial intelligence and machine learning. Data is collected from the Kaggle and analyzes the data for the top ten infected countries, country-wise and state-wise by using Python. This study indicates the spreading pattern of COVID-19 of top countries such as the USA, Russia, Brazil, the UK, Spain, Italy, France, Germany, Turkey, and Iran date-wise.

Table 2 Genera and type of species of coronavirus

Genus	Type of species	Species	References
Alphacoronavirus	Alphacoronavirus 1	Human coronavirus 229E, human coronavirus NL63, Miniopterus bat coronavirus 1, Miniopterus bat coronavirus HKUS, porcine epidemic diarrhea virus, Rhinolophus bat coronavirus HKU2, Scotophilus bat coronavirus 512	[57]
Betacoronavirus	Murine coronavirus (MHV)	Betacoronavirus 1 (bovine coronavirus and human coronavirus OC43), Hedgehog coronavirus 1, human coronavirus HKUl, Middle East respiratory syndrome-related coronavirus, marine coronavirus, Pipistrellus bat coronavirus HKU5, Rousettus bat coronavirus HKU9, severe acute respiratory syndrome-related coronavirus (SARS-CoV, SARS-CoV-*2),* Tylonycteris bat coronavirus HKU4	[58]
Gammacoronavirus	Avian coronavirus (IBV)	Avian coronavirus, Beluga whale coronavirus SW1	[5]
Deltacoronavirus	Bulbul coronavirus HKU11	Bulbul coronavirus HKU11, porcine coronavirus HKU15	[1, 5]

2 Literature Review

Paper [33] analyzes the data, finds the top 10 most infected countries in the world, and predicts the future confirmed active and death cases by using the prophet algorithm of Facebook. The first case of COVID-19 was found in India on January 30, 2020, but till 25 March 2020 numbers of cases are very less [34, 35]. As of May 10, 2020, the total confirmed cases observed in India are 61,000 with 472 recovered cases and 166 deaths [36]. In the test, two people were found corona positive in Qom city on February 19, 2020, but after that in 31 states of Iran, coronavirus spread rapidly, and within two months there were 85,996 confirmed cases and 5391 deaths [37, 38]. Undoubtedly, statistical forecasting models are useful for the control and prediction of this global pandemic [39–41].

Autoregressive integrated moving average (ARIMA) model helps to forecast the trend of COVID-19 pandemic, and this model is also known as the Box–Jenkins methodology [42]. Paper [43] analyzes the effect of coronavirus in Italy by using the

ARIMA model method. They predict the effect of the virus in Italy after 60 days by discounting the effect of lockdown. Totally, there were 105,792 confirmed and 15,726 death cases till 31 March 2020 in Italy. Paper [44] analyzes the effect of coronavirus in India by using the susceptible, infected, and recovered (SIR) epidemic model and predicts the future case in India. They consider the effect of lockdown in India advice social distancing play a measure role to control the outbreak. Paper [45] predicted the confirmed cases by using long short-term memory (LSTM) algorithm in India for the next 30 days.

3 Data Collection and Preprocessing

The scholar collected data from the kaggle sites [10] and performed the experiments to studies the cases of coronavirus worldwide, top infected countries of the world state-wise, and date-wise by using the python language in Jupyter notebooks. "COVID-19" affects approximately 188 countries with 5,193,967 confirmed cases, 1,882,498 recovered cases, 3,129,348 active cases, and 323,413 deaths. We study the confirmed, recover, death, and active cases worldwide. We also study the spreading pattern, recovery rate, death rate, infection rate, active cases, and confirmed cases of top countries such as the USA, Russia, Brazil, the UK, Spain, Italy, France, Germany, Turkey, Iran, and India. We analyze the infection country-wise as well as date-wise. Figure 1 shows the packages of Python language which is used for reading data, analysis of data, and plotting. Pandas and NumPy are the packages that are used to read a file and help to process numerical operation on a multi-dimensional array. For reading a data, we used the "pd.read_csv()" command because we are using comma separated value (CSV) file for data analysis. Data was collected from January 22, 2020, to May 20, 2020, a total of 120 days data with 32,065 row and eight columns. Rename the column name by using the rename command, and find active cases shown in Fig. 2. Province/States column most of the data null value, replaced with space because null value creates a problem in data analysis.

```
import numpy as np
import pandas as pd
import plotly.graph_objects as go
import plotly.express as px
import plotly.io as pio
pio.templates.default = "plotly_white"
from plotly.subplots import make_subplots
```

```
 #   Column          Non-Null Count  Dtype
---  ------          --------------  -----
 0   Province/State  9680 non-null   object
 1   Country/Region  32065 non-null  object
 2   Lat             32065 non-null  float64
 3   Long            32065 non-null  float64
 4   Date            32065 non-null  datetime64[ns]
 5   Confirmed       32065 non-null  int64
 6   Deaths          32065 non-null  int64
 7   Recovered       32065 non-null  int64
```

Fig. 1 Packages and data type

```
cleaned_data.rename(columns={'ObservationDate': 'date',
                    'Province/State':'state',
                    'Country/Region':'country',
                    'Last Update':'last_updated',
                    'Confirmed': 'confirmed',
                    'Deaths':'deaths',
                    'Recovered':'recovered'
                   }, inplace=True)
# Active Case = confirmed - deaths - recovered
cleaned_data['active'] = cleaned_data['confirmed'] - cleaned_data['deaths'] - cleaned_data['recovered']
```

Fig. 2 Rename column and calculate the active cases

4 Algorithm Used

Machine learning algorithms are implementing in this chapter on coronavirus data to find the top 10 infected countries and predict future cases by using deep learning algorithms and prophet algorithm. Machine learning algorithm descriptions are given below:

Linear Regression: Regression is the part of machine learning and artificial intelligence which is used to draw a continuous graph. Linear regression is the simplest algorithm of supervised machine learning which finds the relation between two variables such as dependent and independent variables. The linear equation is "$y = mx + c$"; here, y (output) is dependent variable, x (input) is independent variable, m is the slope, and c is the intercept.

Support Vector Machine (SVM): SVM is generalized from the maximum margin classifier. It is used for classification and regression problems which maximize the accuracy of the algorithm, avoiding the overfitting of data. It is used for a single feature to multi-class classification. SVM efficiently performed the classification by using the kernel; kernel may be linear or nonlinear. Hyper-plain is the line that divides the data into two classes, and hyper-plain created from the data point is also known as support vector. Two lines are also drawn parallel to support vector which is equidistance from the support vector, area between these lines is called margin, and maximum margin hyper-plain is the best classifier. Equation of SVM is

$$B_0 + B_1X_1 + B_2X_2 + \ldots\ldots\ldots\ldots\ldots B_nX_n = 0$$

Bayes Theorem: It is the supervised machine learning classification algorithm. It is assumed that features are not related (independent) to each other in the same class. Bayes theorem is the probability theorem and used for binary class or multi-class classification problems. The formula of Bayes theorem is

$$P(A/B) = P(B/A) * P(A)/P(B)$$

Here, A is the hypothesis, B is the evidence, $P(A/B)$ is the posterior probability, and $P(A)$ is the prior probability. Prior probability means event not happened, and posterior probability means event already happened.

Long Short-Term Memory (LSTM): LSTM is the recurrent neural network that is used for many tasks. In 1997, Hochreiter and Schmidhuber introduced the LSTM algorithm used for image processing, speech recognition, and language translation. LSTM used the logic gate to remember the old information for the long term and maintain the connection between old information and new information. LSTM is made from the collection of cells, these cells store the value, and three types of gates are input gate, output gate, and output gate which regulate the information in the LSTM algorithm.

ARIMA: ARIMA stands for autoregressive integrated moving average model which followed an approach by Box–Jenkins. ARIMA model is analyzed to forecast a future that is time-dependent, i.e., time series. ARIMA model was formed by a combination of three models: autoregressive (AR), integrated (I), and moving average (MA) models, respectively [39, 45].

Prophet: Prophet is the Facebook time series prediction algorithm and freely available to all. It is a very simple algorithm and need not tune the parameters just like other time series algorithms. Trend, seasonality, and holiday are the components of the prophet algorithm as shown in Eq. 1.

$$y(t) = g(t) + s(t) + h(t) + \varepsilon t \tag{1}$$

Here, $g(t)$ is the liner or logistic growth curve, $s(t)$ is the periodic change or seasonality change, $h(t)$ is the effect of holiday, and εt is the error. A prophet is used for both linear and nonlinear models. The parameter is used in trend (growth, changepoints, n_changepoints, changepoints_prior_scale), seasonality (yearly, weekly, daily seasonality), and holidays (holidays, holidays_prior_scale).

5 Result and Discussion

For the data analysis, Python is the best language with a large number of packages that help for data analysis and visualization. Find the most infected countries in the world, group the data by using the "groupby" command, and sum the data to find the total confirmed, death, active, and recovered cases till May 20, 2020. Figure 3 shows the top 10 infected countries with coronavirus confirmed cases. "px.bar", "px" is the shorter name of plotly express for creating a horizontal bar chart between countries and confirmed cases, arranging the 10 countries' confirmed case in descending order. The title represents the title of the graph, height depicts the height, X, Y depict the x-axis and y-axis, and below figure shows that USA has the maximum number of confirmed cases (1,577,147), followed by Russia (317,554), Brazil (310,087), UK (252,246), Spain (233,037), Italy (228,006), France (181,951), Germany (179,021), Turkey (153,548), Iran (129,341) (Fig. 4).

Figure 5 depicts the confirmed (5,102,418), recovered (1,895,640), death (332,924), and active (2,873,854) cases worldwide. Sum and group the data by date using the "groupby" function and sum by "sum()" function, and reset the index.

```
fig = px.bar(latest_grouped.sort_values('confirmed', ascending=False)[:10][::-1],
             x='confirmed', y='country',
             title='Confirmed Cases Worldwide', text='confirmed', height=1000, orientation='h')
fig.show()
```

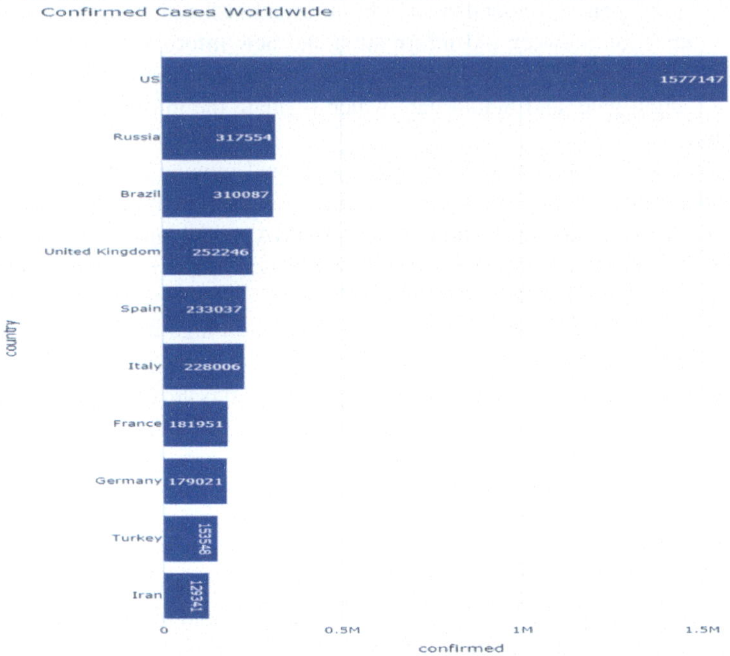

Fig. 3 Top 10 infected countries' confirmed cases

```
grouped = data.groupby('date')['date', 'confirmed', 'recovered','deaths','active'].sum().reset_index()
temp1 = grouped.melt(id_vars="date", value_vars=['confirmed','recovered', 'deaths', 'active'],
                 var_name='case', value_name='count')
fig = px.line(temp1, x="date", y="count", color='case',
             title="Worldwide Confirmed, Recovered, Deaths, Active Cases with Time",
              color_discrete_sequence = ['black','blue', 'red', 'green'])
fig.show()
```

Fig. 4 Code for drawing worldwide cases and other cases

Group by data and cases by date melted in a variable temp1, and draw a line graph by using line() function using a different color (Fig. 4).

Split the data by creating the country-wise group by using a comparison operator, and then split the data by using the "groupby()" function on the base of date for all 10 infected countries [Fig. 7]. Plot the line graph by using the line function of plotly package for all top 10 countries by changing the parameters [Fig. 3]. Figures 6, 7, 8, 9, 10, and 11 depict cases of USA, Russia, Brazil, and UK with confirmed (1,577,147, 317,554, 310,087, 252,246), active (1,184,027, 221,774, 16,408, 214,988), recovered (298,418, 92,681, 12,596, 1134), and death (94,702, 3099, 20,047, 36,184), respectively. In UK and USA epidemic started after 15 March, but in Russia and

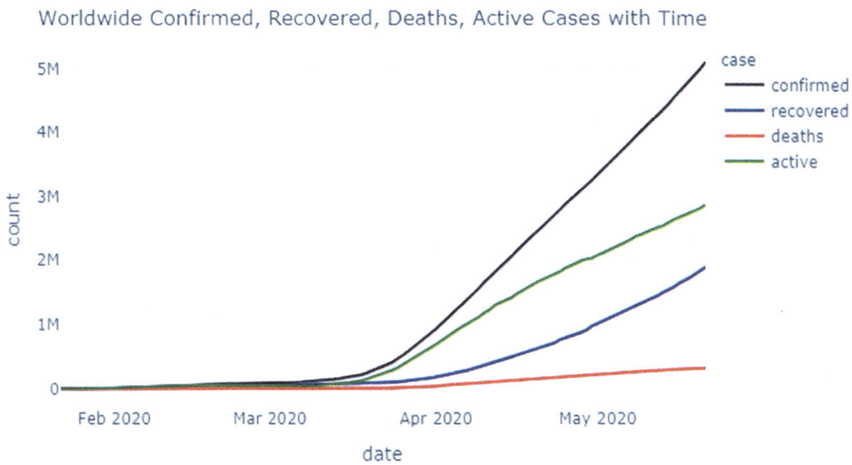

Fig. 5 World confirmed, recovered, deaths, active

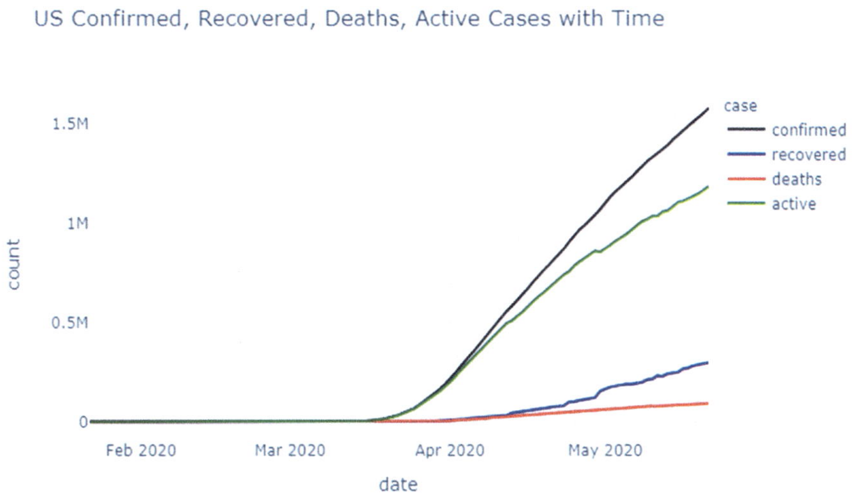

Fig. 6 Confirmed, recovered, deaths, active in the USA

Brazil epidemic started on March 29, 2020. Recovery in patients is minimum in the UK but maximum in the UK, and deaths of patients are minimum in Russia but maximum in the USA. Figures 12, 13, 14, and 15 represent the cases of Spain, Italy, France, and Germany with confirmed (233,037, 228,006, 181,951, 179,021), active (54,721, 60,960, 89,757, 12,731), recovered (150,376, 134,560, 63,976, 158,087), and death (27,940, 32,486, 28,218, 8203), respectively. Figures 16, 17, and 18 show the confirmed (15,348, 129,341, 1,540,480), recovered (114,990, 100,564, 654,894), death (4249, 7249, 70,607), and active (34,309, 21,529, 814,979) cases in Turkey,

```
grouped_us = data[data['country'] == "US"].reset_index()
grouped_us_date = grouped_us.groupby('date')['date', 'confirmed', 'recovered','deaths','active'].sum().reset_index()

grouped_rus = data[data['country'] == "Russia"].reset_index()
grouped_rus_date = grouped_rus.groupby('date')['date', 'state','confirmed', 'recovered','deaths','active'].sum().reset_index()

grouped_bra = data[data['country'] == "Brazil"].reset_index()
grouped_bra_date = grouped_bra.groupby('date')['date', 'confirmed', 'recovered','deaths','active'].sum().reset_index()

grouped_uk = data[data['country'] == "United Kingdom"].reset_index()
grouped_uk_date = grouped_uk.groupby('date')['date', 'confirmed', 'recovered','deaths','active'].sum().reset_index()

grouped_spain = data[data['country'] == "Spain"].reset_index()
grouped_spain_date = grouped_spain.groupby('date')['date', 'confirmed', 'recovered','deaths','active'].sum().reset_index()

grouped_italy = data[data['country'] == "Italy"].reset_index()
grouped_italy_date = grouped_italy.groupby('date')['date', 'confirmed', 'recovered','deaths','active'].sum().reset_index()

grouped_fran = data[data['country'] == "France"].reset_index()
grouped_fran_date = grouped_fran.groupby('date')['date', 'confirmed', 'recovered','deaths','active'].sum().reset_index()

grouped_ger = data[data['country'] == "Germany"].reset_index()
grouped_ger_date = grouped_ger.groupby('date')['date', 'confirmed', 'recovered','deaths','active'].sum().reset_index()

grouped_tur = data[data['country'] == "Turkey"].reset_index()
grouped_tur_date = grouped_tur.groupby('date')['date', 'confirmed', 'recovered','deaths','active'].sum().reset_index()

grouped_iran = data[data['country'] == "Iran"].reset_index()
grouped_iran_date = grouped_iran.groupby('date')['date', 'confirmed', 'recovered','deaths','active'].sum().reset_index()

grouped_rest = data[~data['country'].isin(['Russia', 'Italy', 'US', 'Turkey','Iran', 'Germany', 'United Kingdom', 'Brazil',
                                           'France', 'Spain'])].reset_index()
grouped_rest_date = grouped_rest.groupby('date')['date', 'confirmed', 'recovered','deaths','active'].sum().reset_index()
```

Fig. 7 Splitting the data country-wise and group the data date-wise

```
us = grouped_us_date.melt(id_vars="date", value_vars=['confirmed','recovered', 'deaths', 'active'],
                 var_name='case', value_name='count')

fig = px.line(us, x="date", y="count", color='case',
             title=f" {plot_titles[2].upper()} Confirmed, Recovered, Deaths, Active Cases with Time",
              color_discrete_sequence = color1)
fig.show()
russia = grouped_rus_date.melt(id_vars="date", value_vars=['confirmed','recovered', 'deaths', 'active'],
                 var_name='case', value_name='count')

fig = px.line(russia, x="date", y="count", color='case',
              title=f"{plot_titles[0].upper()} Confirmed, Recovered, Deaths, Active Cases with Time",
             color_discrete_sequence = color1)
fig.show()
iran = grouped_iran_date.melt(id_vars="date", value_vars=['confirmed','recovered', 'deaths', 'active'],
                 var_name='case', value_name='count')

fig = px.line(iran, x="date", y="count", color='case',
             title=f" {plot_titles[4].upper()} Confirmed, Recovered, Deaths, Active Cases with Time",
              color_discrete_sequence = color1)
fig.show()
brazil = grouped_bra_date.melt(id_vars="date", value_vars=['confirmed','recovered', 'deaths', 'active'],
                 var_name='case', value_name='count')

fig = px.line(brazil, x="date", y="count", color='case',
              title=f"{plot_titles[7].upper()} Confirmed, Recovered, Deaths, Active Cases with Time",
             color_discrete_sequence = color1)
fig.show()
turk = grouped_tur_date.melt(id_vars="date", value_vars=['confirmed','recovered', 'deaths', 'active'],
                 var_name='case', value_name='count')

fig = px.line(turk, x="date", y="count", color='case',
              title=f"{plot_titles[3].upper()} Confirmed, Recovered, Deaths, Active Cases with Time",
             color_discrete_sequence = color1)
fig.show()
```

Fig. 8 Code for plotline graph by using plotly express package

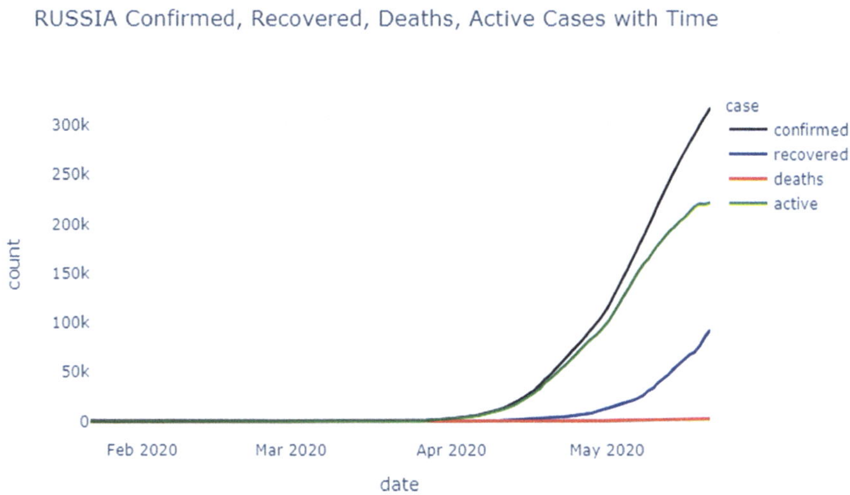

Fig. 9 Confirmed, recovered, deaths, active in Russia

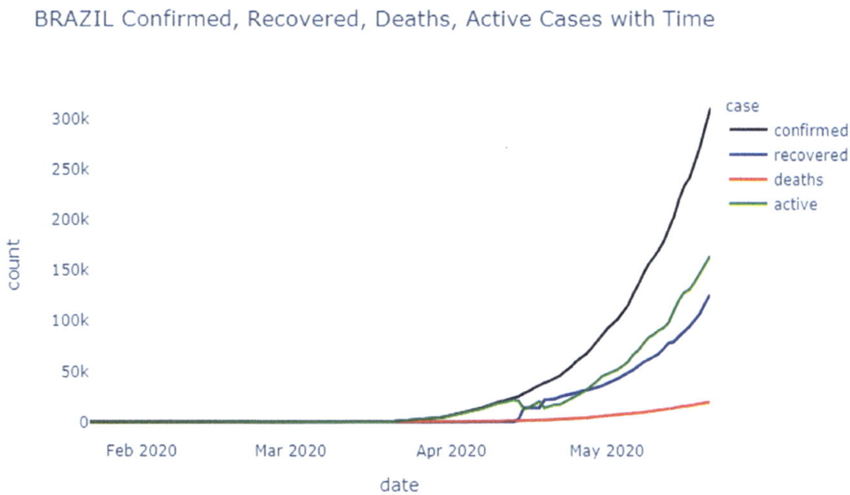

Fig. 10 Confirmed, recovered, deaths, active in Brazil

Iran, and rest of the world, respectively. Cutbreak started in Spain, Italy, France, Germany, and Iran on March 15, 2020, but in Turkey started at the end of March. In the rest of the world, epidemic started in the first week of February 2020 in China; now, this epidemic covers the whole world. Figure 8 depicts the code to draw a line graph for all top 10 countries and the rest of the world.

World map is the graphical representation of land, ocean, boundaries, and object on the paper. Here, choropleth map is used to represent the confirmed and death cases

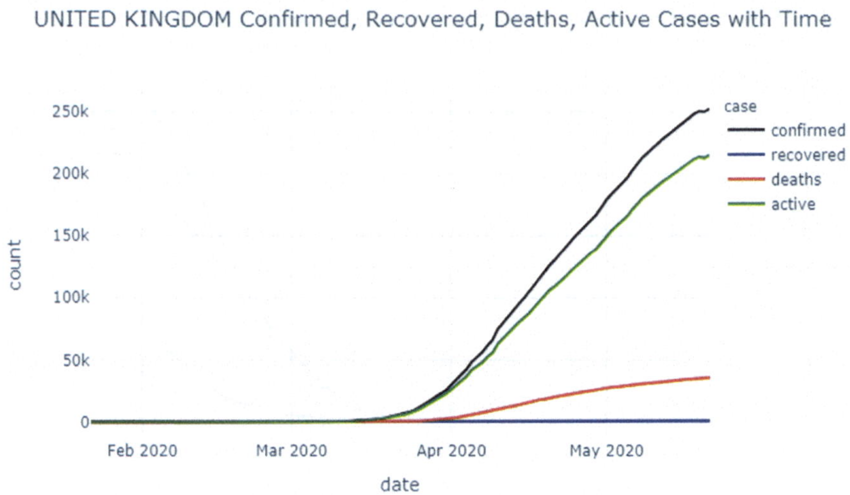

Fig. 11 Confirmed, recovered, deaths, active in UK

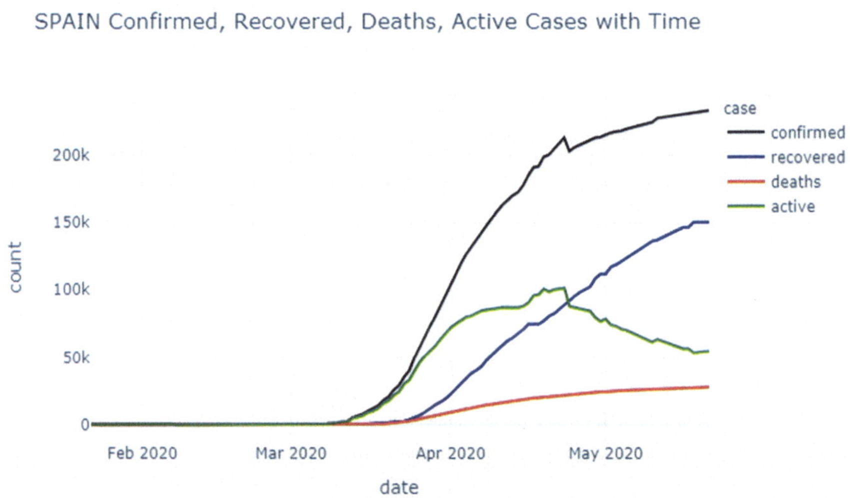

Fig. 12 Confirmed, recovered, deaths, active in Spain

on the map, and thematic map easily shows the confirmed and death case variation on the map with different colors: Light color depicts fewer cases, and dark color depicts more cases. For few countries, state-wise data is available and most of the states with NA replace it with white space by using the "fillna()" function and arrange the data in descending order on the base of a date. In Choropleth function, passing latest_group data, country, location mode is country name, color depends upon the

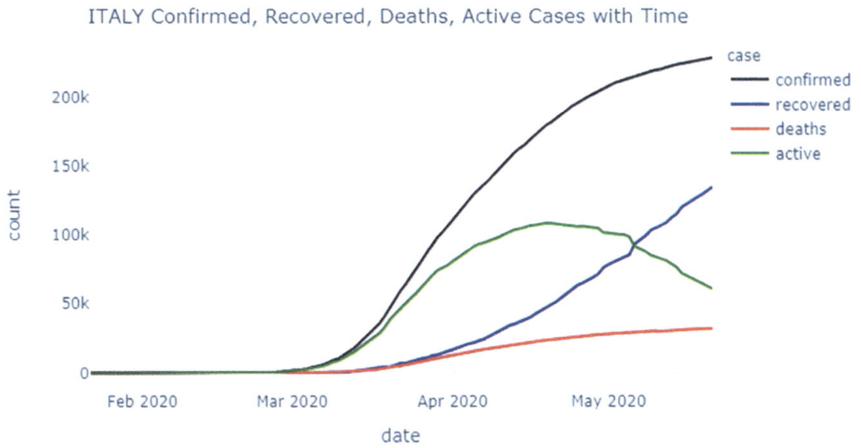

Fig. 13 Confirmed, recovered, deaths, active in Italy

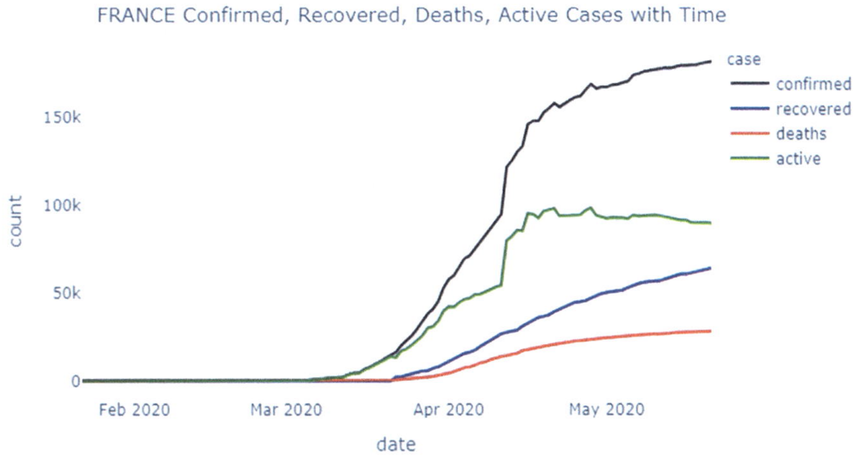

Fig. 14 Confirmed, recovered, deaths, active in France

number of confirmed cases, hover_name is country name, hover_data is the number of confirmed and death cases, range color is 1–5000 cases (Figs. 19, 20, and 21).

Cleaning data is arranged in descending order according to date, group by country data and sum, and reset the index. Mortality rate is calculated, total deaths are divided by total confirmed cases on 1000 confirmed cases, and draw the bar graph of mortality rate by using "px.bar()" function [Fig. 22]. Figure 25 depicts the country name with confirmed and lowest death cases. Belgium has the highest mortality rate, and the Maldives has a minimum mortality rate (Figs. 23, 24 and 26).

Recovery rate is calculated by recovered cases to divide by total infected cases and multiply by 100 to find the percentage [Fig. 27]. Lowest mortality rate and

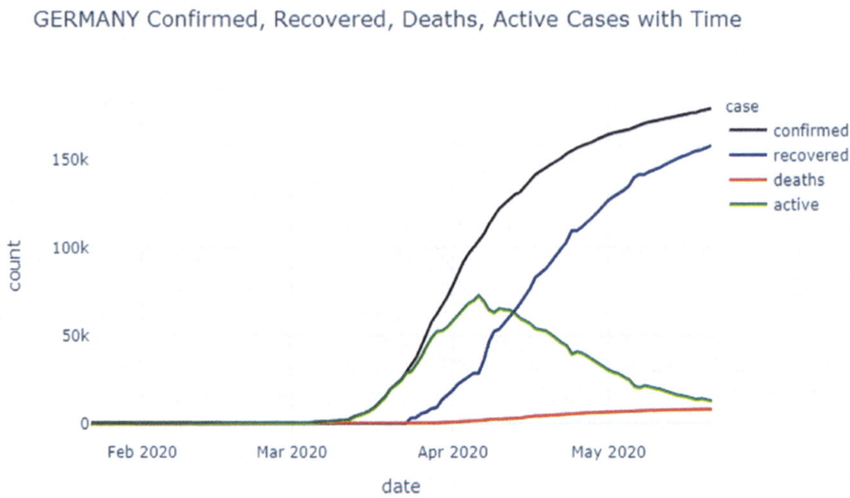

Fig. 15 Confirmed, recovered, deaths, active in Germany

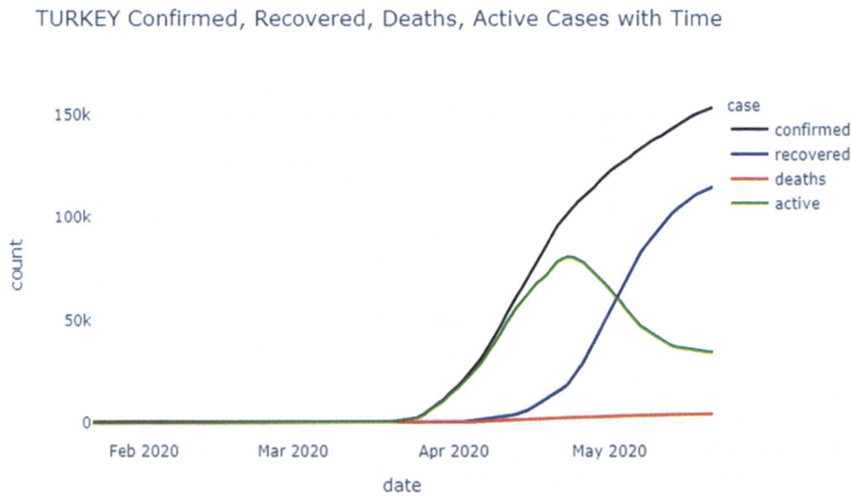

Fig. 16 Confirmed, recovered, deaths, active in Turkey

worst recovery rate with country name are shown in Figs. 25 and 26 by using "style.background_gradient(cmap = 'green') [Fig. 24] and cmap = 'reds' [Fig. 28]", which shows the green and black background color; dark color represents the high death or recovered patients, and light color represents less death or recovered cases. Iceland has a maximum recovery rate, but from the top 10 countries, the USA has maximum recovered cases shown in Figs. 26 and 29.

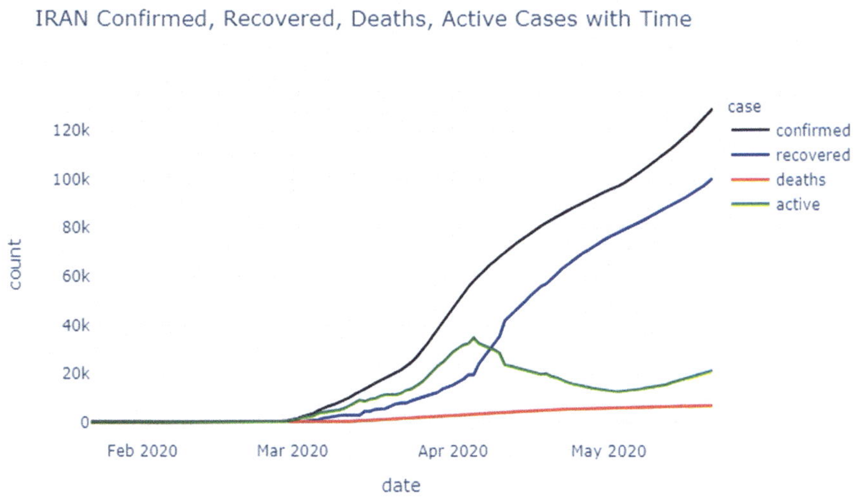

Fig. 17 Confirmed, recovered, deaths, active in Iran

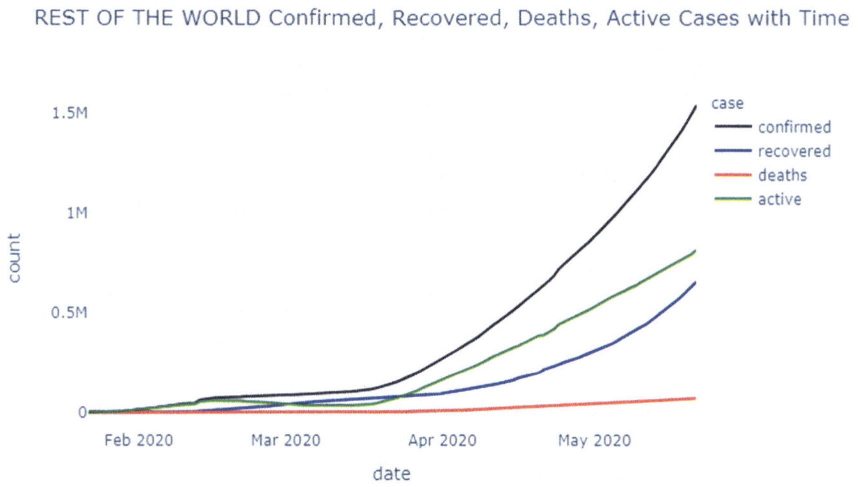

Fig. 18 Confirmed, recovered, deaths, active in rest of world

```
data['state'] = data['state'].fillna('')
temp = data[[col for col in data.columns if col != 'state']]
latest = temp[temp['date'] == max(temp['date'])].reset_index()
latest_grouped = latest.groupby('country')['confirmed', 'deaths'].sum().reset_index()
fig = px.choropleth(latest_grouped, locations="country",
                    locationmode='country names', color="confirmed",
                    hover_name="country",hover_data=["confirmed", "deaths"], range_color=[1,5000],
                    color_continuous_scale="peach",
                    title='Countries with Confirmed Cases')
fig.show()
```

Fig. 19 Code for choropleth map for confirmed and death cases

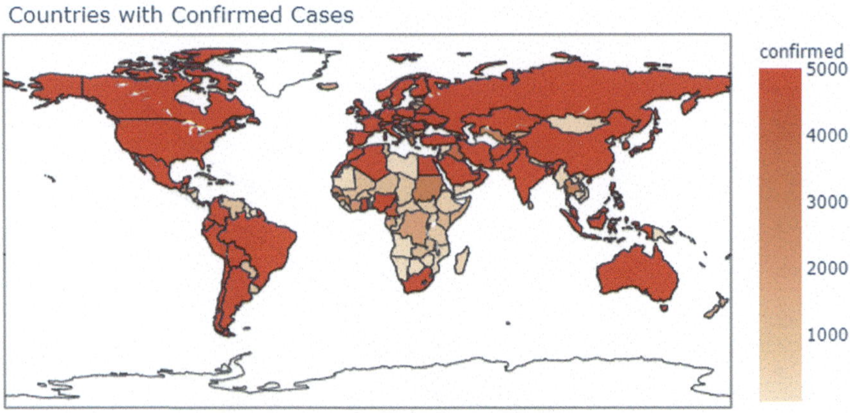

Fig. 20 World map for confirmed cases

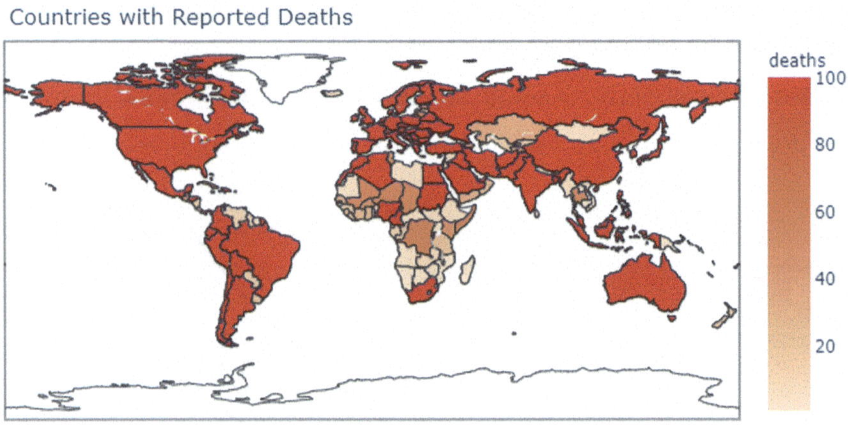

Fig. 21 World map for death cases

```
cleaned_latest = cleaned_data[cleaned_data['date'] == max(cleaned_data['date'])]
flg = cleaned_latest.groupby('country')['confirmed', 'deaths', 'recovered', 'active'].sum().reset_index()

flg['mortalityRate'] = round((flg['deaths']/flg['confirmed'])*100, 2)
temp = flg[flg['confirmed']>1000]
temp1 = temp.sort_values('mortalityRate', ascending=False)

fig = px.bar(temp1.sort_values(by="mortalityRate", ascending=False)[:10][::-1],
             x = 'mortalityRate', y = 'country',
             title='Deaths per 1000 Confirmed Cases', text='mortalityRate', height=800, orientation='h',
             color_discrete_sequence=['darkred']
            )
fig.show()
```

Fig. 22 Code for mortality rate bar graph

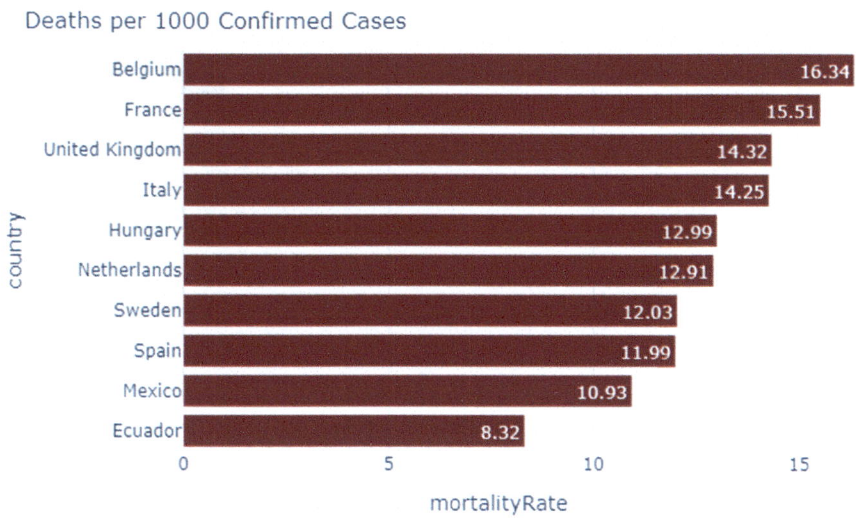

Fig. 23 Bar graph for mortality rate

```
print("Countries with Lowest Mortality Rates")
temp = flg[flg['confirmed']>1000]
temp = temp.sort_values('mortalityRate', ascending=True)[['country', 'confirmed','deaths']][:16]
temp.sort_values('confirmed', ascending=False)[['country', 'confirmed','deaths']][:20].style.background_gradient(cmap='Greens')
```

Fig. 24 Code for lowest mortality rate

Mortality and recovery in most infected countries: Table 3 represents death and recovery rates, minimum recover cases over confirmed cases in the UK (0.45%), followed by Brazil (4.06%), USA (18.92%), and Russia (29.19%), the high recovery rate in Germany (88.31%), the highest mortality rate in France (15.51%), followed by UK (14.34%), Italy (14.25%), Spain (11.99), and lowest mortality rate in Russia (0.98%). The world mortality rate is 6.52%, and rest of the world (excluding 10 infected countries shown in Table 3) is 4.58%; the recovery rate of the world is 37.15%, and the rest of the world is 42.51%.

On comparing the confirmed cases of the top 10 infected countries with the rest of the world by using go object of plotly, draw a figure by using Figure() function, creating an object of go.Figure() function, then add_trace function is used to draw a scatter line graph by passing date and confirmed cases, and name parameter is used to show the name of the country in the graph (Figs. 30 and 31).

Seaborn is an open-source Python library for visualizing the data and part of Matplotlib for visualizing 2D graph. It used visualized statistical relation, plot for categorical data, distribution of dataset, linear relation, and multi-plot grids. Figure 32 depicts the pair plot for scatter graph representation between confirmed and death cases by passing the parameter, data is actual data, x_var and y_vars are confirmed and death cases, the height represents the height of the graph, and kind represents the type of graph which is scattered type (Fig. 33).

Fig. 25 Graph for lowest mortality rate

country	confirmed	deaths
Saudi Arabia	65077	351
Qatar	38651	17
Belarus	33371	185
Singapore	29812	23
Kuwait	18609	129
Bahrain	8174	12
Kazakhstan	7234	35
Oman	6370	31
Ghana	6269	31
Guinea	3067	18
Uzbekistan	2964	13
Djibouti	2047	10
Iceland	1803	10
Gabon	1567	12
Maldives	1216	4

Fig. 26 Graph for worst recovery rates

country	confirmed	recovered
US	1577147	298418
Russia	317554	92681
United Kingdom	252246	1134
France	181951	63976
Canada	82742	0
Belgium	56235	14988
Pakistan	48091	14155
Netherlands	44894	163
Qatar	38651	7288
Ecuador	35306	3557
Sweden	32172	4971
Portugal	29912	6452
Bangladesh	28511	5602
Indonesia	20162	4838
Ukraine	19706	6227
Kuwait	18609	5205

```
flg['recoveryRate'] = round((flg['recovered']/flg['confirmed'])*100, 2)
temp = flg[flg['confirmed']>1000]
temp = temp.sort_values('recoveryRate', ascending=False)

fig = px.bar(temp.sort_values(by="recoveryRate", ascending=False)[:10][::-1],
             x = 'recoveryRate', y = 'country',
             title='Recoveries per 1000 Confirmed Cases', text='recoveryRate', height=800, orientation='h',
             color_discrete_sequence=['#2ca02c']
            )
fig.show()
```

Fig. 27 Code for mortality rate bar graph

```
print("Countries with Worst Recovery Rates")
temp = flg[flg['confirmed']>1000]
temp = temp.sort_values('recoveryRate', ascending=True)[['country', 'confirmed','recovered']][:40]
temp.sort_values('confirmed', ascending=False)[['country', 'confirmed','recovered']][:20].style.background_gradient(cmap='Reds')
```

Fig. 28 Code for mortality rate bar graph

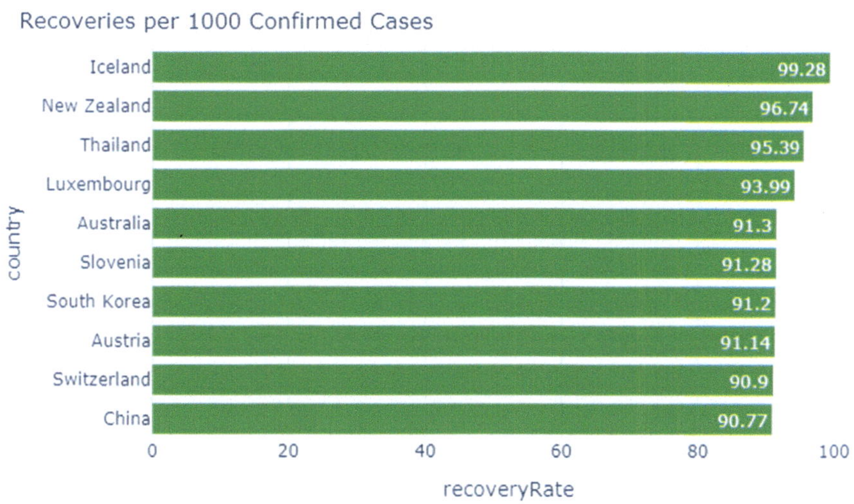

Fig. 29 Horizontal bar graph for recovered cases

Using the linear regression algorithm, X is the input variable that contains confirmed and recovered cases, and y is the output variable that contains death cases. Split the data in X_train, X_test, y_train, and y_test into 70:30, 70 percent for train case (22,445 rows) and 30 percent for the test (9620 rows). For the implementation of the machine learning linear regression algorithm, from the sklearn package import linear regression model, creating an object, and fit the model and prediction for test data [Fig. 34]. The value of the intercept is 0.10,728,098,478,608,672, and the coefficient is 0.05,911,671, 0.02,521,317 (Figs. 35, 36, 37, and 38).

Mean square error and r square error sub-package are imported from the sklearn metrics, and calculate the mean square error (1,237,165.8924) and r square error (0.8539) by passing the test and predicted value [Fig. 39].

Table 3 Death and improvement in the patients of 10 infected countries

S. no.	Country	Confirmed	Recovered	Deaths	Recovery rate	Mortality rate
1	US	1,577,147	298,418	94,702	18.92	6.00
2	Russia	317,554	92,681	3099	29.19	0.98
3	Brazil	310,087	12,596	20,047	4.06	6.46
4	UK	252,246	1134	36,184	0.45	14.34
5	Spain	233,037	150,376	27,940	64.53	11.99
6	Italy	228,006	134,560	32,486	59.02	14.25
7	France	181,951	63,976	28,218	35.16	15.51
8	Germany	179,021	158,087	8203	88.31	4.58
9	Turkey	153,548	114,990	4249	74.89	2.77
10	Iran	129,341	100,564	7249	77.75	5.60
11	Rest_of_World	1,540,480	654,894	70,607	42.51	4.58
12	World	5,102,418	1,895,640	332,924	37.15	6.52

```
fig = go.Figure()
fig.add_trace(go.Scatter(x=grouped_us_date["date"], y=grouped_us_date["confirmed"], name="US",
                    line_shape='linear'))
fig.add_trace(go.Scatter(x=grouped_rus_date["date"], y=grouped_rus_date["confirmed"], name="Russia",
                    line_shape='linear'))
fig.add_trace(go.Scatter(x=grouped_bra_date["date"], y=grouped_bra_date["confirmed"], name="Brazil",
                    line_shape='linear'))
fig.add_trace(go.Scatter(x=grouped_iran_date["date"], y=grouped_iran_date["confirmed"], name="Iran",
                    line_shape='linear'))
fig.add_trace(go.Scatter(x=grouped_tur_date["date"], y=grouped_tur_date["confirmed"], name="Turkey",
                    line_shape='linear'))
fig.add_trace(go.Scatter(x=grouped_uk_date["date"], y=grouped_uk_date["confirmed"], name="United Kingdom",
                    line_shape='linear'))
fig.add_trace(go.Scatter(x=grouped_fran_date["date"], y=grouped_fran_date["confirmed"], name="France",
                    line_shape='linear'))
fig.add_trace(go.Scatter(x=grouped_spain_date["date"], y=grouped_spain_date["confirmed"], name="Spain",
                    line_shape='linear'))
fig.add_trace(go.Scatter(x=grouped_ger_date["date"], y=grouped_ger_date["confirmed"], name="Germany",
                    line_shape='linear'))
fig.add_trace(go.Scatter(x=grouped_italy_date["date"], y=grouped_italy_date["confirmed"], name="Italy",
                    line_shape='linear'))
fig.add_trace(go.Scatter(x=grouped_rest_date["date"], y=grouped_rest_date["confirmed"], name="Rest of World",
                    line_shape='linear', marker_color='red'))
fig.update_traces(hoverinfo='text+name', mode='lines')
fig.update_layout(title='Confirmed Cases in Top 10 countries and Rest of World',
                   xaxis_title='Date',
                   yaxis_title='Number of Confirmed Cases',legend=dict(x=1,y=1, traceorder='reversed', font_size=16))
fig.show()
```

Fig. 30 Source code for the confirmed cases for ten infected countries and rest of the world

Using Bayes theorem algorithm is the part of sklearn library, import by using the command "from sklearn.naive_bayes import GaussianNB", Gaussian naïve Bayes theorem importing. "gnb" is the object of Gaussian Bayes theorem, "gnb.fit(X_train, y_train)" trained the model, and X_train and y_train are the training datasets. For prediction, "gnb.predict()" function is used by passing the test dataset and prediction store in the y_pred variable [Fig. 40]. To find the accuracy precision, f1-score and recall, import the "classification_report" package. The accuracy of this algorithm is 56 percent. The confusion matrix is the table that tells the performance of an algorithm, and it is also known as an error matrix. True positive (TP), true negative

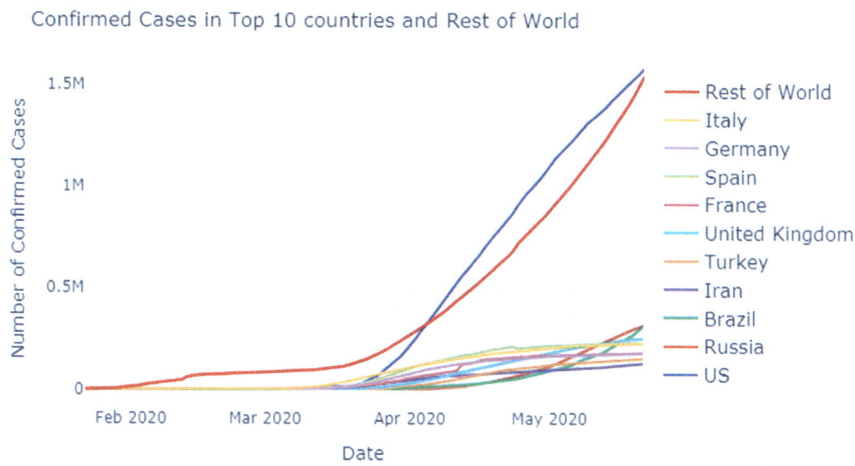

Fig. 31 Depict the line graph of ten infected countries

```
import seaborn as sns
sns.pairplot(data, x_vars=['confirmed'], y_vars='deaths',height=9, aspect=1.5, kind='scatter')
```

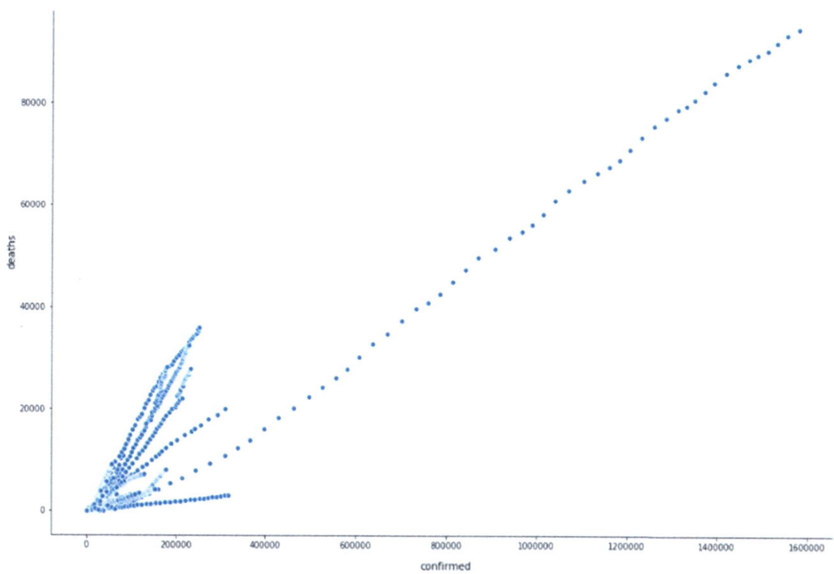

Fig. 32 Pair plots between confirmed cases and death cases

(TN), false positive (FP), and false negative (FN) are the terms that are used to find the accuracy of the algorithm [Fig. 41].

SVM is a part of the sklearn library, import by using "from sklearn import SVM" creating the object or classifier "clf", using the linear kernel, and train the model by

```
X=data[['confirmed','recovered']]
y=data['deaths']
from sklearn.model_selection import train_test_split
X_train, X_test, y_train, y_test = train_test_split(X, y, train_size=0.7 , random_state=100)
print(X_train.shape)
print(y_train.shape)
print(X_test.shape)
print(y_test.shape)
```

Fig. 33 Prepare and splitting of data

```
# import LinearRegression from sklearn
from sklearn.linear_model import LinearRegression
# Representing LinearRegression as lr(Creating LinearRegression Object)
lr = LinearRegression()
# Fit the model using lr.fit()
lr.fit(X_train, y_train)
print(lr.intercept_)
print(lr.coef_)
# Making predictions on the testing set
y_pred = lr.predict(X_test)
```

Fig. 34 Implementation of the linear regression model

```
import matplotlib.pyplot as plt
c = [i for i in range(1,9621,1)]         # generating index
fig = plt.figure()
plt.plot(c,y_test, color="blue", linewidth=2.5, linestyle="-")
plt.plot(c,y_pred, color="red",  linewidth=2.5, linestyle="-")
fig.suptitle('Actual and Predicted', fontsize=20)
plt.xlabel('Confirmed', fontsize=18)
plt.ylabel('Deaths', fontsize=16)
```

Fig. 35 Code to draw actual and predicted cases

```
c = [i for i in range(1,9621,1)]
fig = plt.figure()
plt.plot(c,y_test-y_pred, color="blue", linewidth=2.5, linestyle="-")
fig.suptitle('Error Terms', fontsize=20)
plt.xlabel('Confirmed', fontsize=18)
plt.ylabel('ytest-ypred', fontsize=16)
```

Fig. 36 Code for error term for death case

passing the train dataset. Predict function is used for prediction by passing the test dataset [Fig. 42] (Fig. 43).

LSTM deep learning algorithm is imported by using the TensorFlow and Keras library. MinMaxScaler() function is used to translate each feature of the train and test dataset into 0 and 1, and convert the data into a time series dataset by using the time series generator function. Sequential is the API that implements one network at a time. LSTM is the head of the network which implements a single layer, LSTM with

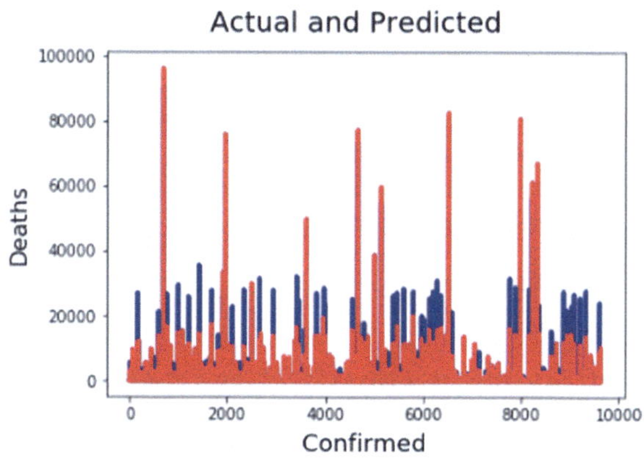

Fig. 37 Plot actual and predicted cases

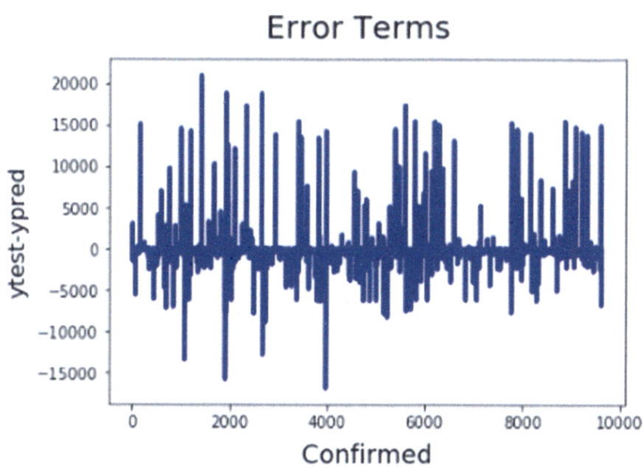

Fig. 38 Plot error in test and predicted value

```
from sklearn.metrics import mean_squared_error, r2_score
mse = mean_squared_error(y_test, y_pred)
r_squared = r2_score(y_test, y_pred)
print('Mean_Squared_Error :' ,mse)
print('r_square_value :',r_squared)
```

```
Mean_Squared_Error : 1237165.8924227783
r_square_value : 0.8539360212537134
```

Fig. 39 Mean square and r square error

dropout removes the overfitting of training data, dropout in this program is 0.2, and run the program 50 epochs. Dense is the fully connected output layer, and optimizer function is "adam" and mean square error [Fig. 44]. LSTM is used to predict the confirmed cases for the next 10 days shown in Figs. 46 and 45.

```python
from sklearn.naive_bayes import GaussianNB
#Create a Gaussian Classifier
gnb = GaussianNB()
#Train the model using the training sets
gnb.fit(X_train, y_train)
#Predict the response for test dataset
y_pred = gnb.predict(X_test)
```

Fig. 40 Implementation of Bayes theorem

```python
from sklearn.metrics import classification_report, confusion_matrix
print(confusion_matrix(y_test,y_pred))
print(classification_report(y_test,y_pred))
```

```
[[5203   37   99 ...    0    0    0]
 [ 564   45   47 ...    0    0    0]
 [ 273   40   42 ...    0    0    0]
 ...
 [   0    0    0 ...    0    0    0]
 [   0    0    0 ...    0    0    0]
 [   0    0    0 ...    0    0    0]]
              precision    recall  f1-score   support

           0       0.79      0.97      0.87      5370
           1       0.09      0.06      0.08       714
           2       0.07      0.11      0.09       367
           3       0.00      0.00      0.00       306
           4       0.00      0.00      0.00       187
           5       0.00      0.00      0.00       107
           6       0.11      0.19      0.14       239
           7       0.03      0.04      0.04       159
           8       0.12      0.23      0.15       134
           9       0.00      0.00      0.00        83
          10       0.01      0.01      0.01        95
```

```python
from sklearn import metrics

# Model Accuracy: how often is the classifier correct?
print("Accuracy:",metrics.accuracy_score(y_test, y_pred))
```

```
Accuracy: 0.5607068607068607
```

Fig. 41 Confusion matrix and accuracy, precision, recall, and f1-score

Forecasting is the method which takes previous data as input and predicts the future data as output, and find the trend of data. Forecasting is the common task of a data scientist but forecasting required more experience for accurate forecasting, and the accuracy of forecasting decides a vital role in company policy, goal, and planning. The time series prophet and ARIMA model are

```
from sklearn import svm
#Create a svm Classifier
clf = svm.SVC(kernel='linear') # Linear Kernel
#Train the model using the training sets
clf.fit(X_train, y_train)
#Predict the response for test dataset
y_pred = clf.predict(X_test)
plt.plot(y_pred)
```

Fig. 42 Implementation of support vector machine

```
Confusion Matrix and Statistics

          Reference
Prediction Negative Neutral Positive
  Negative      806     152      162
  Neutral       158     478      157
  Positive      176     172      857

Overall Statistics

               Accuracy : 0.6867
                 95% CI : (0.67, 0.7029)
    No Information Rate : 0.3772
    P-Value [Acc > NIR] : <2e-16

                  Kappa : 0.5234

 Mcnemar's Test P-Value : 0.7103
```

```
from sklearn.metrics import classification_report, confusion_matrix
print(confusion_matrix(y_test,y_pred))
print(classification_report(y_test,y_pred))
```

```
[[4707    8    0 ...    0    0    0]
 [ 221   15    0 ...    0    0    0]
 [ 121    2    0 ...    0    0    0]
 ...
 [   0    0    0 ...    0    0    0]
 [   0    0    0 ...    0    0    0]
 [   0    0    0 ...    0    0    0]]
              precision    recall  f1-score   support

           0       0.90      1.00      0.94      4715
           1       0.17      0.06      0.09       236
           2       0.00      0.00      0.00       123
           3       0.00      0.00      0.00        69
           4       0.00      0.00      0.00        43
           5       0.00      0.00      0.00        23
           6       0.00      0.00      0.00        55
           7       0.00      0.00      0.00        20
           8       0.00      0.00      0.00        16
           9       0.00      0.00      0.00         5
          10       0.00      0.00      0.00         0
```

Fig. 43 Confusion matrix of SVM

```
from sklearn.preprocessing import MinMaxScaler
from tensorflow.keras.preprocessing.sequence import TimeseriesGenerator

scaler = MinMaxScaler()
scaler.fit(train_data)
scaled_train_data = scaler.transform(train_data)
scaled_test_data = scaler.transform(test_data)
n_input =5
n_features =1

generator = TimeseriesGenerator(scaled_train_data,scaled_train_data, length=n_input, batch_size=1)

lstm_model = Sequential()
lstm_model.add(LSTM(units = 50, return_sequences = True, input_shape = (n_input, n_features)))
lstm_model.add(Dropout(0.2))
lstm_model.add(LSTM(units = 50, return_sequences = True))
lstm_model.add(Dropout(0.2))
lstm_model.add(LSTM(units = 50))
lstm_model.add(Dropout(0.2))
lstm_model.add(Dense(units = 1))
lstm_model.compile(optimizer = 'adam', loss = 'mean_squared_error')
lstm_model.fit(generator, epochs = 50)
```

Fig. 44 LSTM algorithm implementation

```
106/106 [==============================] - 6s 56ms/step - loss: 0.0020
Epoch 35/50
106/106 [==============================] - 4s 40ms/step - loss: 0.0032
Epoch 36/50
106/106 [==============================] - 5s 44ms/step - loss: 0.0026
Epoch 37/50
106/106 [==============================] - 5s 47ms/step - loss: 0.0025
Epoch 38/50
106/106 [==============================] - 4s 39ms/step - loss: 0.0024
Epoch 39/50
106/106 [==============================] - 4s 35ms/step - loss: 0.0023
Epoch 40/50
106/106 [==============================] - 5s 51ms/step - loss: 0.0029: 0s - loss:
Epoch 41/50
106/106 [==============================] - 7s 63ms/step - loss: 0.0024
Epoch 42/50
106/106 [==============================] - 5s 43ms/step - loss: 0.0020
Epoch 43/50
106/106 [==============================] - 5s 46ms/step - loss: 0.0036
Epoch 44/50
106/106 [==============================] - 7s 64ms/step - loss: 0.0020
Epoch 45/50
106/106 [==============================] - 7s 67ms/step - loss: 0.0021
Epoch 46/50
106/106 [==============================] - 8s 76ms/step - loss: 0.0024
Epoch 47/50
106/106 [==============================] - 7s 67ms/step - loss: 0.0016
Epoch 48/50
106/106 [==============================] - 6s 57ms/step - loss: 0.0019
Epoch 49/50
106/106 [==============================] - 5s 51ms/step - loss: 0.0025
Epoch 50/50
106/106 [==============================] - 6s 60ms/step - loss: 0.0023
```

Fig. 45 Result of 50 iterations of LSTM

```
lstm_predictions_scaled = []

batch = scaled_train_data[-n_input:]
current_batch = batch.reshape((1, n_input, n_features))

for i in range(len(test_data)):
    lstm_pred = lstm_model.predict(current_batch)[0]
    lstm_predictions_scaled.append(lstm_pred)
    current_batch = np.append(current_batch[:,1:,:],[[lstm_pred]],axis=1)
prediction = pd.DataFrame(scaler.inverse_transform(lstm_predictions_scaled))
prediction.head(10)
```

	0
0	4.182040e+06
1	4.242944e+06
2	4.294091e+06
3	4.336143e+06
4	4.370670e+06
5	4.398095e+06
6	4.432520e+06
7	4.461135e+06
8	4.485502e+06
9	4.507081e+06

Fig. 46 Prediction of LSTM and output

used for forecasting the death, recovery, and confirmed cases. Figures 47, 48, and 49 show the implementation of the prophet algorithm. We import the prophet package from the fbprophet package because it is the part of the Facebook, and command to import the prophet is "from fbprophet import Prophet". Only two-column data is required in the prophet algorithm such as data[ds, y]; "ds" is the date type, and y is the predicted variable. Figures 47 and 48 show the confirmed, recovered, and death cases, respectively. Create the object m of prophet algorithm, fitting the data df2 passing into "m.fit(df2)", predicting for next 14 days by passing the "future"

```
df2 = df1.groupby([data['date'].dt.date]).sum()
df2=df2.reset_index()
df2.rename(columns = {'date':'ds'}, inplace = True)
df2.rename(columns = {'confirmed':'y'}, inplace = True)
df5 = data.drop(['state', 'country', 'Lat','Long','deaths','confirmed','active'],1)
df6 = df5.groupby([data['date'].dt.date]).sum()
df6=df6.reset_index()
df6.rename(columns = {'date':'ds'}, inplace = True)
df6.rename(columns = {'recovered':'y'}, inplace = True)
df6
```

Fig. 47 Preparing the data of confirmed and recovered case in prophet algorithm format

```
df3 = data.drop(['state', 'country', 'Lat','Long','confirmed','recovered','active'],1)
df3.columns
df4 = df3.groupby([data['date'].dt.date]).sum()
df4=df4.reset_index()
df4.rename(columns = {'date':'ds'}, inplace = True)
df4.rename(columns = {'deaths':'y'}, inplace = True)
```

Fig. 48 Preparing the data of death case in prophet algorithm format

```
m = Prophet()
m.fit(df2)
future = m.make_future_dataframe(periods=14)
forecast = m.predict(future)
forecast[['ds', 'yhat', 'yhat_lower', 'yhat_upper']].tail(20)
```

Fig. 49 Prophet algorithm implementation

	ds	yhat	yhat_lower	yhat_upper
115	2020-05-16	4.629593e+06	4.617142e+06	4.641561e+06
116	2020-05-17	4.714235e+06	4.700933e+06	4.726151e+06
117	2020-05-18	4.795589e+06	4.783629e+06	4.807775e+06
118	2020-05-19	4.878121e+06	4.865910e+06	4.891505e+06
119	2020-05-20	4.963758e+06	4.951588e+06	4.976094e+06
120	2020-05-21	5.053639e+06	5.042085e+06	5.066655e+06
121	2020-05-22	5.140490e+06	5.128175e+06	5.152984e+06
122	2020-05-23	5.226158e+06	5.213728e+06	5.238696e+06
123	2020-05-24	5.310800e+06	5.295587e+06	5.325166e+06
124	2020-05-25	5.392153e+06	5.376126e+06	5.409652e+06
125	2020-05-26	5.474686e+06	5.455371e+06	5.494115e+06
126	2020-05-27	5.560322e+06	5.535204e+06	5.585852e+06
127	2020-05-28	5.650404e+06	5.619742e+06	5.681885e+06
128	2020-05-29	5.737055e+06	5.700015e+06	5.777171e+06
129	2020-05-30	5.822722e+06	5.775456e+06	5.868403e+06
130	2020-05-31	5.907364e+06	5.853526e+06	5.959969e+06
131	2020-06-01	5.988718e+06	5.928429e+06	6.051583e+06
132	2020-06-02	6.071251e+06	6.001956e+06	6.142257e+06
133	2020-06-03	6.156687e+06	6.075003e+06	6.240134e+06
134	2020-06-04	6.246969e+06	6.157967e+06	6.339149e+06

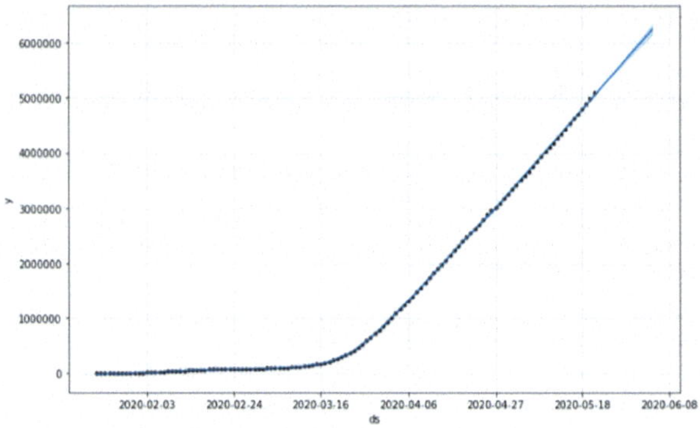

Fig. 50 Prediction output for confirmed and plots the confirmed cases

	ds	yhat	yhat_lower	yhat_upper
111	2020-05-12	290985.900351	289857.338094	292076.918437
112	2020-05-13	296244.088430	295126.339059	297390.213246
113	2020-05-14	301403.270685	300366.508881	302475.095015
114	2020-05-15	306738.238517	305846.624816	307901.015319
115	2020-05-16	311451.066882	310307.592743	312576.161127
116	2020-05-17	315658.818598	314502.865901	316796.056227
117	2020-05-18	320149.859393	319076.786425	321204.931641
118	2020-05-19	325285.837750	324209.684178	326438.170751
119	2020-05-20	330544.025828	329450.443581	331651.748205
120	2020-05-21	335703.208083	334604.320547	336806.417832
121	2020-05-22	341038.175916	339925.196955	342150.737210
122	2020-05-23	345751.004280	344653.052684	346901.978824
123	2020-05-24	349958.755997	348632.562214	351223.284543
124	2020-05-25	354449.796791	353012.660232	356030.173050
125	2020-05-26	359585.775148	357858.713543	361395.683672
126	2020-05-27	364843.963226	362682.907701	367044.979573
127	2020-05-28	370003.145482	367249.186643	372946.275745
128	2020-05-29	375338.113314	372022.220498	378756.899033
129	2020-05-30	380050.941679	376173.156596	384390.825245
130	2020-05-31	384258.693395	379733.755969	389302.829759

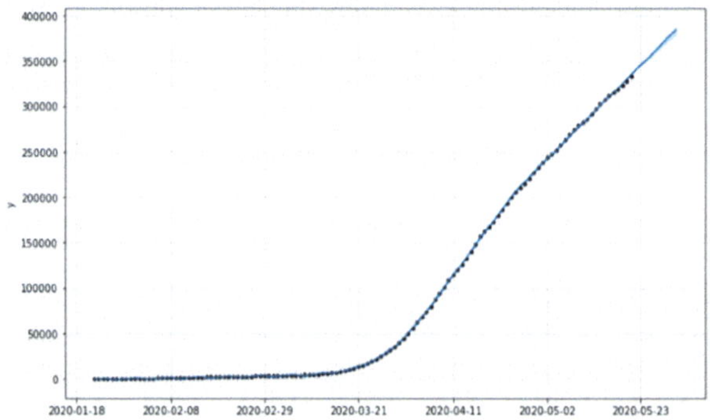

Fig. 51 Prediction output for recovered and plots the recovered cases

argument in the "m.predict(future)" function, and show the prediction for confirmed cases; similarly, we predict the for recovered and death cases by changing the data "df6" and "df4", respectively. Figures 50, 51, and 52 depict the prediction for world confirmed, recovered, and death cases for next 14 days. "ds" is the date, "yhat" is the actual predicted value, and "yhat_lower" and "yhat_upper" represent the lower and upper limits of prediction. "Figure 1 = m.plot(forecast)" command is used to draw the prediction [Fig. 50].

	ds	yhat	yhat_lower	yhat_upper
115	2020-05-16	1.644019e+06	1.633522e+06	1.654868e+06
116	2020-05-17	1.684083e+06	1.673377e+06	1.696082e+06
117	2020-05-18	1.725064e+06	1.713653e+06	1.735630e+06
118	2020-05-19	1.766721e+06	1.755329e+06	1.776919e+06
119	2020-05-20	1.811333e+06	1.800346e+06	1.822433e+06
120	2020-05-21	1.854922e+06	1.844907e+06	1.865670e+06
121	2020-05-22	1.895340e+06	1.884863e+06	1.906600e+06
122	2020-05-23	1.938441e+06	1.927597e+06	1.949453e+06
123	2020-05-24	1.978506e+06	1.966835e+06	1.990947e+06
124	2020-05-25	2.019486e+06	2.006746e+06	2.031725e+06
125	2020-05-26	2.061143e+06	2.048239e+06	2.074605e+06
126	2020-05-27	2.105756e+06	2.092785e+06	2.119913e+06
127	2020-05-28	2.149345e+06	2.134152e+06	2.166116e+06
128	2020-05-29	2.189762e+06	2.171887e+06	2.207068e+06
129	2020-05-30	2.232863e+06	2.212051e+06	2.252532e+06
130	2020-05-31	2.272928e+06	2.251535e+06	2.296649e+06
131	2020-06-01	2.313909e+06	2.288282e+06	2.339197e+06
132	2020-06-02	2.355566e+06	2.325749e+06	2.383600e+06
133	2020-06-03	2.400178e+06	2.367730e+06	2.433451e+06
134	2020-06-04	2.443767e+06	2.410147e+06	2.480012e+06

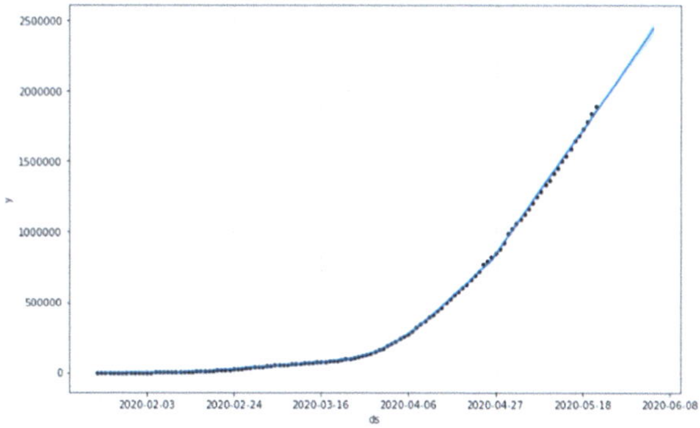

Fig. 52 Prediction output for death and plots the death cases

```
tms=cleaned_data.groupby(['Date'],as_index=False)[['Confirmed']].sum()
tms.set_index('Date')
tms.dtypes
from statsmodels.tsa.arima_model import ARIMA
model = ARIMA(tms['Confirmed'], order=(5,2,0))
model_fit = model.fit()
model_fit.summary()
```

Fig. 53 Data preparation and ARIMA model implementation

Preparing the dataset by taking date and confirmed cases, group by confirmed cases on the base of date, and sum the confirmed cases. ARIMA model is implemented by using the statsmodels library, and ARIMA function is used to implement the ARIMA algorithm by passing data (tms[confirmed]) and order; order contains three values p, d, q, (5,2,0), and fit the model [Fig. 53]. Figure 54 shows the ARIMA model result with 5 p-value, z-value, Akaike information criterion (AIC), and Bayesian information criterion (BIC). Minimum AIC and BIC values are the indicator for the best value of p, d, q. Figure 55 depicts the prediction of an algorithm for next 10 days, first row shows predicted confirmed cases, second row shows the daily variation, and third row represents the upper and lower value of predicted confirmed case.

ARIMA Model Results

Dep. Variable:	D2.Confirmed	No. Observations:	119
Model:	ARIMA(5, 2, 0)	Log Likelihood	-1201.652
Method:	css-mle	S.D. of innovations	5866.810
Date:	Thu, 28 May 2020	AIC	2417.304
Time:	22:20:15	BIC	2436.758
Sample:	2	HQIC	2425.204

	coef	std err	z	P>|z|	[0.025	0.975]
const	841.2687	264.784	3.177	0.001	322.302	1360.236
ar.L1.D2.Confirmed	-0.2463	0.091	-2.711	0.007	-0.424	-0.068
ar.L2.D2.Confirmed	-0.1597	0.092	-1.736	0.083	-0.340	0.021
ar.L3.D2.Confirmed	-0.2933	0.089	-3.303	0.001	-0.467	-0.119
ar.L4.D2.Confirmed	-0.1999	0.092	-2.167	0.030	-0.381	-0.019
ar.L5.D2.Confirmed	-0.1584	0.092	-1.729	0.084	-0.338	0.021

Roots

	Real	Imaginary	Modulus	Frequency
AR.1	0.7923	-0.9996j	1.2755	-0.1433
AR.2	0.7923	+0.9996j	1.2755	0.1433
AR.3	-1.4321	-0.0000j	1.4321	-0.5000
AR.4	-0.7072	-1.4865j	1.6462	-0.3207
AR.5	-0.7072	+1.4865j	1.6462	0.3207

Fig. 54 ARIMA model result, value of AIC, BIC, and Z

```
prediction10=pd.DataFrame(model_fit.forecast(10))
model_fit.forecast(10)

(array([5205890.61742737, 5306751.54319702, 5406507.2429177 ,
        5507473.56752021, 5610206.59703391, 5715281.05141254,
        5821507.11636799, 5928221.45640471, 6035130.92612742,
        6142559.72533723]),
 array([ 5866.81026965, 11843.84209973, 18436.9224253 , 24824.45481519,
        31135.57959907, 37437.14468025, 44263.98198287, 51706.23844585,
        59759.44582846, 68247.29685743]),
 array([[5194391.88059473, 5217389.35426001],
        [5283538.03924298, 5329965.04715107],
        [5370371.53897834, 5442642.94685705],
        [5458818.5301466 , 5556128.60489382],
        [5549181.98238194, 5671231.21168588],
        [5641905.59615523, 5788656.50666985],
        [5734751.30586924, 5908262.92686675],
        [5826879.09127481, 6029563.82153462],
        [5918004.56456756, 6152257.28768728],
        [6008797.48145447, 6276321.96922   ]]))

prediction10
```

	0	1	2	3	4	5	6	7
0	5.20589e+06	5.30675e+06	5.40651e+06	5.50747e+06	5.61021e+06	5.71528e+06	5.82151e+06	5.
1	5866.81	11843.8	18436.9	24824.5	31135.6	37437.1	44264	
2	[5194391.880594733, 5217389.354260008]	[5283538.039242978, 5329965.047151065]	[5370371.538978345, 5442642.946857049]	[5458818.5301466035, 5556128.604893823]	[5549181.982381945, 5671231.211685876]	[5641905.596155226, 5788656.506669853]	[5734751.305869237, 5908262.926866749]	[5826879. 6029563.

Fig. 55 Prediction for next 10 days by using ARIMA model

References

1. Su, S., Wong, G., Shi, W., Liu, J., Lai, A.C., Zhou, J. et al. Epidemiology, genetic recombination, and pathogenesis of coronaviruses. Trends in Microbiology. **24**(6), pp. 490–502 (2016). https://doi.org/10.1016/j.tim.2016.03.003
2. Zhu, N., Zhang, D., Wang, W., Li, X., Yang, B., Song, J. et al.: A novel coronavirus from patients with pneumonia in China, 2019. New England J. Med. **382**(8), pp. 727–733 (2020). https://doi.org/10.1056/nejmoa2001017
3. Estola, T.: Coronaviruses, a new group of animal RNA viruses. Avian Dis. **14**(2), pp. 330–336 (1970). https://doi.org/10.2307/1588476
4. Fabricant, J.: The early history of infectious bronchitis. Avian Dis. **42**(4), pp. 648–650 (1998). https://doi.org/10.2307/1592697
5. McIntosh, K.,: Coronaviruses: a comparative review, current topics in microbiology and immunology. Ergebnisse der Mikrobiologie und Immunitätsforschung, p. 87. Berlin, Heidelberg, Springer, 1974. https://doi.org/10.1007/978-3-642-65775-7_3
6. Kahn, J.S., McIntosh, K.: History and recent advances in coronavirus discovery. Pediatric Infect. Dis. J. **24**(11), S223–S227 (2005). https://doi.org/10.1097/01.inf.0000188166.17324.60
7. Mahase, E.: The BMJ in 1965, BMJ. **369**, pp. 547 (2020). https://doi.org/10.1136/bmj.m1547
8. Tyrrell, D.A., Bynoe, M.L.: Cultivation of viruses from a high proportion of patients with colds. Lancet **1**, 76–77 (1966)
9. Hamre, D., Procknow, J.J.: A new virus isolated from the human respiratory tract. Proc. SocExpBiol. Med. **121**, 190–193 (1966)
10. McIntosh, K., Dees, J.H., Becker, W.B., Kapikian, A.Z., Chanock, R.M.: Recovery in tracheal organ cultures of novel viruses from patients with respiratory disease. Proc. Natl. Acad. Sci. U.S.A. **57**, 933–940 (1967)
11. Tyrrell, D.A., Almeida, J.D., Cunningham, C.H. et al.: Coronaviridae, Intervirology, **5**, 76–82 (1975)
12. Drosten, C., Gunther, S., Preiser, W. et al.: Identification of a novel coronavirus in patients with severe acute respiratory syndrome see comment. N. Engl. J. Med. **348**, 1967–1976 (2003)
13. Ksiazek, T.G., Erdman, D., Goldsmith, C.S., et al.: A novel coronavirus associated with severe acute respiratory syndrome see comment. N. Engl. J. Med. **348**, 1953–1966 (2003)
14. Peiris, J.S., Lai, St, Poon, L.L. et al.: Coronavirus as a possible cause of severe acute respiratory syndrome see comment, Lancet. **361**, 1319–1325 (2003)

15. Centers for Disease Control and Prevention. http://www.cdc.gov/ncidod/sars/index.htm
16. Van der Hoek, L., Pyrc, K., Jebbink, M.F., et al.: Identification of a new human coronavirus. Nat. Med. **10**, 368–373 (2004)
17. Fouchier, R.A., Hartwig, N.G., Bestebroer, T.M., et al.: A previously undescribed coronavirus associated with respiratory disease in humans. Proc. Natl. Acad. Sci. U.S.A. **101**, 6212–6216 (2004)
18. Disease Outbreak News (2014). www.who.int. 8 October 2014
19. Middle East respiratory syndrome coronavirus (MERS-CoV)—Republic of Korea, (2015). www.who.int. 24 May 2015
20. COVID-19: WHO names disease caused by new coronavirus, https://www.aljazeera.com, 11, Feb 2020
21. Woo, P.C., Huang, Y., Lau, S.K., Yuen, K.Y.: Coronavirus genomics and bioinformatics analysis. Viruses **2**, 1804–1820 (2010)
22. Dhama, K., Khan, S., Tiwari, R. et al.: Coronavirus disease 2019–COVID-19, Preprints (2020). https://doi.org/10.20944/preprints202003.0001.v1
23. Geller, C., Varbanov, M., Raphael, E.: Duval human coronaviruses: insights into environmental resistance and its influence on the development of new antiseptic strategies. Viruses **4**, 3044–3068 (2012). https://doi.org/10.3390/v4113044
24. WHO: Novel Coronavirus—Thailand, (2020a). https://www.who.int/csr/don/14-January-2020-novel-coronavirus-thailand-ex-china/en/
25. International Committee on Taxonomy of Viruses (ICTV). October 2018. Archived from the original on 2019–05-14
26. ICTV Taxonomy history: Orthocoronavirinae. International Committee on Taxonomy of Viruses (ICTV) (2020)
27. Fan, Y., Zhao, K., Shi, Z.L., Zhou, P.: Bat coronaviruses in China. Viruses. **11**(3), 210 (2019). https://doi.org/10.3390/v11030210
28. Wertheim, J.O., Chu, D.K., Peiris, J.S., Kosakovsky Pond, S.L., Poon, L.L.: A case for the ancient origin of coronaviruses. J. Virol. **87**(12), 7039–45 (2013). https://doi.org/10.1128/jvi.03273-12
29. Nextstrain, phylogenetic tree of Beta-CoV
30. Liu, P., Shi, L., Zhang, W., He, J., Liu, C., Zhao, C. et al.: Prevalence and genetic diversity analysis of human coronaviruses among cross-border children. Virol. J. **14**(1), 230 (2017). https://doi.org/10.1186/s12985-017-0896-0
31. Kuiken, T., Fouchier, R.A., Schutten, M., Rimmelzwaan, G.F., et al.: Newly discovered coronavirus as the primary cause of severe acute respiratory syndrome. Lancet **362**, 263–270 (2003)
32. Zaki, A.M., Boheemen, S.V., Bestebroer, T.M., Osterhaus, A.D., Fouchier, R.A.: Isolation of a novel coronavirus from a man with pneumonia in Saudi Arabia. N. Engl. J. Med. **367**, 1814–1820 (2012)
33. Yadav, D.; Maheshwari, H.; Chandra, U.: Outbreak prediction of covid-19 in most susceptible countries. Global J. Environ. Sci. Manage. **6**(4), (2020). https://www.gjesm.net/article_39228.html
34. PIB, (2020). https://pib.gov.in/pressreleaseiframepage.aspx?prid=1601095
35. WHO (2020b) World Health Organization website https://www.who.int/health-topics/coronavirus
36. Covid-19.in, (2020). https://www.mygov.in/covid-19/?cbps=1
37. Abdi, M.: Coronavirus disease 2019 (COVID-19) outbreak in Iran; actions and problems. Infect. Control Hosp. Epidemiol. pp. 1–5 (2020)
38. ECDC: European Centre for Disease Prevention and Control (2020). https://www.ecdc.europa.eu/en/publications-data/download-todays-data-geographic-distribution-covid-19-cases-worldwide
39. Chintalapudi, N., Battineni, G., Amenta, F.: COVID-19 disease outbreak forecasting of registered and recovered cases after sixty day lockdown in Italy: a data driven model approach. J. Microbiol. Immunol. Infect. (2020). https://doi.org/10.1016/j.jmii.2020.04.004

40. Roosa, K., Lee, Y., Luo, R., Kirpich, A., Rothenberg, R., Hyman, J.M., Yan, P., Chowell, G.: Real-time forecasts of the COVID-19 epidemic in China from February 5th to February 24th, 2020. Infect. Dis. Model. **5**, 256–263 (2020)
41. Gao, Y., Zhang, Z., Yao, W., Ying, Q., Long, C., Fu, X.: Forecasting the cumulative number of COVID-19 deaths in China: a Boltzmann function-based modeling study. Infect. Control Hosp. Epidemiol. pp. 1–3 (2020)
42. Box, G.E.P., Jenkins, G.M.: Time series analysis: forecasting and control. Revised edition, Holden Day, San Francisco, 1976. https://www.abebooks.com/first-edition/Time-Series-Analysis-Forecasting-Control-Holden-Day/30570957911/bd
43. Gorse, G.J., O'Connor, T.Z., Hall, S.L., Vitale, J.N., Nichol, K.L.: Human coronavirus and acute respiratory illness in older adults with chronic obstructive pulmonary disease. J. Infect. Dis. **199**, 847–857 (2009)
44. Ranjan, R.: Predictions for covid-19 outbreak in India using epidemiological models (2020), medRxiv preprint doi:https://doi.org/10.1101/2020.04.02.20051466
45. Tomar, A., Gupta, N.: Prediction for the spread of COVID-19 in India and effectiveness of preventive measures. Sci. Total Environ. (2020). https://doi.org/10.1016/j.scitotenv.2020.138762
46. Pene, F., Merlat, A., Vabret, A., Rozenberg, F., Buzyn, A., Dreyfus, F., Cariou, A., Freymuth, F., Lebon, P.: Coronavirus 229E-related pneumonia in immunocompromised patients. Clin. Infect. Dis. **37**, 929–932 (2003). https://doi.org/10.1086/377612
47. Vijgen, L., Keyaerts, E., Moës, E., Maes, P., Duson, G., van Ranst, M.: Development of one-step, real-time, quantitative reverse transcriptase pcr assays for absolute quantitation of human coronaviruses OC43 and 229E. J. Clin. Microbiol. **43**, 5452–5456 (2005)https://doi.org/10.1128/jcm.43.11.5452-5456.2005
48. Van der Hoek, L.: Human coronaviruses: what do they cause? Antivir. Ther. **12**, 651–658 (2007)
49. Walsh 2007, E.E., Shin, J.H., Falsey, A.R.: Clinical impact of human coronaviruses 229E and OC43 infection in diverse adult populations. J. Infect. Dis. **208**, 1634–1642 (2013). https://doi.org/10.1093/infdis/jit393
50. The Korean Society of Infectious Diseases: Korean society for healthcare-associated infection control and prevention. an unexpected outbreak of middle east respiratory syndrome coronavirus infection in the Republic of Korea. Infect. Chemother. **47**, 120–122 (2015)
51. McBride, R., Fielding, B.C.: The role of severe acute respiratory syndrome (SARS)-coronavirus accessory proteins in virus pathogenesis. Viruses **4**, 2902–2923 (2012)
52. Jones, B.A., Grace, D., Kock, R., Alonso, S., Rushton, J., et al.: Zoonosis emergence linked to agricultural intensification and environmental change. Proc. Natl. Acad. Sci. USA. **21**, 8399–8340 (2013)
53. Esper, F., Martinello, R.A., Boucher, P. et al.: Evidence of a novel human coronavirus that is associated with respiratory tract disease in infants and young children. J. Infect. Dis. **191**, 492–498 (2005)
54. Arbour, N., Day, R., Newcombe, J., Talbot, P.J.: Neuroinvasion by Human Respiratory Coronaviruses. J. Virol. **74**, 8913–892 (2000)
55. Woo, P.C., Lau, S.K., Lam, C.S., Lau, C.C., et al.: Discovery of seven novel Mammalian and avian coronaviruses in the genus deltacoronavirus supports bat coronaviruses as the gene source of alphacoronavirus and betacoronavirus and avian coronaviruses as the gene source of gammacoronavirus and deltacoronavirus. J. Virol. **86**(7), 3995–4008 (2012)
56. Doucleef, M.: Scientists go deep on genes of SARS-like virus, Associated Press (2012)
57. Decaro, N.: Alphacoronavirus. The Springer Index of Viruses, pp. 371–383. (Springer, 2011). https://doi.org/10.1007/978-0-387-95919-1_56
58. Decaro, N.: Betacoronavirus. The Springer Index of Viruses, pp. 385–401. Springer, 2011. https://doi.org/10.1007/978-0-387-95919-1_57

MML Classification Techniques for the Pathogen Based on Pnuemonia-nCOVID-19 and the Detection of Closely Related Lung Diseases Using Efficacious Learning Algorithms

M. Kannan and C. Priya

Abstract The main purpose of this topic is to provide an excellent classification method for predicting the disease based on the key aspect of the disease. Here, we used a multiclass variable database for the prediction; also the methods, random forest and linear SVC, are used for the classification. Furthermore, based on the confusion matrix, we can know the outcome of the prediction model. In this, all the results are discussed using the confusion matrix. Infectious diseases such as nCOVID-19 cause serious damage to the human body's immune system. It recently emerged from China and affects neighbors' country and flu-like symptoms initially manifest in 89.9%. The disease spreads faster than SARS-CoV and MERS-CoV, and soon, the disease begins to spread from one person to another, with high fever (101.4 F), inhalation or dyspnea, sore throat, sneezing and coughing. In India, as of January 31, 2020, the number of cases was one, and on March 28, 2020, the outrage began to rise to 909. In addition, COVID is also caused by pneumonia-related illnesses. So far, such epidemics have been studied and diagnosed by reverse transcriptase polymerase chain reaction (RT-PCR) and serology laboratory testing. Chest X-ray or computed tomography helps identify damaged and white cells in the affected body, identifying pathogens, and the presence of abundant metagenomic sequence in RNA is a major clinical challenge. Since the vaccine has not yet been announced, the current treatment is supplemental care. In this study, we compared machine learning classification methods such as NN, SVM, MLP, RF and KNN, which are widely used in the healthcare sector to diagnose disease by X-ray. Doctors often prescribe chest radiography to diagnose and/or predict infections, since we have read numerous articles on coronavirus. Further, in the clinical perspective, machine learning plays a

M. Kannan (✉)
PhD Research Scholar, Department of Computer Science, Vels Institute of Science, Technology and Advanced Studies (VISTAS), Chennai, India
e-mail: kannanmuthusamy.research@gmail.com

C. Priya
Associate Professor, Department of Information Technology, Vels Institute of Science, Technology and Advanced Studies (VISTAS), Chennai, India
e-mail: drcpriya.research@gmail.com

© The Editor(s) (if applicable) and The Author(s), under exclusive license to Springer Nature Singapore Pte Ltd. 2020

C. Chakraborty et al. (eds.), *Internet of Medical Things for Smart Healthcare*, Studies in Big Data 80, https://doi.org/10.1007/978-981-15-8097-0_3

vital role in solving the problem of prognosis and, thanks to treatment monitoring, there are effective mechanisms. In the presence of airborne diseases, we need an effective tool such as machine learning to investigate this, because nCOVID is transmitted by sneezing or coughing and/or other pulmonary syndrome. Therefore, this review summarizes the current outbreaks of coronavirus and its closely related lung viruses such as influenza and pneumonia, medical-based machine learning (MML) techniques and comparative analysis of MML for infectious diseases.

Keywords nCOVID-19 · Chest X-ray · Pulmonary diseases · Pneumonia · Medical machine learning · Classification models · Outbreaks · World Health Organization

1 Introduction

The latest nCOVID-19 public health epidemic problem is one of the infectious viral diseases that first erupted in Wuhan, Hubei Territory, China (2019). This is followed by the announcement of a blockade of the world's countries. Day after day, the disease will increase the infection among people. The serious symptoms of COVID are breathing difficulties, in which it occurs within the incubation period of 1–14 days. Furthermore, in a few decades, the World Health Organization-WHO has to continually face many viral diseases. For example [1]: Avian influenza in 1997, SARS-CoV in 2002–2003, H1N1 influenza in 2009, MERS-CoV in 2012 and EZV in 2014. These diseases cause severe acute respiratory syndrome and various lung diseases in the human brain and increase mortality with these new types of viruses; the mortality rate increases, making WHO the top priority in controlling the spread of COVID. Compared to other infectious diseases, nCOVID causes a serious outbreak worldwide. Currently, there are no current vaccines or other supplements against nCOVID due to the lack of scientific and clinical studies. As of April 4, 2020, a total of 205 countries and territories have been reported and about 11,17,860 positive cases have been identified in China and India has 2,902 confirmed cases. In addition, there is a huge increase in people's mortality every day. The disease also has close contact with the flu virus and viral pneumonia, in which the flu causes viral cough in which pneumonia also causes severe respiratory problems. For this reason, in the medical industry, computed tomography [2] is highly recommended for checking and diagnosing disease such as pneumonia. In today's world, the human race is increasingly affected by combinations of pandemic and epidemic diseases. Most of these viruses are infected with low resistance levels or the main airways of the human body. According to a report published by pathologists [3] so far, COV is known to cause more germs in the respiratory tract and intestinal tract, as well as other bacterial diseases such as influenza. Thus, the WHO named the "corona" from the family Coronoviridae and is divided into four categories: α, β, γ, δ by various pathologists. The human body contains a multitude of RNA-filled blood cell proteins and DNA culture. Any viral disease can easily occur through the blood immunity cell. In the medical industry, blood cell count is also important test and tremendous. Basically, the hemocytometer and some chemical compounds will count the blood cells. Therefore, it is a tedious task to count all infected and low immunity blood cells. For this reason, Mahmudhul Alam and Taqual Isam proposed a "YOLO" ("only seen once") method for automatic blood cell counting in 2019 [4] (Tables 1 and 2).

The Centers for Disease Control and Prevention (CDC) have reported that the contagious respiratory swine flu virus or H1N1 is one of the most serious public health problems and that humans can easily become infected with fever, cough and chills. As a result, the type-A influenza virus is influenced by pigs. It is classified into avain, pig, pandemic, seasonal. The human-mammalian (avian) transaction scenario is rare, but compared to other flu types, the avian influenza virus and COV have a similar structure along with the infectious stages, https://www.cdc.gov/flu/pdf/avianflu/avian-flu-transmission.pdf. The human gene is constructed as a multiple cell sequence, which is sensitive and can be easily influenced by bacteria and other pandemic viruses, such as influenza disease, if the gene contains low immunity. Machine learning methods are very effective in the multidisciplinary area, including

Table 1 Total number of suspected cases [31]—2020

Country	1st May	2nd May	3rd May	4th May	5th May	6th May	7th May	8th May
Afghanistan	2171	2335	2469	2704	2894	3224	3392	3563
Algeria	4006	4154	4295	4474	4648	4838	4997	5182
Australia	6762	6767	6783	6801	6825	6849	6875	6896
Austria	15,424	15,458	15,470	15,538	15,569	15,586	15,651	15,673
Bangladesh	7667	8238	8790	9455	10,143	10929	11719	12425
Brazil	85,380	91,589	96,559	101,147	107,780	114,715	125,218	135,106
Canada	53,236	55,061	56,714	59,474	60,772	62,046	63,496	64,922
China	83,956	83,959	83,961	83,964	83,966	83,968	83,970	83,976
France	**129,581**	**130,185**	**130,979**	**131,287**	**131,863**	**132,967**	**137,150**	**137,779**
Germany	**159,119**	**161,703**	**162,496**	**163,175**	**163,860**	**164,897**	**166,091**	**167,300**
Ghana	2074	2074	2169	2169	2719	2719	3091	3091
India	35,043	37,336	39,980	42,533	46,433	49,391	52,952	56,342
Indonesia	10,118	10,551	10,843	11,192	11,587	12,071	12,438	12,776
Iran	94,640	95,646	96,448	97,424	98,647	99,970	101,650	103,135
Ireland	20,612	20,833	21,176	21,506	21,722	21,983	22,248	22,385
Israel	15,946	16,101	16,185	16,208	16,246	16,289	16,310	16,381
Japan	14,281	14,544	14,839	15,057	15,231	15,354	15,463	15,547
Mexico	19,224	20,739	22,088	23,471	24,905	26,025	27,634	29,616
Netherlands	39,316	39,791	40,236	40,571	40,770	41,087	41,319	41,774
Pakistan	16,817	18,114	19,103	20,186	21,501	22,550	24,073	25,837
Paraguay	266	333	370	396	415	431	440	462
Peru	36,976	40,459	42,534	45,928	47,372	51,189	54,817	58,526
Philippines	8488	8772	8928	9223	9485	9684	10,004	10,343
Poland	12,877	13,105	13,375	13,693	14,006	14,431	14,740	15,047
Portugal	24,987	25,351	25,190	25,524	25,524	25,702	26,182	26,715
Puerto Rico	1539	1575	1757	1808	1843	1924	1968	2031

(continued)

Table 1 (continued)

Country	1st May	2nd May	3rd May	4th May	5th May	6th May	7th May	8th May
Qatar	13,409	14,096	14,872	15,551	16,191	17,142	17,972	18,890
Romania	12,240	12,567	12,732	13,163	13,512	13,837	14,107	14,499
Russia	**106,498**	**114,431**	**124,054**	**134,687**	**145,268**	**155,370**	**165,929**	**177,160**
Saudi Arabia	22,753	24,097	25,459	27,011	28,656	30,251	31,938	33,731
Singapore	16,169	17,101	17,548	18,205	18,778	19,410	20,198	20,939
South Africa	5647	5951	6336	6783	7220	7572	7808	8232
Spain	**215,216**	**216,582**	**217,466**	**218,011**	**219,329**	**220,325**		**221,447**
Turkey	**120,204**	**122,392**	**124,375**	**126,045**	**127,659**	**129,491**	**131,744**	**133,721**
United Arab Emirates	12,481	13,038	13,599	14,163	14,730	15,192	15,738	16,240
United Kingdom	**171,253**	**177,454**	**182,260**	**186,599**	**190,584**	**194,990**	**201,201**	**206,715**
United States	**1,069,826**	**1,103,781**	**1,133,069**	**1,158,041**	**1,180,634**	**1,204,475**	**1,228,603**	**1,256,972**

immunology, virology, microbiology and other health testing laboratories, the ability to split big data into multiple test data sets and training for the prediction model of illnesses. Computed tomography (CT) and X-rays tests are crucial medical features [5] that are used to identify pneumonia. With the spread of infectious diseases such as COVID fever and pneumonia, it is very difficult to diagnose their true disease, and doctors are analyzing the true impact of the disease with a chest X-ray.

Today, with the large amount of data, descriptive or statistical analysis is sometimes confusing and also creates an arduous task that includes understanding and extracting knowledge. One of the efficient applications of the machine learning methodology and its techniques helps many other industries; even the clinical industry uses it widely and quickly. Machine learning, a subfield of AI [6], allows the system to read data for multiple uses. The collected data set is divided into training and test data sets for future forecasting. Therefore, ML techniques are mainly used for classification and prediction with three different learning methods: supervised, unsupervised and reinforcement. Each of them has unique diagnostic benefits. Furthermore, in the medical field, early disease prediction is a rather difficult task, the disease and related data can only be viewed by experienced doctors. Sometimes, it even confuses the experts. But machine learning has the ability to build a prediction model together with the previously available original dataset. They are increasingly used in the health industry, such as EEG, ECG and radiology (Table 3 and Fig. 1).

2 Recent Pandemic

In recent decades, China has faced several infectious diseases, such as human-zoonotic viral infection, including severe acute respiratory syndrome and Middle East respiratory syndrome. Coronavirus-19 is a family of Coroviridae/RNA virus. Virulent diseases such as SARS and MERS [7] identified with zoonotic animals; therefore,

Table 2 Death cases [31]—2020

Country	1st May	2nd May	3rd May	4th May	5th May	6th May	7th May	8th May
Afghanistan	64	68	72	85	90	95	104	106
Algeria	450	453	459	463	465	470	476	483
Australia	92	93	93	95	95	96	97	97
Bangladesh	168	170	175	177	182	183	186	199
Brazil	5901	6329	6750	7025	7321	7921	8536	9146
Canada	3184	3391	3566	3682	3854	4043	4232	4408
China	4637	4637	4637	4637	4637	4637	4637	4637
France	**24,376**	**24,594**	**24,760**	**24,895**	**25,201**	**25,531**	**25,809**	**25,987**
Germany	6288	6575	6649	6692	6831	6996	7119	7266
Ghana	17	17	18	18	18	18	18	18
India	1147	1218	1301	1373	1568	1694	1783	1886
Indonesia	792	800	831	845	864	872	895	930
Iran	6028	6091	6156	6203	6277	6340	6418	6486
Ireland	1232	1265	1265	1303	1319	1339	1375	1403
Israel	222	225	229	232	235	238	239	240
Italy	**27,967**	**28,236**	**28,710**	**28,884**	**29,079**	**29,315**	**29,684**	**29,958**
Mexico	1859	1972	2061	2154	2271	2507	2704	2961
Netherlands	4795	4893	4987	5056	5082	5168	5204	5288
Pakistan	385	417	440	462	486	526	564	594
Paraguay	10	10	10	10	10	10	10	10
Peru	1051	1124	1200	1286	1344	1444	1533	1627
Philippines	568	579	603	607	623	637	658	685
Poland	644	651	664	678	698	716	733	755
Portugal	1007	1007	1023	1063	1063	1074	1089	1105
Puerto Rico	92	94	95	97	97	99	99	102
Qatar	10	12	12	12	12	12	12	12
Romania	717	744	771	780	803	827	858	876
Russia	1073	1169	1222	1280	1356	1451	1537	1625
Saudi Arabia	162	169	176	184	191	200	209	219
Singapore	15	16	17	18	18	18	20	20
South Africa	103	116	123	131	138	148	153	161
Spain	**24,824**	**25,100**	**25,264**	**25,428**	**25,613**	**25,857**		**26,070**
Turkey	3174	3258	3336	3397	3461	3520	3584	3641
United Arab Emirates	105	111	119	126	137	146	157	165
United Kingdom	**26,771**	**27,510**	**28,131**	**28,446**	**28,734**	**29,427**	**30,076**	**30,615**
United States	63,006	65,068	66,385	67,682	68,934	71,078	73,431	75,670

Table 3 The strong correlation of the two previous epidemic diseases: Information on these data has collected from the World Health Organization

Influenza	COVID
It causes respiratory disease, asymptomatic	It causes basic, respiratory disease and asymptomatic
Transmitted through droplets, cough	Also transmitted through droplets, sneeze, direct contact
The interval range of this disease is 3 days	The incubation period of this disease is 1–14 days
It shows mild symptoms only	It will also show mild symptoms
Mortality ranges is (0.1%) lower	The mortality ratio between 3–4%
Children are highly affected	Adult cases are more
Antivirals and vaccine are available	No vaccine or therapeutic

According to this disease, the coronavirus and the flu virus have a certain similarity, which will be represented in the above table

they cause low morbidity and transmission between people. In contrast, nCOVID-19 has wreaked havoc with humans. The result of this high mortality varies with the short term. Therefore, the zoonotic virus, SARS-CoV, was transmitted through bats and civet cats and originated in 2002. Probably in 2012, MERS-CoV was identified, which is transmitted through bats to the camel. The clinical manifestation of both viruses is fever, chills, dyspnoea, myalgia, respiratory problems, diarrhea, general malaise, dilemma and pneumonia. Compared to other zoonotic diseases, nCOVID-19 has tremendous vigor. The 0th death case of MERS-CoV [8] is reported in Saudi Arabia (Jeddah); this virus is belonging to the lineage C of the *betacoronavirus* in which it causes severe respiratory illness to the people. In July 2013, total, 91 cases were identified from the Arab peoples and the fatality range is 50%. Simultaneously,

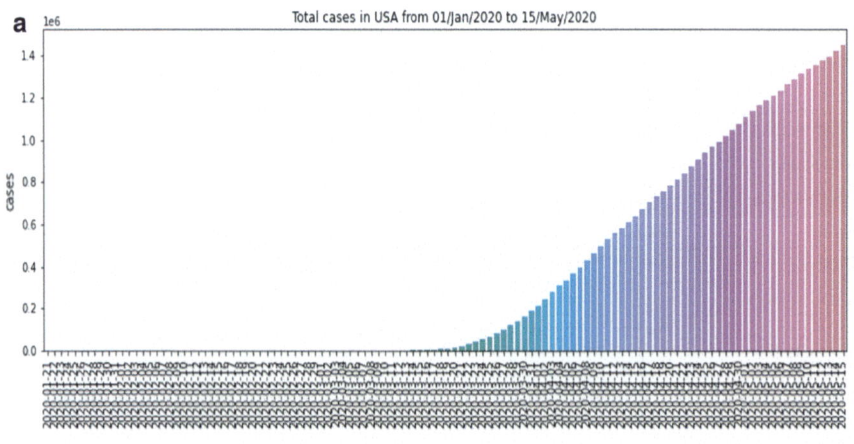

Fig. 1 **a**. USA COVID + cases **b**. USA death cases

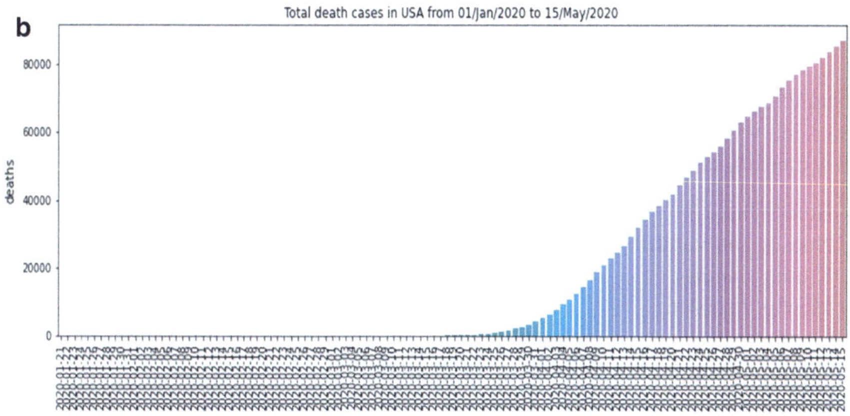

Fig. 1 (continued)

another 27 International countries including UK, France, Italy, Germany also have found and reported to the World Health Organization.

The MERS-CoV infected person is strongly confirmed by the laboratory test; for this in the medical industry, a sample of sputum [9] is collected from the infected person and then the samples are tested by using real-time RT-PCR laboratory method. In 2009, influenza family viruses [10], termed airborne diseases, threatened people. And these have made its connection to the population through droplets that usually come from sneezing. Along with respiratory viruses, H1N1, H5N1 and H5N7 are also included. And these are related in SARS and MERS. We obtained the data through several online sources. Their data list and associated mortality rates are explained in further sections (Table 4).

Table 4 Specimen ranges. https://apps.who.int/iris/bitstream/handle/10665/331329/WHO-COVID-19-laboratory-2020.4-eng.pdf

Type of the specimens collected from the infected/suspected cases	Temperature range to store the collected specimens
Nasopharyngeal/Oropharyngeal	2–8°C if ≤ 5 days–70°C (dry ice) if > 5 days
Sputum	2–8°C if ≤ 2 days–70°C (dry ice) if > 2 days
Serum	2–8°C if ≤ 5 days–70°C (dry ice) if > 5 days
Blood	2–8°C if ≤ 5 days–70°C (dry ice) if > 5 days
Urine	2–8°C if ≤ 5 days–70°C (dry ice) if > 5 days
Stool	2–8°C if ≤ 5 days–70°C (dry ice) if > 5 days

3 Pneumonia Infection

Pneumonia, which is caused by some fungi or negative bacteria in the human body, is attacked by various soft parts of the body such as the throat, lungs and blood vessels. They cause a variety of diseases. These include the following.

- Breathless
- Nausea and vomiting
- Kidney damage
- Mental disorder
- Coughing
- Color changes in many organs of the body
- Chest pain
- Cancer (Fig. 2).

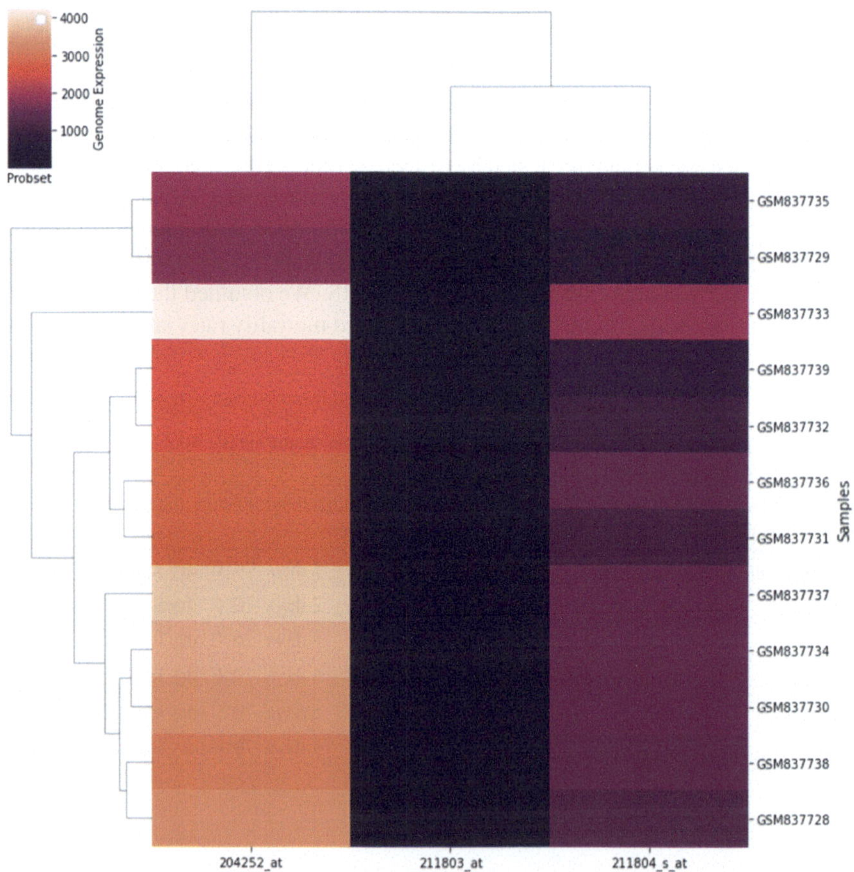

Fig. 2 The probable sequence of genomes for lung cancer [29, 30]

Pneumonia is also one of the routes to travel the infectious disease (Coronavirus) from one person to another through the droplets, simultaneously. Clinicians prefer chest X-ray test to diagnose the active pneumonia from the respirator. As the proof of, a study published by Sufang Tian et al. in Journal of Thoracic Oncology (IASLC Special Report) found that two people had coronavirus from lung cancer.

4 Pneumonia with COVID-19

Initially, the two cases were discovered from the province of china. At first, both patients are admitted for the lung cancer treatment [11]. First, an 84-year-old woman was admitted to Wuhan, China, for treatment of lung cancer due to increased stress, and doctors prescribed a CT-scan for the patient. Pneumonia infection in the lung was detected by scan report. Because of this, the patient was transferred to the special ward and the medical test was carried out with the swap spaceman. At the end of the report, it was revealed that the patient was infected with coronavirus.

Next, a 73-year-old man was admitted to lung cancer surgery. He was slightly healed and discharged in a few weeks. Shortly thereafter, coughs with fever were frequent, and she was taken back to the hospital for examination, and CT scans and nucleic acid tests revealed that she and her pneumonia had been affected. In the end, both patients were diagnosed with hypertension at an early age, comparing the outcome. The below Fig. 3a the normal and COVID-19 patient lung X-ray image, which are collected from, https://github.com/ieee8023/covid-chestxray-dataset/tree/master/images [31].

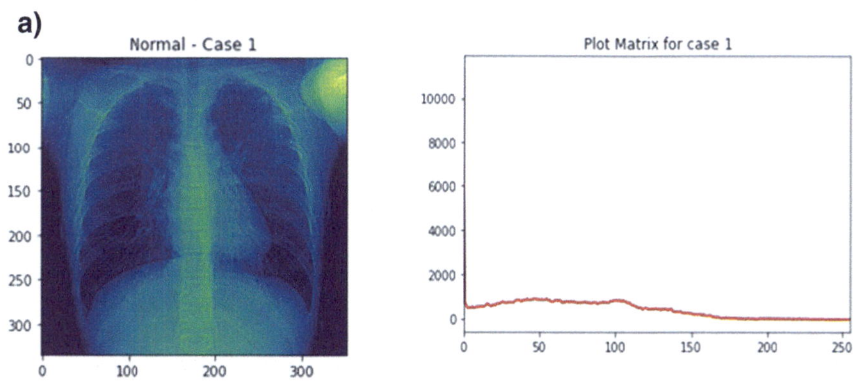

Fig. 3 **a**, **b**, **c**. Graphical representation of chest X-ray test image with plot matrix

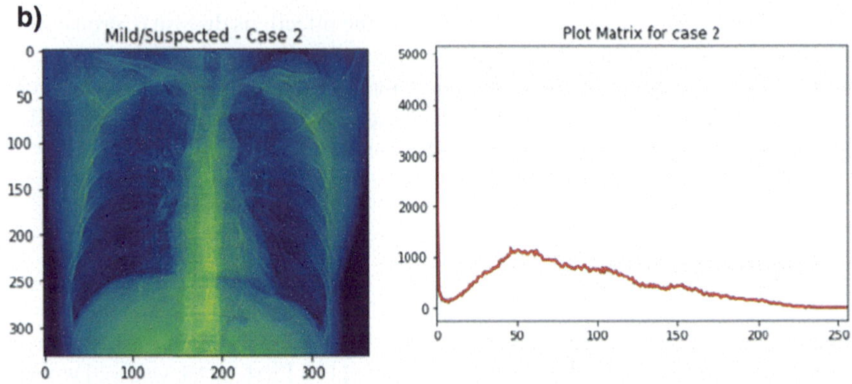

Fig. 3 (continued)

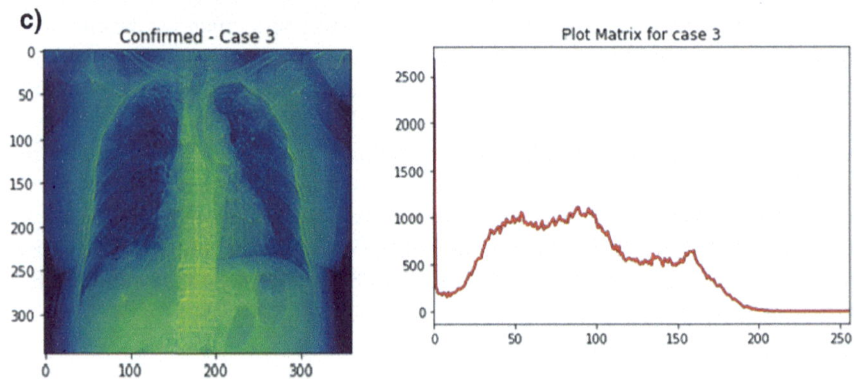

Fig. 3 (continued)

5 Related Literature in ML with Healthcare

For COVID-19 in viral infections, most medical examiners prefer X-ray testing to detect pathogens or pneumonia. Day by day, infectious disease is becoming more and more unpredictable in humans. In the medical field, chest X-ray is an important clinical trial that can be very useful for pathogen identification. Machine learning and deep learning enable examiners to identify the disease in its early stages using the confident accuracy of scan reports. Here, we reviewed the literature on the CAD-based predictive model. The literature helps to understand the reality of ML and DL prognostic models in the medical field (Fig. 4).

Anuja Kumar and Rajalakshmi [12] have proposed an automated detection model to identify pneumonia from chest X-ray imaging using deep Siamese NN. In chest X-ray, all viral pneumonia is captured as a white substance. The pathogen can spread to the left lung or to the right side. The convolution neural network has come into

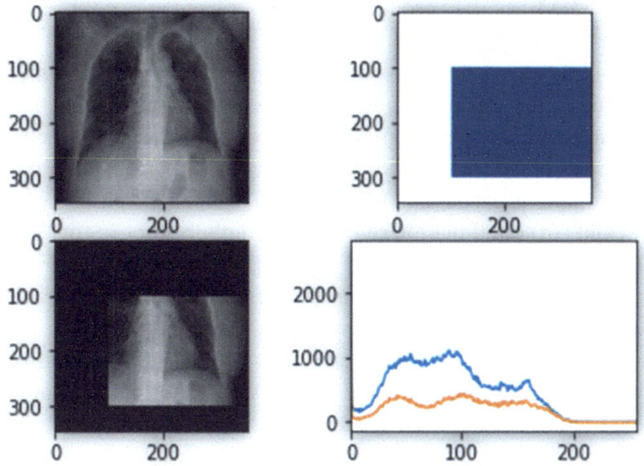

Fig. 4 COVID + lung X-ray with histo plot

the picture to extract image pixels. Initially, the CXR image is retrieved from the original image (mm) pixel size. After that, the transformed image is divided into two sections, like the left and the right. The Siamese network model has been used to calculate the end of the segment. To increase the efficiency of the proposed model, the author approaches the K-fold CV technique to divide the model into k-values. Furthermore, AUROC is used to identify the overall performance of the proposed model. Furthermore, the authors divide the problem into three categories, namely normal image, viral pneumonia picture and bacterial pneumonia.

Sebastian Gundel et al. [13] have proposed an abnormal classification based on deep learning using scan image. The model operates on a different task, such as division, abnormality and regional classification.

In the modern and e-technological world, wearable devices are the most common and most useful electronic devices for humans. These devices automatically detect human health situations such as headache, fever, BMI, heart rate, blood pressure, etc., based on the monitoring sensors. Paulo Resque et al. [14] investigate five main ML algorithms, such as: support vector machine, random forest, naive Bayes, KNN and neural network for the health problem of the epileptic seizure problem. Analysis-based work is performed using the patient's EEG dataset. For the implementation of the model, the R language was used to calculate the model. In the result of the evaluation of the model is calculated based on accuracy. Here, kappa statistics have also been used for comparison of results. The kappa statistics will be calculated using the formula [14] [Paulo et al.].

$$\text{KAPPA} = \frac{\text{Observed Accuracy} - \text{Expected Accuracy}}{1 - \text{Expected Accuracy}}.$$

Finally, the SVM model produces 97.31% accuracy with computational complexity O (n^3).

Ibrahim Almubark et al. [15] discussed the prediction of Alzheimer's disease using neuropathological patient data. Alzheimer's disease is a disease that primarily attacks the human neurological system. To improve the accuracy of the classification, the neurophysiological data set was used. The datasets are grouped into three parts: (i) common neurological test data, (ii) mild cognitive data indicating the reaction and response time, and (iii) combination of both. The authors choose four classification algorithms, namely SVM, RF, GB and AB are used to classify the data. For these three types of data, a total of three experiments are performed and fivefold cross-validations and leave-one-out are used to evaluate the model.

In the healthcare sector [16], computed tomography and mammography are the most used for making decisions, as if the patient was in normal or abnormal conditions. SVM and image processing are the techniques in which image processing plays a key role in the medical science to detect lung cancer through the acquired image. In today's life, most people admitted because of the cancer-oriented problem, the mortality rate also increases. Up to now, anticipation is much more important. The author explains "How are computed tomography images used to detect the defect?". Image processing techniques are used here to clean the X-ray image such as acquisition, feature extraction, segmentation, noise reduction, filter, etc. SVM is one of the supervised techniques; it helps to identify and classify the + ve and -ve ratio of cancer patients. For this application, the Java framework and JSP were used to build the application model.

We can say that chronic diseases are lifelong illnesses. Decision trees, random forest and SVM [17] [Swetha Ganikar] have been used to test whether or not the patient is infected. Chronic diseases such as diabetes, liver and heart disease are collected from an open database. All data were used for each method. The RF generates 98% accuracy in the benchmarking phase.

Thirunavukarasu et al. [18] discussed the prognosis of liver disease. Because of the length of health records, the author uses machine learning classification techniques to find the hidden area for the best predictive model. Supervised learning methods, such as KNN, LR, and SVM, were used to predict the disease. Therefore, the performance of the proposed models is calculated using the confusion matrix of the proposed model.

Muhammad Imran Faisal et al. [19] used machine learning classifiers and ensemble classification techniques to detect lung cancer based on its symptoms. The UCI reference dataset is used for this analysis. 10-fold cross validation of training and testing data after the initial data preprocessing phase. The data are applied to each ML method and set the classifier to choose the best classifier for the problem.

Israeli AI-Tauraika [20] and others have discussed MERS-CoV, a family of Coronaviridae, which mainly affects animals. The authors use data mining techniques to develop a predictive model of MERS virus. Approximately, 1082 records of patient data were collected to create the model. The NB classifier and J48 methods were used to validate the model. After processing the data, the collected data will be applied to the selected sample. J48 and NB is a well-known classifiers and supervised learning methods for creating tree-like image after classification. Using the WEKA software tool, the predictive model has been successfully built, and with the use of 10-fold cross-validation techniques, both the stability model and the recovery model yield the most accurate result. The stability model provides 55.69% accuracy for the J48 method compared to NB and J48. The patient recovery model provides 71.58% accuracy for the NB classification.

6 Roles of Machine Learning

Artificial intelligence is a computer-based technology, also known as "machine intelligence." Artificial intelligence is more powerful for making multitrack decisions and can learn the data set itself to predict the future. Today, AI technologies are used in multiple industries. Artificial intelligence extends the technique to machine learning. Hence, ML is also called as a subset of AI. It also further expands another subset called "deep learning." Artificial intelligence aims to develop and build the computer, and efficiently learn large amounts of data. The technology helps machine learning to extract the relevant functionality of the large synthetic data set. The term "machine learning" was coined by the computer scientist "Arthur Samuel" in 1959, who was the developer of the artificial intelligence model. The main role of ML is to learn any type of data. Machine learning has the ability to predict the future, so it plays on multiple disciplines. It is also possible to perform automatic operations such as data extraction, data grouping, data classification, etc.

Artificial intelligence and machine learning are an emerging technology, currently used by the era all over the world, especially in the medical field with the name of medical image analysis, including magnetic resonance imaging, X-rays and/or computed tomography. We know that in the hospital sector, computer scanners are used to diagnose the level of disease along with the patient's clinical symptoms. Sometimes, the result can lead to low accuracy due to the medical report. This is the problem that will normally occur in the medical area.

The era of machine learning technology offers numerous classification and prediction algorithms to determine the most accurate result of severely infected cases. Recently, coronavirus has caused major outbreaks on earth. Many people have been seriously affected, so the graphical representation of the report will be shown in Fig. 1a, b. In the pandemic situation, research-oriented results will be the most common need. The main strength of this document is to discuss the role of the machine learning techniques most used in bioinformatics (Figs. 5 and 6).

As mentioned earlier, ML is a subset of AI, taking the initiative to learn the data itself. It plays a key role in medical forecasting using the statistical and probabilistic classification technique. For example, in the medical field, early diagnosis of the disease is a difficult task. But in machine learning, it offers many classification and prediction techniques to predict disease at an early stage. In addition, in the recent pandemic, viral disease is a COVID-19 that spreads through the flu drops and is

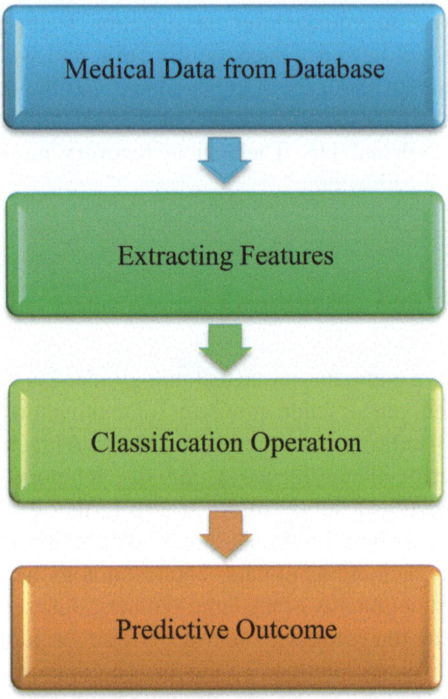

Fig. 5 Disease prediction using machine learning

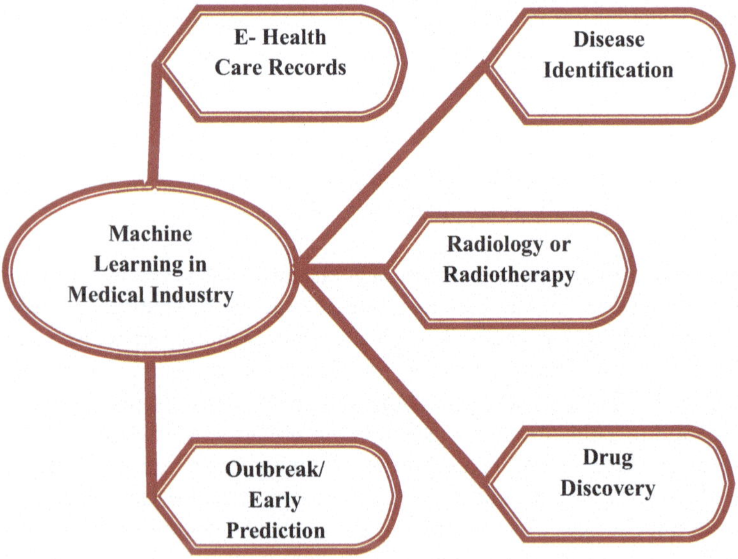

Fig. 6 ML in medical

mainly infected in the chest and lung areas. For this, clinical examiners suggest tests and radiographic results to diagnose the infection.

Although due to the lack of small medical imaging problems, we sometimes get low precision results. For this, machine learning helps to avoid this problem during the disease detection phase. Machine learning uses several methods to process data, including [21], supervised, unsupervised, semi-supervised, strengthening, multi-tasking, ensembles, neural networks and instance-based learning. Primarily, it can be divided into two parts, (i) supervised learning and (ii) unsupervised learning. These two methods are the most used in medical diagnosis.

6.1 Supervised Learning

Supervised learning is one of the machine learning methods used to perform some statistical operations based on classification and regression. Structured data called "*labeled data*" was used to train the model. In the supervised learning model, the data structure is already known. The data will be separated according to the known characteristics. For example, consider the DNA sequence [22]. We know that the human cell contains numerous proteins. Each of them has a unique sequence or type. The chromosome is unique and varies from one human model to another. Based on the sequence module, the algorithm will classify the genome. The learning model is further divided into two subparts.

- Regression
- Classification.

Work flow:

- Data collection/Preprocessing and data preparation
- Extract the data
- Data split up
- Apply the model and evaluate the performance
- Train the model again and again for better accuracy.

Example:

- Data classification—To classify, suspected versus infected case.

6.2 Unsupervised Learning

It is one of the learning models. When we are entering into unsupervised learning method, the label is not mandatory of the data. Basically, unsupervised learning does not know about the data. Based on the data correlation, the data will be segregated. Major operations are,

- Clustering
- Association.

In other words, the cluster-based analysis method is majorly used to get the several types of data and it makes as a group. The supervised learning is working under the specific rules, which is clearly defined. Unlike, unsupervised learning methods are working under the condition-based rules, or in other words, it observes the information from the unlabeled data.

Work flow:

- Data preparation
- To learn the information from the preprocessed data
- Set the centroid point
- Make the similar data as a group
- Assign the cluster of data to each centroid.

Example:

- Doctors and ward boys—the method will work based on the similar feature.

6.3 Semi-supervised Learning

Semi-supervised learning is a one kind of machine learning approach in which the method will handle both labeled and unlabeled data, for example, like in the ration of 40:60 approximately. In other words, it contains a small number of labeled data and huge amount of unlabeled data. So that this learning method is referred as a combination of supervised and unsupervised learning. The fruit-full applications like, speech analysis, web content classification and cell protein sequence classification are working under the semi-supervised learning methods. Multiple literature [22] reviewed, semi-supervised methods are most useful for the findings and also provide better accuracy due to have the capability to learn combined data, than the supervised model.

6.4 Reinforcement Learning

Machine learning distributes a unique category of learning methods called reinforcement learning, is an automated decision-making process. The model will learn the data by using the past experience, environment and it works under the reward based system, unlike supervised and unsupervised. In the artificial intelligence, it is a type of dynamic programming, has the capability to train the model, while in the case of data is absent. Suppose the result is not satisfied after the training phase, then the model can take up the punishment/or the reward to train the model one again. Until, the process will continue, till the model gets the correct result based on the reward value. For this, the model is simply referred as an agent-reward-based model.

6.5 Neural Networks Learning

In general, the neural network is known as ANN, which is one of the learning processes. The main feature of ANN is the processing of the input elements, which automatically read the input data based on the characteristics. It is a revolutionary neural network that contains multiple layers of nodes, which will be treated like a neuron, used for pattern recognition. These are divided into three levels, namely: input layer (receive input), hidden layer (calculation) and the output layer (check the signal result). In general, the perceptron network is developed for the huge data set consisting of numerous attribute classes. This model contains the weight values of each neuron. The model will be trained until no error occurs. MLP levels are interconnected to synaptic links called edges which have some weight values for the calculation (Fig. 7).

The hidden layer receives input signals from the input layer through the communication link. For the purpose of processing values, each link will be assigned some weight values. Here, weight values are input information. After this process, the layer will calculate the net input value for the future process. It will be sent to the release layer called output layer. If the network is unable to give the desired output, the model will be re-trained with different weight values.

7 Methodology

7.1 Naïve Bayes Classifier

Based on the Bayes theorem, the naive Bayes algorithm will evaluate the probability of the class. The model is helpful, even if the attribute of the data belongs to some other attribute. Therefore, in machine learning, this model is also called "probability classifier." Finally, it will return the result based on the predicted class.

$$\text{Bayes theorem, } \frac{P(H|E) = P(E|H).P(H)}{P(E)}$$

The NB classification is categorized into three parts: GaussianNB, MultinomialNB and Bernoulli model.

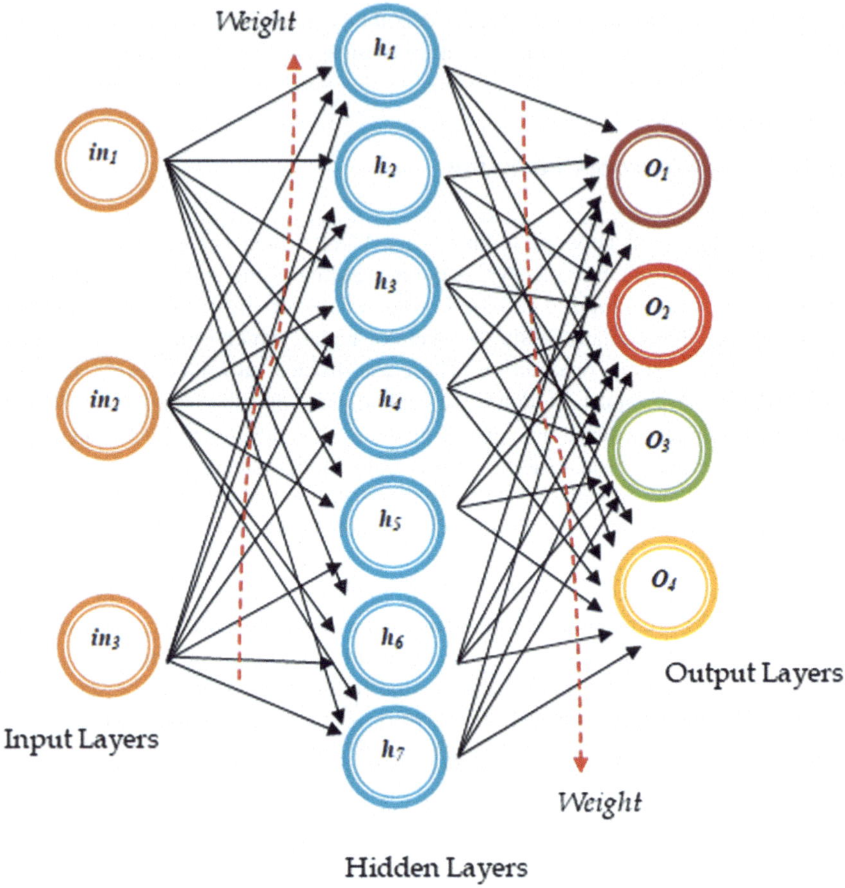

Fig. 7 Simple N-network architecture

Example:

Sweating	Vomiting	Dehydration	Fever	Fever (Multiclass)
Y	Y	Y	Y (1)	High
Y	N	Y	Y (1)	Medium
N	N	Y	N (0)	Normal
Y	N	N	N (0)	Normal
N	Y	Y	Y (1)	Prob
Y	Y	N	Y (1)	Prob
N	N	Y	N (0)	Normal

- ***Gaussian Model***: Typically, the model is used when the data are in numeric format
- ***Multinomial Model***: It deals with multiclass variables, which is why this model is called multinomial, which is suitable for text-based data.
- ***Bernoulli Model:*** This model is used, while the data are in vector-based (binary values) format.

7.2 *Random Forest*

It is an ensemble classification model, one of the supervised techniques. It can create multiple decision trees to classify attributes using "bagging." The model also separates the relevant features for classification. Once the model is trained, the output of each tree is integrated into a single group. The model predicts the final result based on the high number of votes cast on the tree. This is an ensemble classifier, which means that the properties are more deeply divided than a normal decision tree. This random forest classification does not allow for excessive matching (overfitting) of the data, which is a major advantage compared to other classifiers.

7.3 *Linear SVC*

Support vector clustering is a method that is commonly used for the hierarchical clustering problem. It is a non-parametric classification model, which automatically calculates the value with its method, regardless of the format of the data. Like the support vector machine, the kernel function is used to compile data. This method works by using a decision boundary or a hyperplane to separate the data points.

7.4 *Feature Selection*

The selection of characteristics is an important step in the problem of classification and forecasting. The feature selection model allows the machine to classify the variable for training. Manually, specific attributes cannot be extracted during big data. In other words, we do not know which class is associated with which class. Assuming that the decision is made by man, the model will have errors during the training phase. In addition, selecting an important class is also a complicated task. Therefore, machine learning provides a feature selection method (such as PCA) to extract relevant variables/attributes from large amounts of data. For example: Data classification, if the data set contains multiple variables, the machine needs preliminary knowledge to extract the feature to increase the degree of precision. The method is designed to,

(1) Reduce the processing time
(2) Simplify the problem
(3) Reach best accuracy score
(4) Reduce the data length
(5) Choose the best fit and data correlation.

8 Experimental Setup

For this experimental analysis, we collected primary tumor [32] data from the open dataset repository, which is a UCI repository in CSV format. The dataset contains 18 attributes (including age and gender) and 339 instances. In addition, the data set consists of a multiclass variable. So we import the MultinomialNB classifier from the sklearn. Based on the dataset we have, the most common type of cancer known as "adeno" is known to be the most pathogenic when looking at which histological type is most harmful (Figs. 8 and 9).

Python and Sklearn have been used for testing. Machine learning provides several useful guidelines for clinical prognosis. Sometimes, based on the data, the model will provide less accuracy during the training phase. To avoid such a problem, we initially conducted a general performance analysis of ML models (RF, Linear SVC, LR, and NP) with our clinical dataset. All models achieved full accuracy score (Fig. 10). To ensure this, we select two classifier models such as SVM and RF for the training phase.

As we have noted above, there are many types of histologic variants in the primary tumor database. Therefore, we have the responsibility of extracting the feature from

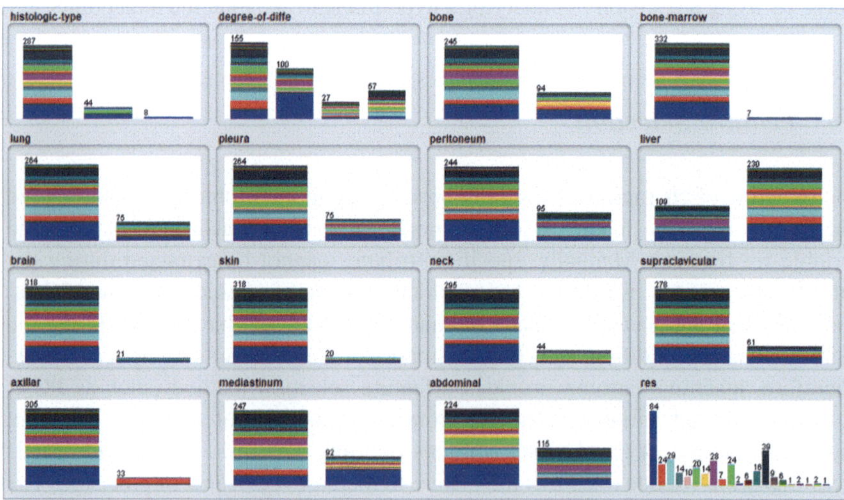

Fig. 8 Visualization of data attributes

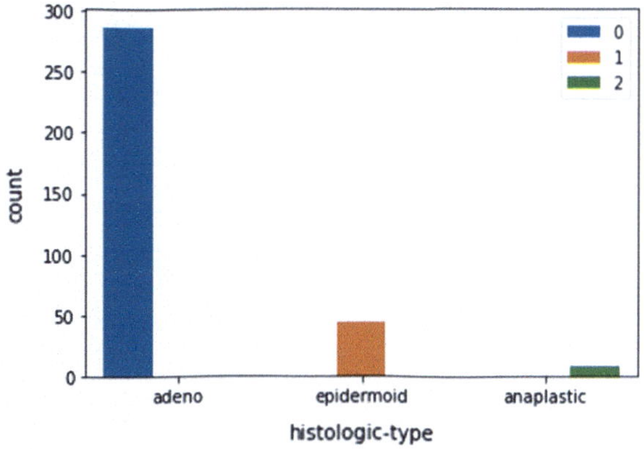

Fig. 9 Total count of histologic-type

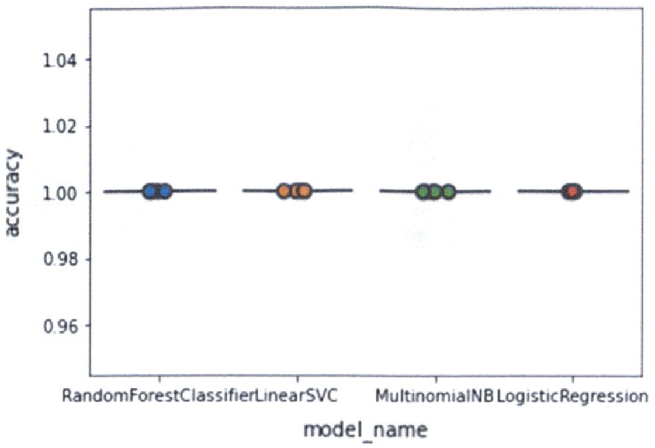

Fig. 10 Total accuracy of the selected model

the histologic (cancer type) type. Here, TfidfVectorizer and CountVectorizer are used to convert text data into a matrix format [33]. In this unique performance, we choose the random forest and linear support vector machine classifier to demonstrate model accuracy with the primary tumor dataset. After the two models work equally well, we obtain the same confusion matrix of the RF and linear SVC classifier (Figs. 11, 12).

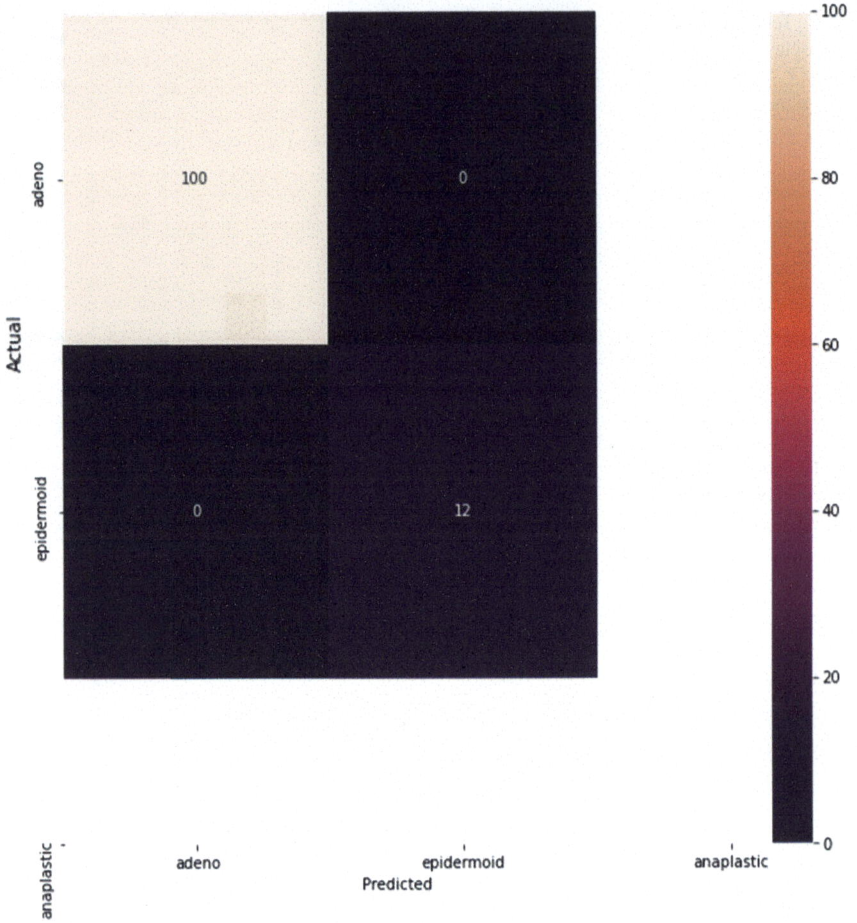

Fig. 11 Confusion matrix–linear SVC

Fig. 12 Confusion matrix–random forest

Predicted Species	Lungs	Class
Actual Species		
Lungs	12	0
Class	0	100

9 Publications Relevant to ML and DL for Medical Imaging

Author(s)	Aim	Model description	Methodology	Performance evaluator	Result and accuracy
Jie Ren, Kai Song et al. [23]	Discovering virus of metageonomic sequence data	Proposed "reference-free" and "alignment-free" method to disassemble the virus. DeepVirFinder has used to find the sequence of the viral genome (DNA)	Machine learning and deep learning-convolutional neural networks	AUROC	1. Viral seq (500): 95% 2. Viral seq (1000): 97% 3. Viral seq (3000): 98%
Zhenyu Tang, Wei Zhao et al. [24]	The assessment model to detect the COVID patients complication	Based on the quantitative features of the Coronavirus, the data have trained the model. Using lung CT images and the main features is helping the RF model to detect, if the infected patient is in severe or normal condition.	Random forest	AUC curve	1. Total accuracy: 87% 2. Accuracy in AUC: 91%
Ghanshyam Verma et al. [25]	Infected gene classification for viral respiratory infection	Early stage detection of viral infection using top most viral genes	KNN, linear SVM, RF and SVM with RBF	10-fold, hold-out	1. Overall accuracy in 10-fold: SVM with RBF 2. Overall accuracy in hold-out: Random forest
Okeke Stephen et al. [26]	Classification and detection of pneumonia infection in chest X-ray	The Convloutional neural network method has approached to analyze the pneumonia in the X-ray image using several network layers	Deep learning	Epochs for training and loss	1. Average accuracy of training set: 95% 2. Average accuracy of validation set: 93%
Dhiraj Dahiwade et al. [27]	General disease prediction with symptoms	The work was carried on the Java platform. The general disease patient dataset is used for the prediction. Based on the ML preprocessing, the training dataset is created for the problem analysis	KNN and CNN	–	1. Best algorithm: KNN 2. Best Time Complexity: CNN
Amani Yahyaoui et al. [28]	Diabetes prediction	Based on the decision support system (DSS), the ML and DL model has approached to predict the diabetes. The performance analysis of ML and DL has also conducted	SVM, RF and CNN	Kappa Co-efficient	1. Class Diabetic-82% (RF) 2. Class Non-diabetic-86.7% (SVM)
Shuaijing Xu, Hao Wu and Rongfang Bie [34]	Anomaly detection on chest X-ray	CXNet-m1 is a proposed network structure, was used to train the model and Softmax cross_entropy has approached to classify the X-ray image due to the format of binary	Deep neural network	F1 Score and AUC	1. Accuracy rate in old data: 67.6% 2. Accuracy rate in new data: 84.4% 3. Accuracy rate in OpenI: 93.6%

10 Conclusion and Future Work

COVID-19 is a serious viral problem, and early detection of this virus is a complex task because it is directly or indirectly linked to other viral genome proteins. Since December 2019, many countries have been enslaved by the disease and have killed countless human species. We have found many positive literature to solve such a genetic classification problem. Computer-assisted diagnosis (CAD) is one of the medical techniques that play a major role in the problem prediction area. The medical key findings of this disease are the human lungs that are the major influences. So, clinicians suggest X-ray or CT scans for medical examination to find the cause of the infection. Nowadays, many high quality technology and medical disciplines are helping to identify drugs and vaccines for this. However, systematic research on this is being carried out and implemented.

Through the daily COVID-19 statistics, we know that many people infected with the virus have reduced and fully recovered, despite the deaths caused by this quarantine or infection. Immunity is the first of all parts of the human body. Such diseases attack the body through immune deficiency. Early detection of viral immunity may prevent infection. For this purpose, in the pharmaceutical industry, the method of "immunotherapy" is being manipulated. In some cases, these methods may not be effective due to the high viral component. Therefore, in the near future, we will be working with machine learning and deep learning to make these computational models more important to a clinician in order to meet their difficulties and increase their accuracy.

References

1. Li, J., et al.: Machine learning methods for predicting human-adaptive influenza a viruses based on viral nucleotide compositions. Mol. Biol. Evol. **37**(4), 1224–1236 (2020). https://doi.org/10.1093/molbev/msz276
2. "Title Page," J. Sex. Med. **14**(5), e205 (2017), https://doi.org/10.1016/s1743-6095(17)31143-8
3. Madjid, M., Safavi-Naeini, P., Solomon, S.D., Vardeny, O.: Potential effects of coronaviruses on the cardiovascular system: a review. JAMA Cardiol. **10**, 1–10 (2020). https://doi.org/10.1001/jamacardio.2020.1286
4. Alam, M.M., Islam, M.T.: Machine learning approach of automatic identification and counting of blood cells. Healthc. Technol. Lett. **6**(4), 103–108 (2019). https://doi.org/10.1049/htl.2018.5098
5. Abbas, A., Abdelsamea, M.M., Gaber, M.M.: Classification of COVID-19 in chest X-ray images using DeTraC deep convolutional neural network, 2020, [Online]. Available: http://arxiv.org/abs/2003.13815
6. Luo, Y., et al.: Machine learning for the prediction of severe pneumonia during posttransplant hospitalization in recipients of a deceased-donor kidney transplant. Ann. Transl. Med. **8**(4), 82–82 (2020). https://doi.org/10.21037/atm.2020.01.09
7. Meo, S.A., et al.: Novel coronavirus 2019-nCoV: prevalence, biological and clinical characteristics comparison with SARS-CoV and MERS-CoV. Eur. Rev. Med. Pharmacol. Sci. **24**(4), 2012–2019 (2020). https://doi.org/10.26355/eurrev_202002_20379

8. Salamatbakhsh, M., Mobaraki, K., Sadeghimohammadi, S., Ahmadzadeh, J.: The global burden of premature mortality due to the middle east respiratory syndrome (MERS) using standard expected years of life lost, 2012 to 2019. BMC Publ. Health **19**(1), 1–7 (2019). https://doi.org/10.1186/s12889-019-7899-2
9. Cho, S.Y., et al.: MERS-CoV outbreak following a single patient exposure in an emergency room in South Korea: an epidemiological outbreak study. Lancet **388**(10048), 994–1001 (2016). https://doi.org/10.1016/S0140-6736(16)30623-7
10. Ramanathan, K., et al.: Transmission of SARS and MERS coronaviruses and influenza virus in healthcare settings: the possible role of dry surface contamination. J. Hosp. Infect. **92**(January), 235–250 (2020)
11. Tian, S., Hu, W., Niu, L., Liu, H., Xu, H., Xiao, S.Y.: Pulmonary pathology of early-phase 2019 novel coronavirus (COVID-19) pneumonia in two patients with lung cancer. J. Thorac. Oncol. **15**(5), 700–704 (2020). https://doi.org/10.1016/j.jtho.2020.02.010
12. Acharya, A.K., Satapathy, R.: A deep learning based approach towards the automatic diagnosis of pneumonia from chest radio-graphs. Biomed. Pharmacol. J. **13**(1), 449–455 (2020). https://doi.org/10.13005/bpj/1905
13. S. Guendel et al.: Multi-task learning for chest X-ray abnormality classification on noisy labels, pp. 1–10 (2019), [Online]. Available: http://arxiv.org/abs/1905.06362
14. Resque, P., Barros, A., Rosario, D., Cerqueira, E.: An investigation of different machine learning approaches for epileptic seizure detection. 15th Int. Wirel. Commun. Mob. Comput. Conf. IWCMC **2019**, 301–306 (2019). https://doi.org/10.1109/IWCMC.2019.8766652
15. Almubark, I., Chang, L.C., Nguyen, T., Turner, R.S., Jiang, X.: Early detection of alzheimer's disease using patient neuropsychological and cognitive data and machine learning techniques. Proc.–2019 IEEE Int. Conf. Big Data, Big Data 2019. **2**(Mci), 5971–5973 (2019), https://doi.org/10.1109/bigdata47090.2019.9006583
16. Rahane, W., Dalvi, H., Magar, Y., Kalane, A., Jondhale, S.: Lung cancer detection using image processing and machine learning healthcare. Proc. 2018 Int. Conf. Curr. Trends Towar. Converging Technol. ICCTCT 2018, pp. 1–5 (2018). https://doi.org/10.1109/icctct.2018.8551008
17. Ganiger, S., Rajashekharaiah, K.M.M.: Chronic diseases diagnosis using machine learning. 2018 Int. Conf. Circuits Syst. Digit. Enterp. Technol. ICCSDET 2018. pp. 1–6 (2018). https://doi.org/10.1109/iccsdet.2018.8821235
18. Thirunavukkarasu, K., Singh, A.S., Irfan, M., Chowdhury, A.: Prediction of liver disease using classification algorithms. 2018 4th Int. Conf. Comput. Commun. Autom. ICCCA 2018. **6**(9), 1–3 (2018). https://doi.org/10.1109/ccaa.2018.8777655
19. Faisal, M.I., Bashir, S., Khan, Z.S., Hassan Khan, F.: An evaluation of machine learning classifiers and ensembles for early stage prediction of lung cancer. 2018 3rd Int. Conf. Emerg. Trends Eng. Sci. Technol. ICEEST 2018. pp. 1–4 (2019). https://doi.org/10.1109/iceest.2018.8643311
20. Al-Turaiki, I., Alshahrani, M., Almutairi, T.: Building predictive models for MERS-CoV infections using data mining techniques. J. Infect. Public Health **9**(6), 744–748 (2016). https://doi.org/10.1016/j.jiph.2016.09.007
21. Dey, A.: Machine learning algorithms: a review. Int. J. Comput. Sci. Inf. Technol. **7**(3), 1174–1179 (2016). [Online]. Available: www.ijcsit.com
22. Libbrecht, M.W., Noble, W.S.: Machine learning applications in genetics and genomics. Nat. Rev. Genet. **16**(6), 321–332 (2015). https://doi.org/10.1038/nrg3920
23. Ren, J., et al.: Identifying viruses from metagenomic data using deep learning. Quant. Biol. **8**(1), 64–77 (2020). https://doi.org/10.1007/s40484-019-0187-4
24. Tang, Z. et al.: Severity assessment of coronavirus disease 2019 (COVID-19) using quantitative features from chest CT images. **2019**, pp. 1–18 (2020). [Online]. Available: http://arxiv.org/abs/2003.11988
25. Verma, G., Jha, A., Rebholz-Schuhmann, D., Madden, M.G.: Using machine learning to distinguish infected from non-infected subjects at an early stage based on viral inoculation. Lect. Notes Comput. Sci. (including Subser. Lect. Notes Artif. Intell. Lect. Notes Bioinformatics). **11371 LNBI**(November), 105–121 (2019). https://doi.org/10.1007/978-3-030-06016-9_11

26. Stephen, O., Sain, M., Maduh, U.J., Jeong, D.U.: An efficient deep learning approach to pneumonia classification in healthcare. J. Healthc. Eng. **2019**, (2019). https://doi.org/10.1155/2019/4180949
27. Dahiwade, D, Patle, G., Meshram, E.: Designing disease prediction model using machine learning approach. Proc. 3rd Int. Conf. Comput. Methodol. Commun. ICCMC 2019. Iccmc, 1211–1215 (2019). https://doi.org/10.1109/iccmc.2019.8819782
28. Yahyaoui, A., Jamil, A., Rasheed, J., Yesiltepe, M.: A decision support system for diabetes prediction using machine learning and deep learning techniques. 1st Int. Informatics Softw. Eng. Conf. Innov. Technol. Digit. Transform. IISEC 2019—Proc. 2, 1–4 (2019). https://doi.org/10.1109/ubmyk48245.2019.8965556
29. https://www.kaggle.com/paultimothymooney/coronavirus-genome-sequence
30. Human lung cancer genomes, http://biogps.org/dataset/tag/lung%20cancer/
31. Total death and confirmed cases-COVID-19, Github, https://github.com/datasets/covid-19/tree/master/data
32. Dataset-Primary Tumor, https://datahub.io/machine-learning/primary-tumor
33. Scikit-learn.org
34. Xu, S., Wu, H., Bie, R.: CXNet-m1: anomaly detection on chest X-Rays with image-based deep learning. In: IEEE Access, vol. 7, pp. 4466–4477 (2019). https://doi.org/10.1109/ACCESS.2018.2885997

Diagnosing COVID-19 Lung Inflammation Using Machine Learning Algorithms: A Comparative Study

Abbas M. Ali, Kayhan Zrar Ghafoor, Halgurd S. Maghdid, and Aos Mulahuwaish

Abstract In this paper, we performed a comparative analysis using machine learning algorithms named support vector machine (SVM), decision tree (DT), k-nearest neighbor (kNN), and convolution neural network (CNN) to classify pneumonia level (mild, progressive, and severe stage) of the COVID-19 confirmed patients. More precisely, the proposed model consists of two phases: first, the model computes the volume and density of lesions and opacities of the CT images using morphological approaches. In the second phase, we use machine learning algorithms to classify the pneumonia level of the confirmed COVID-19 patient. Extensive experiments have been carried out and the results show the accuracy of 91.304%, 91.4%, 87.5%, 95.622% for kNN, SVM, DT, and CNN, respectively.

Keywords Pneumonia · COVID-19 · Machine learning algorithms · Level of COVID-19 severity

---

A. M. Ali (✉) · K. Z. Ghafoor
Department of Software Engineering, Salahaddin University-Erbil, Erbil, Iraq
e-mail: abbas.mohamad@su.edu.krd

K. Z. Ghafoor
e-mail: kayhan@ieee.org

K. Z. Ghafoor
School of Mathematics and Computer Science, University of Wolverhampton, Wulfruna Street, Wolverhampton WV1 1LY, UK

H. S. Maghdid
Department of Software Engineering, Faculty of Engineering, Koya University, Koysinjaq, Kurdistan Region, Iraq
e-mail: Halgurd.Maghdid@koyauniversity.org

A. Mulahuwaish
Department of Computer Science and Information Systems Saginaw, Valley State University, 7400 Bay Rd, Science East 174 University Center, Itta Bena, MI 48710, United States
e-mail: amulahuw@svsu.edu

© The Editor(s) (if applicable) and The Author(s), under exclusive license to Springer Nature Singapore Pte Ltd. 2020

C. Chakraborty et al. (eds.), *Internet of Medical Things for Smart Healthcare*, Studies in Big Data 80, https://doi.org/10.1007/978-981-15-8097-0_4

1 Related Work

In this section, we review the existing methods that are used for the diagnosis of novel COVID-19. There are many methods that are utilized to distinguish viral pneumonia in dubious cases.

Today, the coronaviruses is impacting over hundreds of countries around the globe. The first confirmed coronavirus case is found in Wuhan city, Huanan Seafood, which is large comprehensive market, includes frozen seafood. In December 30, 2019, Wuhan health commission issued a notice on the continues occurrence of pneumonia cases due to COVID-19 at Huanan Seafood Market. This notice received public attention about the epidemic. On January 26, 2020, the institute of virology of China announced that 33 out of 585 cases were found to contain novel the coronavirus nucleic acid. Thus, health officials concluded that Huanan Seafood Market being the suspected source of the epidemic [1, 2].

The fast transmission of COVID-19 and the increase in demand for diagnosis has encouraged researchers to evolve more intelligent, highly sensitive, and effective diagnostic methods to help stem the spread of coronavirus disease 19. The diagnosis method which is managed by the radiologists is the manual measure of the lung infection quantity. Furthermore, AI-based automated pneumonia diagnosis is used to distinguish the density, size, and opacities of the lesions in COVID-19 confirmed cases. These algorithms are capable to analyze CT scan images outcome in a little while comparing to other available ways [2].

Because of the new existence of COVID-19, there is a scarcity of existing literature in this field. In an effort, the researchers used deep learning based on an AI engine to identify COVID-19 by using high resolution CT images [2]. However, their suggested model exclusively depends on CT images. In reliance on the latest research [3], the detection of COVID-19 is more credible when multiple methods are used together. In another attempt, a smart reading system for CT image, developed by Ping An Insurance Company of China Ltd [4, 5] which can read and examine in a short period of time.

There was an important arguement in [2], related to the importance of CT scan images in the detection of COVID-19 cases, which can be deemed a lot faster way in comparison with the traditional method utilizing the nucleic acid detection. Besides its effectiveness in diagnosing the disease, it can assess the severity level of pneumonia [6, 9]. With all 140 laboratory-confirmed COVID-19 cases, CT results were reported positive. Moreover, CT scan was capable to identify these positive cases even within their early stage, which shows its effectiveness in detecting symptoms of pneumonia level [7, 8]. Thus, developing a diagnosis tool of COVID-19, lung inflammation level is a pressing need in order to detect the severity stage of the pneumonia.

In this chapter, we performed a comparative analysis using machine learning algorithms named support vector machine (SVM), decision tree (DT), k-nearest neighbor (kNN), and convolution neural network (CNN) to classify pneumonia level (mild, progressive, and severe stage) of the COVID-19 confirmed patients. More precisely, the proposed model consists of two phases: first, the model computes the volume and density of lesions and opacities of the CT images using morphological approaches. In the second phase, we use machine learning algorithms to classify the pneumonia level of the confirmed COVID-19 patient. Extensive experiments have been carried out and the results show the accuracy of 91.304%, 91.4%, 87.5%, 95.622% for kNN, SVM, DT, and CNN, respectively.

2 The Proposed Approach

The proposed approach comprises three main parts; in first part, the weight for CT images has been computed for confirmed COVID-19 patient utilizing morphological methodology, and the second subsequent technique classifies the pneumonia level of the confirmed COVID-19 patient and internal representation for the CT images. To accomplish the exact classification of lung inflammation, a modified CNN has been utilized and some other traditional classifications. The following sections are showing the three phases.

2.1 Preprocessing of CT Images

This phase related to pre-handling and clustering of the salient features for the phases of COVID-19 infection virus CT image to be determined and feed to the CNN and other traditional machine learning algorithms. This procedure was to fragment the lesions in the lung using segmentation process, and afterward to improve the image concentration on this area. Then, extracting significant features for the lungs containing lesion areas. These features simply were joining together to improve the feature depiction of the tainted lung. The proposed algorithm steps for extracting important features vectors for the images are outlined in Fig. 2. The procedure will apply for the all images that expected to train the framework on the COVID-19 cases. This is to recognize different cases, which depends on the trained images. Preprocessing of the images is significant and makes the morphological operation to remember many features for CT scan images as early, progressive and sever together with noncovid case. This process depends on weight pixels looked in the two sides of lung. Figure 1 shows the training machine learning algorithms on the CT images COVID-19 stages

The greater parts of morphological operations have done to make the sores places in the lungs to be clearer; this will impact on the abstraction of the feature vectors. The implementation of morphological procedure on the original images and the outcome it will adjust the lesion areas produced by COVID-19 to be white pixels inside a black lung quarters, this let determining of the affected areas by the virus infection become extremely basic. Figure 3 illustrates the resulted image after applying the steps which are mentioned in Fig. 2. The two calculations HOG and EOH are extracted the

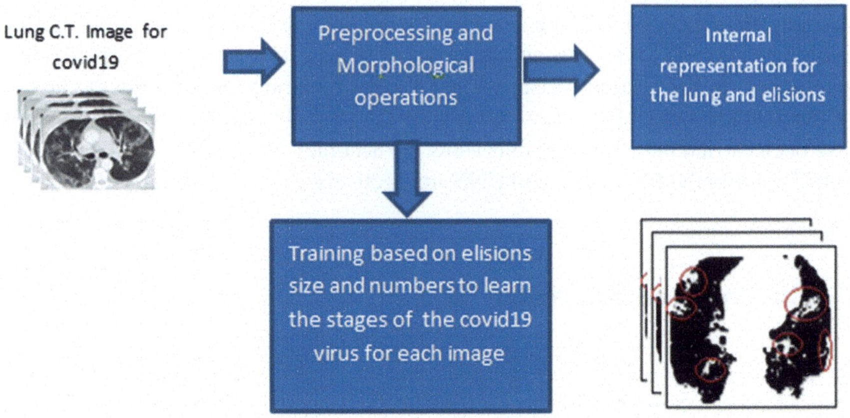

Fig. 1 Training machine on COVID-19 patient and internal representation

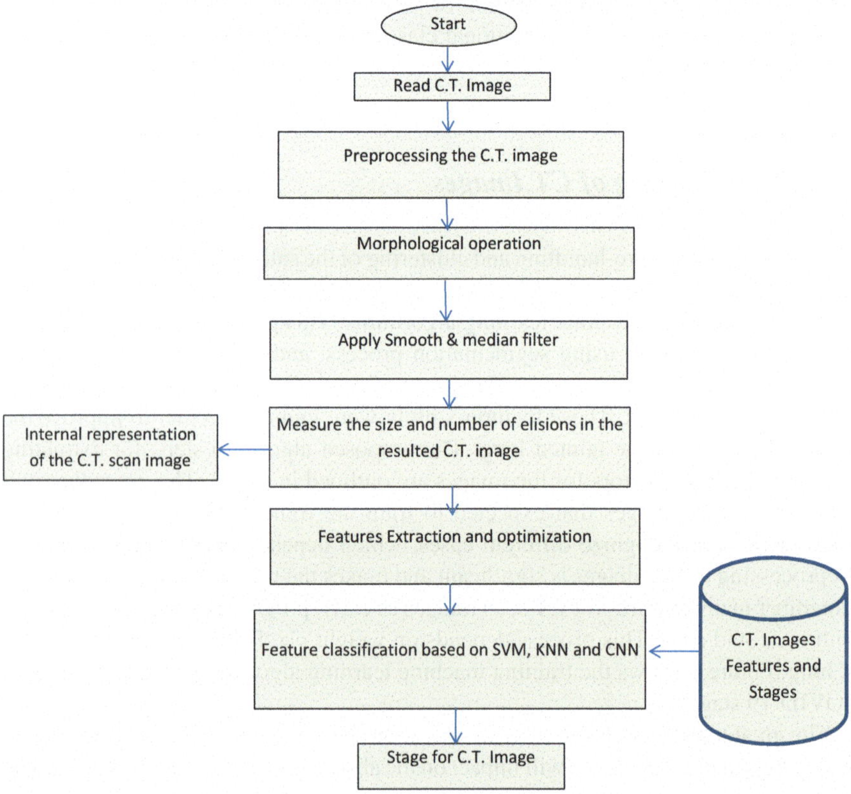

Fig. 2 CT scan image classification

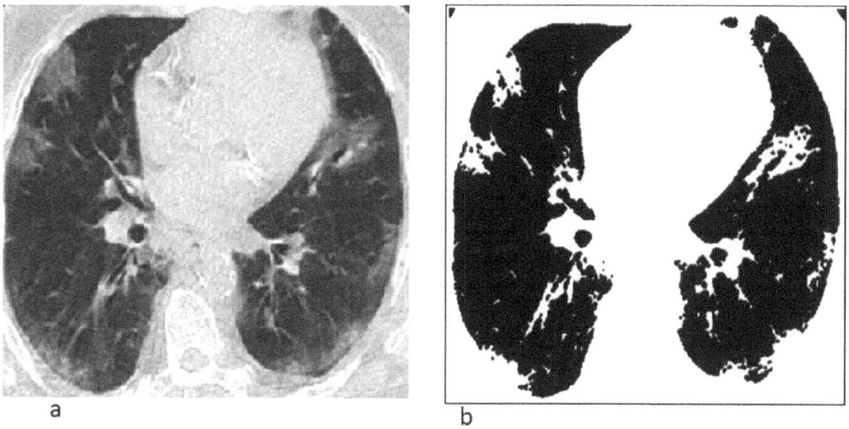

Fig. 3 CT scan images after morphological operation a: before processing, b: after processing

important features to be taken care of to the CNN and other learning algorithms. The portion of the elisions inside the different sides of lung will be relative to the phases of the COVID-19 infection inside the patient body. For instance, the lung image containing small areas in size, a number will point to beginning stage of the virus. While the large lesion areas inside the lung show to sever stage for the patient.

(a) Histogram of Gradient (HOG) [10]

The CT scan images are partitioning into windows of images (cells), these windows state to small windows or districts (cells) spatially related, the histograms for every region will produce a local histogram of these segment gradient directions which will be gathered together. The combined histograms of these districts independently will shape the entire image representation. The normalization for these neighborhood histograms could be built up or applying some valuation on these local histograms to separate the local reactions for the CT images considered.

This leads to more prominent spatial district that can be abused for standardized significant descriptors like histogram of oriented gradient. The procedure has been utilized by [1, 2]. The promising results and acknowledgment of these descriptors drove the authors to utilize it in such analyzing of these kinds of images and joining it naively with EOH includes after some morphological tasks to extract more powerful descriptor for elisions areas inside the lung. Figure 4 shows the distribution of features creation for the image. The CT image will be partitioned into cells inside small zones and these zones are associated with one another. Every cell containing pixels throwing channel direction dependent on came about estimation of slope calculation. From 0 to 180 degrees, the channels of the histogram are spreading similarly. At that point, the assortment of these histograms of gradient directions produces the image's features vector.

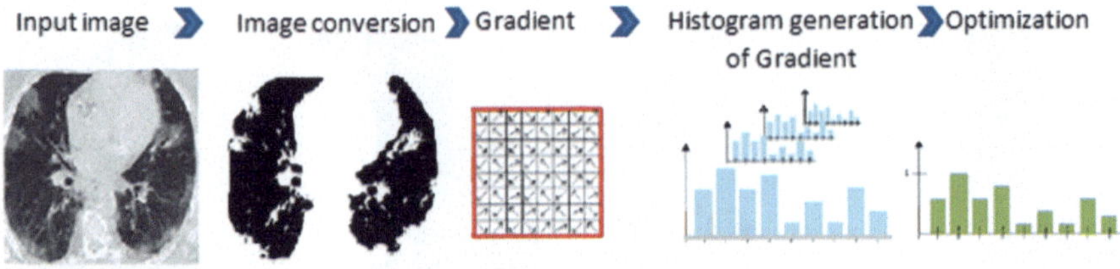

Fig. 4 HOG descriptor

(b) Edge of Histogram (EOH) for the CT images

The orders of edges inside the CT scan images provide a significant features where it can show some additional elisions inside the lung and this originating from local direction of edges inside CT image which can consider it as descriptors. Edge direction histograms (EOH) is utilized in this work to promote features for representing the sides of the lung. The histograms are assembled by starting with ascertaining the direction of the edges inside the image. This will be achieved by filtering process for the edge in the image. This filtering utilizes two kernels: [− 1 0 1] and [− 1 0 1] to get filtered CT images is coordinated by d*x* and d*y* individually. Two parameters will be thought of, the magnitude (*M*) and the direction α and for the edge's pixels inside the image. These are registered by Eqs. 1 and 2 separately.

$$\alpha = \arctan(\mathrm{d}y/\mathrm{d}x) \tag{1}$$

$$M = \mathrm{SQRT}\left(d_x^2 + d_y^2\right) \tag{2}$$

The bins identified with edge direction inside the histogram are equally scattered through orientation of the edge. The quantity of histogram bins relies upon the edge magnitude; at that point, the computation of the histogram will be identified with the weighted vote [3]. Figure 5 illustrates the effect of implementing edge detection on the lung images for the normal and COVID-19 virus infection.

Naively combining HOG and EOH features learning for visual elision recognition is building more distinct features for the lung as stated in Eq. 3:

$$(x, f1 : nm) = Hg(1 : n), Eh(1 : m) \tag{3}$$

where *x* is the CT image handled morphologically, Hg is the features for histogram of oriented gradient, and *Eh* is the features for edge histogram.

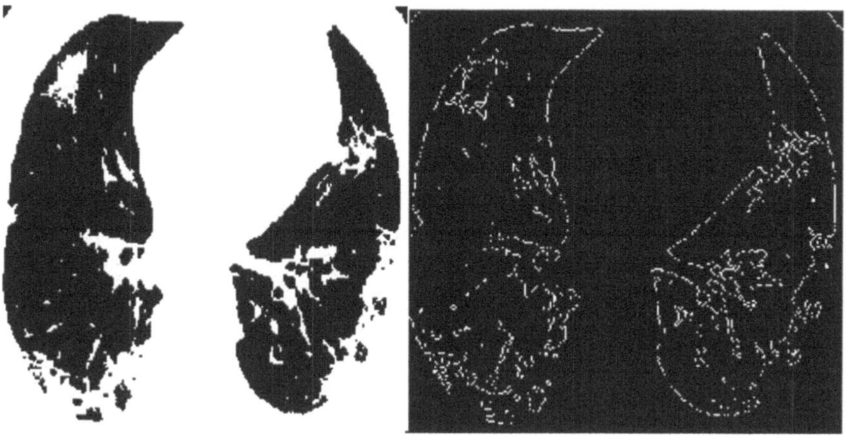

Fig. 5 Edge descriptions for CT scan image

3 Classification of COVID-19 Pneumonia Level

This phase is to classify the CT images based on the features extracted from the CT image, in this work, the classification for these features has done based on CNN, KNN, SVM, and decision tree. The following sections some explaining for these algorithms which are used:

(a) **Convolutional Neural Network (CNN)**

The second phase of the proposed work is that the constructed element vectors (NV) which are computed are rearranged to a square grid then entered to the CNN for training based on these kinds of feature vectors. For CNN testing, the CT test image will be handled as same procedure in Fig. 2, the achieved features from morphological stage rearranged to be entered into the CNN. In the training phase, 15 layers CNN from scratch have been utilized. These layers involve, 1 layer used for input, 3 layers used as convolution filtered by 3×3 size, 2 layers used for max pooling, 3 layers used for bunch standardization, 3 layers used for rectified linear unit, and 3 layers used for (completely associated, softmax, and classification). Coming up next are some descriptions of the layers:

1. **Input layer**: Pass features for CT images after resizing them to feed it into the next layers [11]
2. **Convolution layers**: These are known as filter values. In each layer, convolutions and kernels are there in addition to a stable stride is running on the CT complete image. Here, the features inside the images will be recognized and passed to the pooling layer [12]. The convolution operation is expressed in Eq. (4):

$$y^j = \max\left(0, b^j + \sum_i k^{ij} * x^i\right) \tag{4}$$

k^{ij} is the kernel for convolution between ith output of map and input x map, while the * sign points to convolution operation.

3. **Max Pooling Layer**: In this layer, the big sized CT images are shrinking down with keeping most important information in them. In each window, greatest value will be reserved; finally, the finest fits will be reserved of each element in the window [12]. The maximum pooling process is outlined in Eq. (5) [5].

$$\underset{yj,k}{i} = \max_{0 \le m,n \le r}\left(x^i_{jxr+m,kxr+n}\right) \tag{5}$$

4. **Rectified Linear Units Layers (ReLU)**: The result of negative numbers from the pooling layer will be noticed as zeros. This layer provides the CNN steady mathematically [12]. It is expressed by Eq. (6) underneath:

$$F(x) = \max(0, x) \tag{6}$$

5. **Batch normalization layer**: The setting of this layer can be placed in the model, for example, fully connected layer. It applies the results from the previous layer as input feed-forwarding to calculate gradients with respect to the parameters.
6. **Softmax layer**: It is a function to provide the property of deep learning to give an answer for classification issue. This layer identifies the discrete likelihood P allocation for K classes. This can be demonstrated by $\sum_{k=1}^{k} pk$. Assume x is the activation, and θ indicate to weight parameters at the softmax layer, at that point, o is considered as input to the softmax layer,

$$F(x) = \sum_i^{n-1} \theta i x i \tag{7}$$

Then,

$$pk = \frac{\exp(o_k)}{\sum_{k=0}^{n=1} \exp(o_k)} \tag{8}$$

Thus, the calculation of the class would be $\hat{y}$

$$\hat{y} = \underset{i \in 1 \ldots N}{\arg\max} \quad pi \tag{9}$$

4 Traditional Classification Methods

In this section, some traditional classifications which have been used in this work to check the performance accuracy for recognizing the COVID-19 stages from the CT images

(a) **K-Nearest Neighbors Classifier (kNN)**

It is simple and common method to categorize the natural scene objects whose supervised learning algorithm. The process is built on one notion that the similarity between observations and groups which are relating to each other [13]. The algorithm has two phases in its working, which are training and testing. The process of training phase is building the training dataset by means of a set of cases holding training pattern with its related class.

In the process of testing phase, the query begins with a given unlabeled point and the algorithm generates a set of k closest or nearest (results) scores corresponding to the trained input patterns. The similarity results of two feature vectors are estimated by using distance measure such as Euclidian or Manhattan. Finally, the classification or decision is established by tagging the class of a tested pattern based on the majority voting method.

(b) **Support Vector Machine (SVM)**

One of the supervised learning algorithms for classification is the support vector machine which was introduced by AT&T Bell Laboratories members Vapnik and others [14]. Since an excellent performance results with the researchers today's SVM is used widely with the efficient way in implementation of classification problems.

The binary SVM classification was extended to take multi-class problems. SVM finds the optimal separating hyper-plane and separates the classes negative (-1) from the positive (+1) ones. The classification is done by maximizing the biggest margin between the classes. The main idea is shown in Fig. 6. The optimal hyper-plane separation is in the middle of the margin.

(c) **Decision tree classification (DT)**

A decision tree is a device for classification support that utilizes a tree-like model of results and their possible values, comprising chance event results, resource costs, and utility. It is one way to show an algorithm that only covers conditional control statements.

Decision trees are widely used in operations research and machine learning, especially in decision analysis, to help reaching the goal. It helps determine expected, best, and worst values for unlike scenarios.

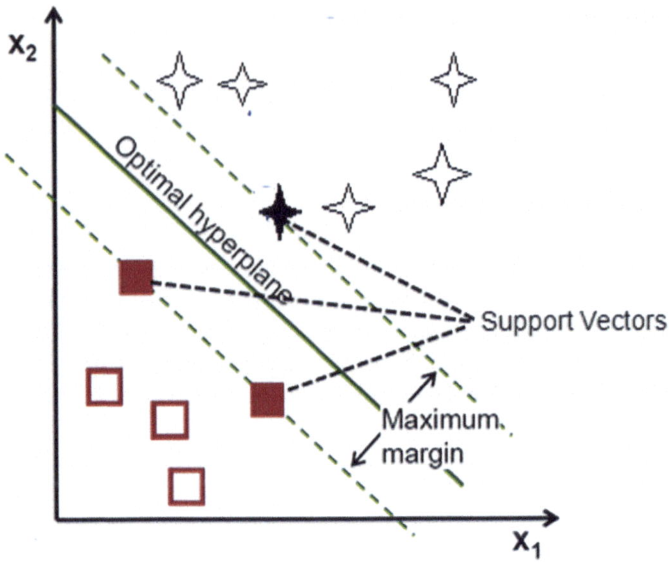

Fig. 6 SVM classification

5 Infected Lung Severity Level

Since Coronavirus Disease 2019 (COVID-19) quickly spread worldwide specially in early 2020, causing the researchers of the world to think of detection and representation of lung infections from CT images in many different ways. Since a huge of CT images transferred and stored for the COVID-19 stages; which in turn leads to consuming more time for processing like transmitting the image and more space needing to store in memory. Furthermore, CT image faces some challenges, containing high disparity in infection appearances, and low contrast intensities between infection areas and normal tissues in the lung.

The authors proposed an internal representation for the segmented image using morphological operations. The CT scan image for lung segmented into two parts the first part boundary is that containing holes and the second part without holes. Figure 7 shows the two parts in two colors red and green.

It is clear that the green region of the CT image is boundary which containing holes.

Representing these features as a text instead of image is better to store. Thus, representing the CT image is aggregating of partial representations of the regions features and generates a global representation for the whole CT lung. This gives an implicit representation for the explicit illusion-attention is exploited to shape the boundaries and enhance the representations. The function can be expressed in

$$\mathrm{IR} = \mathrm{bwboundaries(holes)} + \mathrm{bwboundaries(no\,holes)} \tag{10}$$

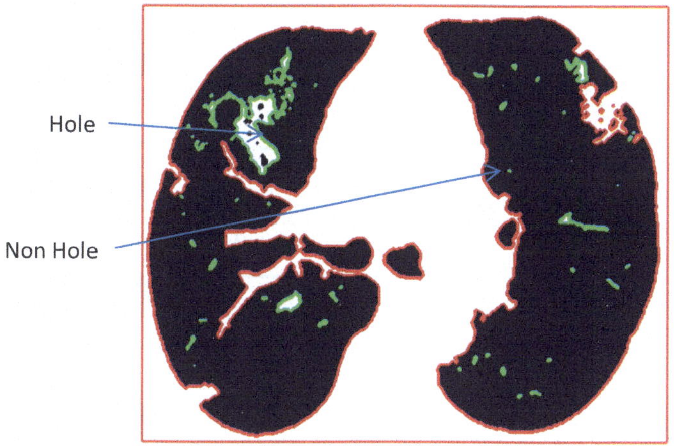

Fig. 7 Two parts boundaries

6 Experimental Setup

The feature vectors are developed naively to be 89 features (81 HOG and 8 EOH). In this work, the practical experimental has been conducted in two ways. CT scan images dataset has been used that is accessible in a GitHub store [15]. It was built by a group in [15] on a number of confirmed COVID-19 patients. The COVID-19 dataset contains 186 CT scan images of pneumonia lungs. Specifically, the images are clearly show the variety of lung inflammation over the span of COVID-19 patient between 1–21 days. The scanned images size is 346 × 442 × 3 uint8. Obviously, we currently do not have a lot of COVID-19 images openly accessible to the research community to lead extreme investigation and there is a need to gather more radiology images which can be available by the research community.

COVID-19 severity classification, the experiment has done based on some traditional machine learning algorithms like k-nearest neighbor (KNN), SVM, and decision tree. The results of the experiment are done by testing arbitrary CT images. These images are not trained by the chosen algorithms. In Fig. 8, the result distances of tested CT scan image's feature vectors based on Euclidean's distance with the other CT image's feature vectors. These distances sorted in ascending order, from small to large value, the smallest distance value is more similar to the tested CT image. The results of testing the query image and based on the KNN algorithm implemented on the dataset. The precision (p) of the N retrieved CT images for the query (Q) CT image is expressed in Eq. 10

$$p(Q, N) = \frac{|Ir|\text{Rank}(Q, Ir) \leq N \text{ such that Ir} \in g\,(Q)\}||}{N} \tag{11}$$

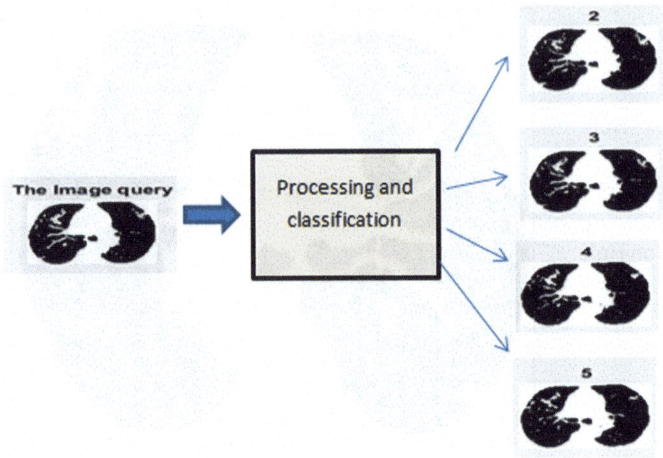

Fig. 8 Distances between query image and CT images answer

Table 1 COVID-19 confirmed patient pneumonia stage accuracy diagnosing

Classification	Results
kNN	91.304
SVM	91.3
DT	87.5
CNN	95.622

where $g(Q)$ denotes to the virus's group stage for the query image and Ir is the retrieved CT image. The results for all constructed distance feature values are arranged in ascending order; at that point, the best matching virus stage is the minimum value.

The results of performance accuracy based on Weka software results implemented to all algorithms listed in Table 1.

BSTI dataset comprises CT images is isolated into two categories to check the proposed strategy. For this reason, a multilayer perceptron's Weka implemented deep learning Rj has been utilized for checking the accuracy of the proposed procedure. Table 1 shows the consequence of the accuracy performance to find the virus stages. Further, Fig. 9 shows the proposed method result of the perceived stages of the question image fed into the program. The number over the CT image demonstrates to zone size of the elision inside both sides lung.

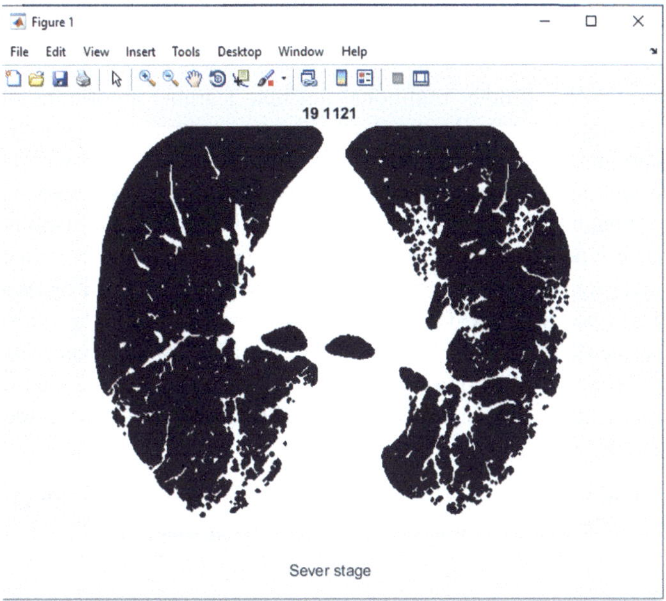

Fig. 9 Patient's stage of COVID-19 recognition

7 Results and Discussion

In this work, the accuracy performance of pneumonia stage detection during a course of confirmed COVID-19 patient has been computed. For this purpose and to attain this goal, morphological operations and deep learning with traditional learning algorithms are applied on the extracted feature vectors by using HOG and EOH. GitHub dataset repository is exploited to extract feature vectors. GitHub COVID-19 dataset includes a set of CT scan images for confirmed COVID-19 patients, whereby the whole images containing two sides lungs for the patients, the dataset consists of several stages (early stage, progressive, and sever) collected from different patients. The dataset composed of 186 CT images of size 372 × 556 × 3 uint8. Morphological operations are applied to convert the dataset to logical images. In this operation, noises within the images are filtered out to make the lesions and opacities on the infected lungs appear more clearly. The feature vector is constructed from HOG and EOH to get higher invariant features for classification. When CNN is used to the severity stage of the lung infection, we obtained the accuracy of 95.6%. Furthermore, the results for KNN and SVM were 91.3, while DT was 87.5 when CNN applied on HOG features without EOH, we achieved 82.608%, which is lower accuracy while EOH achieved less than the others, which is 34.782%. Table 1 presents the detection accuracy of different features used for classification. The results assure the improvement of detection accuracy through changing the features and classification methods. As shown in Table 1, CNN outperforms the other classification algorithms using HOG with EOH.

8 Conclusion

In this paper, CNN and other traditional machine learning algorithms like KNN, SVM, and DT have been used to recognize the stage of pneumonia in the lung by using CT scan images. This work is adopted to improve the accuracy of diagnosing lung in inflammation severity in confirmed COVID-19 patient. We build a complete pre-processed dataset of CT scan images which are taken from GitHub repository. After extensive experiments, the results show that the proposed CNN with combined HOG and EOH significantly outperforms the other approaches. Furthermore, when morphological operation based on EOH is used, the result is not promising. This indicates that multi-scale features for medical image recognition are better than a single scale features. The morphological operation is more useful to filter out noises and unnecessary features in the classification, which results in high accuracy of lung in inflammation detection.

Submission Guidelines: Prospective contributors are invited to submit chapter proposal to *cchakrabarty@bitmesra.ac.in* with the subject "IoMTSH-2020"

References

1. Huang, C., Wang, Y., Li, X., Ren, L., Zhao, J., Hu, Y., Zhang, L., Fan, G., Xu, J., Gu, X., et al.: Clinical features of patients infected with 2019 novel coronavirus in wuhan, china. The Lancet **395**(10223), 497–506 (2020)
2. Chen, J., Wu, L., Zhang, J., Zhang, L., Gong, D., Zhao, Y., Hu, S., Wang, Y., Hu, X., Zheng, B. et al.: Deep learning-based model for detecting 2019 novel coronavirus pneumonia on high-resolution computed tomography: a prospective study, medRxiv, 2020
3. Cnn health, https://edition.cnn.com/2020/03/11/health/coronaviruspandemic-world-health-organization/index.html, Accessed in March, 2020
4. Maghdid, H. S., Ghafoor, K.Z.: A smartphone enabled approach to manage COVID-19 lockdown and economic crisis. arXiv.org. arXiv:2004.12240
5. Wang, D., Hu, B., Hu, C., Zhu, F., Liu, X., Zhang, J., Wang, B., Xiang, H., Cheng, Z., Xiong, Y. et al.: â€œClinical characteristics of 138 hospitalized patients with 2019 novel coronavirusâ€“infected pneumonia in wuhan
6. Zu, Z.Y., Jiang, M.D., Xu, P.P., Chen, W., Ni, Q.Q., Lu, G.M., Zhang, L.J.: Coronavirus disease 2019 (covid-19): a perspective from China, Radiology, p. 200490, 2020
7. Huang, C., Wang, Y., Li, X., Ren, L., Zhao, J., Hu, Y., Zhang, L., Fan, G., Xu, J., Gu, X. et al.: Clinical features of patients infected with 2019 novel coronavirus in wuhan, China. The Lancet. **395**(10223), 497–506 (2020)
8. Chen, N., Zhou, M., Dong, X., Qu, J., Gong, F., Han, Y., Qiu, Y., Wang, J., Liu, Y., Wei, Y. et al.: Epidemiological and clinical characteristics of 99 cases of 2019 novel coronavirus pneumonia in wuhan, China: a descriptive study. The Lancet. **395**(10223), 507–513 (2020)
9. Shan, F., Gao, Y., Wang, J., Shi, W., Shi, N., Han, M., Xue, Z., Shen, D., Shi, Y.: Lung infection quantification of covid-19 in ct images with deep learning, arXiv preprint arXiv:2003.04655, 2020
10. Jiang, Y.-G., Ngo, C.-W., Yang, J.: Towards optimal bag-of-features for object categorization and semantic video retrieval. In Proceedings of the 6th ACM international conference on image and video retrieval, 2007, pp. 494–501

11. Sharma, N., Jain, V., Mishra, A., An analysis of convolutional neural networks for image classification. Proc. Comput. Sci. *132*, 377–384 (2018)
12. Chen, Z., Jacobson, A., Â hauf, N.S., Liu, B.L., Shen, C., Reid, I., Milford, M.: Deep learning features at scale for visual place recognition. In 2017 IEEE international conference on robotics and automation (ICRA). IEEE, 2017, pp. 3223–3230
13. Bin Abdullah, A.: Supervised learning algorithms for visual object categorization. Universiteit Utrecht, 2010
14. Cortes, C., Vapnik, V.: Support-vector networks. Mach. Learn. **20**, 273–297 (1995)
15. Cohen, J.P., Morrison, P., Dao, L.: Image data collection, arXiv 2003.11597, vol. 6 (2020)

Abbas M. Ali is currently working as associate professor at the department of software engineering, Salahaddin university-Erbil. He received PhD degree from National University of Malaysia in 2013.

Kayhan Zrar Ghafoor [S'10, M'15, SM'19] is currently working as an associate professor at the Salahaddin University-Erbil and visiting scholar at the University of Wolverhampton. Before that, he was a postdoctoral research fellow at Shanghai Jiao Tong University, where he contributed to two research projects funded by National Natural Science Foundation of China and National Key Research and Development Program. He is also served as a visiting researcher at University Technology Malaysia. He received the B.Sc. degree in electrical engineering, the M.Sc. degree in remote weather monitoring and the Ph.D. degree in wireless networks in 2003, 2006, and 2011, respectively. He is the author of 2 technical books, 7 book chapters, 65 technical papers indexed in ISI/ Scopus. He is the recipient of the UTM Chancellor Award at the 48th UTM convocation in 2012.

Factors Affecting the Success of Internet of Things for Enhancing Quality and Efficiency Implementation in Hospitals Sector in Jordan During the Crises of Covid-19

Malik Mustafa and Sharf Alzubi

Abstract The rapid growth of Internet of things (IoT) has vigorously affected healthcare applications over the last decade particularly in the health information technology sector. This is done through improving healthcare delivery by increasing efficiency, reducing cost and time involved. However, the applicability of DeLone and McLean IS success model achievement model for health welfare implementation in IoT remains unknown. Thus, this research amid to establish the significance of IS application and its associations with user intention, client fulfilment and net advantages of IoT in five hospitals in a developing country such as Jordan. Furthermore, this research emphasized on the technological and infrastructural facilities factors that are considered imperative in improving the social healthcare procedures of resident's health care. Hope that this discovery would convince the administration of hospitals to focus on important viewpoints that impact the utilization of Internet of things (IoT) in healthcare services. The fundamental of this research is to determine the variables that impact the achievement of Internet of things (IoT) in the execution of human services from the viewpoint of medical clinic residents in Jordan. The fundamental point of the current paper was to examine the features that impact the achievement of Internet of things (IoT) in the implementation of health care from the perspective of hospitals in Jordan. An aggregate of 700 questionnaires will be circulated to five (5) hospitals in various regions in Jordan, out of which 417 questionnaire surveys returned, representing a response rate of between 50 and 60 per cent. This study presented elements of technological and infrastructural features of technological and infrastructural factors in the DeLone and McLean success model data framework and how these variables impacted user intention and citizen satisfaction as parts of medicinal healthcare services in Internet of things (IoT). This research used the PLS-SEM analysis techniques to test fourteen hypotheses. Variables are technological and infrastructural factors, estimation of data, framework quality and

M. Mustafa (✉)
Gulf College, Seeb, Oman
e-mail: malikjawarneh@gmail.com

S. Alzubi
Jordan University of Science and Technologym, Irbid, Jordan
e-mail: sharaf_alzoubi@yahoo.com

© The Editor(s) (if applicable) and The Author(s), under exclusive license to Springer Nature Singapore Pte Ltd. 2020

C. Chakraborty et al. (eds.), *Internet of Medical Things for Smart Healthcare*, Studies in Big Data 80, https://doi.org/10.1007/978-981-15-8097-0_5

nature of administration. The research results supported technological and infrastructural factors, quality of the data and system service quality as significant aspects affecting the successful implementation of the Internet of things (IoT) for health care in Jordan. The study extended the DeLone and McLean IS success model by implementing variables of technological and infrastructural facilities factors impact that are critical factors in the Arab regions.

Keywords Internet of things · Covid-19 · Health care · Jordan

1 Introduction

According to Worldometer, the population of the world is rising at a rapid pace. As of May 2020, the current total population is 7.8 billion, as explained by the most recent United Nations [1]. The total population will peak at 9.22 billion in 2075, based on a UN report [2]. In contrast, the asset is not boundless, there is a sure deficiency of the absolute most significant common assets overall. For example, new water, non-renewable energy sources, petroleum gas and precious metal. What is more, the irregular circulation of the population is exacerbated by more than 50% of the total population packs in urban communities and urban centres. The distinction in volume of the populations is a thousand-overlay. There are subsequently megacities with a population of more than 10 million such as Tokyo, Shanghai and New York [3]. Without a doubt, there are various issues related to metropolitan territories. For example, overwhelming contamination, clog, wasteful utilization of energy and assets.

In order to adapt to the circumstances, a number of activities were undertaken. Observably, the United Nations has defined the term "Sustainable Development" as a reference model and direction for every single human movement on Earth. As indicated in the report of the United Nations World Commission on Environment and Development 1987 (Brundtland Report), economic growth is characterized as "a step forward that discusses the needs of the present generation without compromising future generations' ability to overcome their own problems down the line" [2]. From the whole point on, a huge amount of ideas and philosophies tried to present the possibility of "sustainable development" or "sustainable development".

2 Research Background

Today, fifty percentage (50%) of the world's citizens live in cities and towns. The pattern is expected to continue, helping to bring urban residents to around 75% of the total population by 2050. [4]. There are a few explanations behind this, including better access to human services, diversion, media transmission and transportation. Notwithstanding, from the city authorities' perspective, urbanization is meeting new expectations and opportunities. City officials are relied upon to face a range of emerging issues, ranging from technical, social, physical to hierarchical, brought by the overcrowded population in a geologically constrained region. Congested driving conditions, environmental contamination (air, water, noise, light and radioactivity), high crime rate, wasteful use of energy and assets, and waste disposal are problems in a major urban area.

The point is to analyse Covid-19 prior and to improve its treatment by applying clinical innovation, the "COVID-19 Intelligent Diagnosis and Treatment Assistant Program (NCAP)" in view of the Internet of things (IoT). Terminal eight (8) capacities can be actualized continuously online correspondence with the "cloud" through the page choice key. As per existing information, surveys and check results, the determination is naturally created as affirmed, suspected or dubious of 2019 novel coronavirus (2019-nCoV) contamination. This arranges patients to mellow, moderate, extreme or basic pneumonia. NCapp can likewise build up an online Covid-19 continuous update database, and it refreshes the model of analysis progressively dependent on the most recent genuine case information to improve symptomatic precision. Moreover, nCapp can manage treatment. Forefront doctors, specialists and directors are connected to perform discussion and anticipation. nCapp additionally adds to the long-haul line up of patients with Covid-19. A definitive objective is into empower various degrees of Covid-19 finding and treatment among various specialists from various medical clinics to move up to the national and worldwide by through the insightful help of the nCapp framework. Along these lines, we can square ailment transmission, keep away from doctor disease and plague anticipation and control as quickly as time permits [5].

As the coronavirus extends its effect from China, growing its catchment into encompassing locales and different nations, expanded national and universal measures are being taken to contain the flare-up. The putting of whole urban communities in "lockdown" straightforwardly influences urban economies on a multi-sidelong level, including from social and monetary points of view. This is being stressed as the episode makes strides in different nations, driving towards a worldwide well-being crisis, and as worldwide joint effort is looked for in various quarters. Be that as it may, while powerful conventions concerning the sharing of well-being information are stressed, urban information, then again, explicitly identifying with urban well-being and safe city ideas, is still seen from a patriot viewpoint as exclusively profiting a country's economy and its monetary and political impact. This point of view paper thought of one month after location and through the flare-up, overviews the infection episode from an urban viewpoint and advances how brilliant city systems have to progress in the direction of improving normalization conventions for expanded information partaking in case of flare-ups or fiascos, prompting better worldwide comprehension and the board of the equivalent [6].

3 Theories and Models of Successful IS Implementation

Currently, a noticeable issue circulating among associations is the significance of putting resources into new data frameworks design and foundation. The requirement for the venture is driven by the need to give predominant items and administrations through powerful flexibly chains.

Therefore, business administrators have started searching for approaches to evaluate their financial-related allocation of IS at three levels: strategic, operative and strategic tactical.

Moreover, administrators are concerned with their capability to appraise IS investments before leveraging their fiscal and emotional capitals [7].

3.1 IS Success Theory

The primary causes to provide a sense of description of the information structure framework have been faced with difficulty due to the complex, dependent and multidimensional nature of the estimates. This issue was addressed during the period 1981–1987, as a result of which the scientific classification of IS was successful [8]. The model structure is introduced in Fig. 1.

3.2 Information Systems (IS) Effectiveness Concept

Seddon [10] revised DeLone and McLean's [8] model framework. Primary differentiation among the two was the grouping and significance of IS utilization. As per Seddon et al. [10], IS use as conduct offers anticipation for net advantages from the utilization of IS. Subsequently, the model of IS use comes from conduct of IS achievement. This new formulation of DeLone and McLean's perspective into other two restricted change models caused difficulties in the evaluation dimension. Indeed, the first idea to explain IS's hypothesis was simplicity.

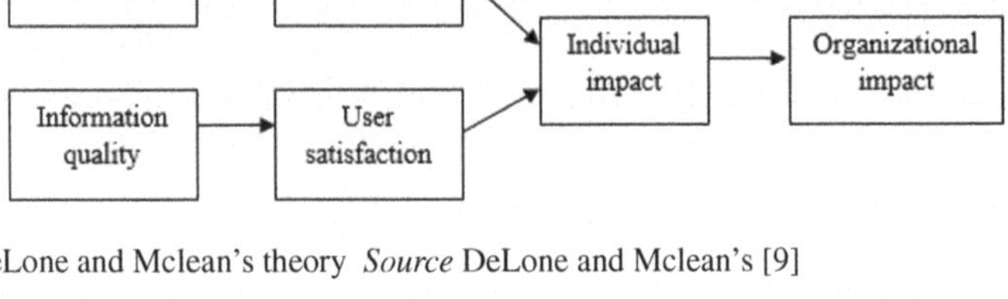

Fig. 1 DeLone and Mclean's theory *Source* DeLone and Mclean's [9]

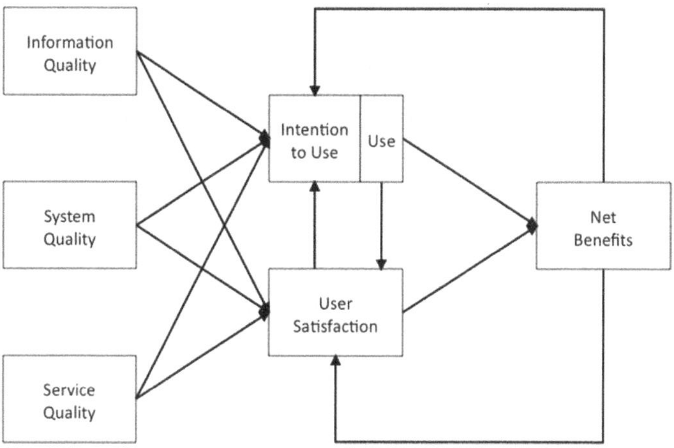

Fig. 2 DeLone and McLean Theory *Source* DeLone and McLean's [11]

3.3 Extended of Information Systems (IS) Success Theory

It is a refinement of DeLone and McLean's original theory [9], which they considered several disparagements and recommendations for enhancement. The improved concept is presented in Fig. 2, in which the arrows depict influences. This new formulation of DeLone and McLean's perspective into other two restricted change models caused difficulties in the evaluation dimension. Indeed, the first idea to explain IS's hypothesis was simplicity, redetermination of the construct connections and expansion of the idea of administration quality.

3.4 Systems Dynamic Theory of Information Systems (IS) Success

Wang and Liu [12] integrated the DeLone and McLean theory with the technology reception framework (proposed by Venkatesh et al. [13]) and proposed a new model that is presented in Fig. 2.6.3. Their effort became known as The framework dynamics model of IS success and includes two steady circles and a single adjusting circle. Figure 2.8 shows the influence diagram with response associations. A response connection refers to a closed-loop circle hover of circumstances and logical effect. In addition, response circles can be considered as relationship-generating and goal-seeking behaviour while behaviour remains core action in which the entire dynamic schemes interact.

Goal maintains the course of conditions within a system. In case of deviation, feedback relationships bring about corrective actions to return the process to its correct direction. Feedback relationships are of two types, namely negative (counteracting) and positive (reinforcing). The former is designated as B, while the latter is designated as R. In case any concept in a negative loop is transformed, the loop drives the readjustment of the construct in the opposite way. The negative loop generates a self-correcting mechanism. Wang and Liu [12] emphasis that the main support, loop R1, which arises from the IS benefits, uses the modification loop that arises from the benefits of IS, will be the dominant element in the model's behaviour.

However, the complexity of this model makes it challenging to test and validate. On top of this, the response loops contribute to the strain of semantic testing. Wang and Liu [12] acknowledged this complexity and noted that they tested the model on the basis of a small response size. They proceeded to recommend a thorough and expansive review of literature to refine their model. They further acknowledged that the lack of practical test and a minimal data set made the constructs difficult to test successfully.

3.5 Sabherwal's Theory

Sabherwal et al. [14] took Rai et al. [15] observations into consideration and developed a theory for IS success. They presented two novel constructs in their theory, which is top administration support and simplifying conditions. The senior executives' positive attitudes are towards IS, whereas the latter reflects processes and resources enabling individuals use of IS. With top management supporting IS, considerable resources may be appropriated for their development and support in improving facilitating conditions [14].

This theory has disadvantages. The primary disadvantage is the fact that it is based on conveyed info obtained after a significant quantity of disparate pragmatic studies. The theory proposes that combining findings on the basis of various constructs and measures throughout different empirical studies is reasonable, which, in fact, may not be appropriate [14]. Another drawback lies in the constructs prior research has validated such as information qualities that were largely ignored. In addition to this, moderating effects were also excluded owing to the incapability of testing [14]. They concluded through contending that the developing structure created from the hypothesis best suits the post-execution circumstances with reverence to data frameworks towards associations.

3.6 Information Systems-Impact Success Theory

According to DeLone and McLean's [9] theory, Gable et al. [16] claimed that an encompassing measure for surveying IS usage includes scopes covering the regressive feature (impacts) and the frontward aspects (quality). According to them, the IS-Impact of Information Systems considers a sum at a point in spell of the net assistance created by information system as perceived by key client user groups as state of the art and expected. They accepted that this model's validity and development were carried out with the help of data from the Australian public sector, and they are unclear as to the citations' completeness and the suitable representation of information system. Besides Gable et al.'s [16] study, the model has been largely untested.

3.7 Information Systems Success Research

This section presented a review of literature that has examined successful implementation of IS, most specifically in relationship to the D&M's model. Prior studies have examined and evaluated the various dimension of IS success and investigated how the dimension affects organizational attributes.

The original work of DeLone and McLean is referred to IS accomplishment literature. Somewhere in the range of 1993 and 2002, their paper was referred to in excess of 285 companion evaluated articles and gathering procedures. The DeLone and McLean's [9] model provides detailed elements of IS achievement factors [17, 18]. Some help of the model is that it offers a setting depending on the orders of the few accomplishment methodology. Also, the model shows that the interrelationships among the achievement intermediaries are not lasting and that the connections are easy going [9]. In the interim, disagreeing sees in regard to DeLone and McLean model exist most particularly as that model identifies with the collaborations inside the model, including relationship among the measurements, and the intermediaries used to speak to the different measurements. The fundamental work of D&M's is habitually cited in IS achievement writing. Somewhere in the range of 1993 and 2002, their paper was referred to in excess of 285 friend looked into articles and meeting procedures. The DeLone and McLean's [9] model gives definite components of IS achievement factors [17, 18]. A few commitments of the model are that it gives a system that is dependent on the arrangements of the different achievement measures. Likewise, the model shows that the interrelationships among the achievement intermediaries are not perpetual and that the connections are easy going [9]. Meanwhile, contradicting view concerning DeLone and McLean is most likely to occur as the model structure contributes to the connections in the model, and crucial relationship between the degrees and intermediaries used to represent measurements system framework.

More than 29 lessons have been thoroughly examined in the relations between the two constructs in the model as well as findings of these studies are consistent. Generally, these studies either use the entire construct in the model or select some of the constructs to suit a specific context. Some researchers are enlarging the framework by adding or removing variables from the model. For example, Pitt, Watson, & Kavan [19] and Wilkin and Hewitt [20] presented the quality of service, a design model from advertising to the model framework. In addition, Van Dyke, Kappelman, & Prybutok [21] and Seddon [18] challenged the inclusion of service value in the model and excluded them from their studies.

3.8 Summary of IS Success Theories

An aggregate of six achievement speculations was given the point of picking one for usage to suit the setting of a developing nation. A synopsis of the examinations between the hypotheses is introduced in Table 2.9. The inference of elements to look at changed speculations of IS achievement was taken from Garity and Sanders (1998) and Petter & McLean [8]. The top measures for choosing a model system to utilize are that clients must be sure about the hypothesis and for this to occur, the hypothesis must be well tested and authorized (Petter and McLean [8].

Another basis for speculations is the domain of utilization in a manner of speaking where the level at which the model structure is used. The solicitation zone alludes to the hypothesis' adaptability of work to the investigation level that the specialist regards to be generally huge. Simplicity makes reference to the opportunity from trouble and is regularly connected with the difficulties that a thought ventures and on the person, who is attempting to get it. Something that is straightforward is basic while that which is difficult to comprehend is unpredictable [22]. Adaptability is characterized as the adjusting capacity (getting appropriate) towards an accurate condition or use [22]. IS can be evaluated by more than three statures [23]. These levels are firm or hierarchical-level proportions of accomplishment, capacity or procedure-level proportions of accomplishment, lastly singular proportions of achievement. At the hierarchical level, IS accomplishment can be surveyed for the most part through systems identifying with basic execution including an expanded piece of the overall industry or productivity, working proficiency, working expenses and profit for value and stock. At the capacity or procedure level, IS can be assessed as far as skilled asset use and the minimization of procedure cycles. At the individual or client level, information systems (IS) can be measured as far as client recognitions concerning viability and fulfilment [23].

Among the six concepts revised, the DeLone and McLean [9] and [24] theories have extensively verified and authorized (i.e. by [8, 12]. The top challenges faced by most developed countries are lack of educated users [25]. Therefore, a concept to be employed in a emerging nation needs to be modest. Simplicity has been attributed to DeLone and McLean's theories [9, 24], Sabherwal et al.'s theory [14] and Gable et al.'s theory [16].

Seddon et al.'s theory [10] is considered to be among the most complex of the theories. The most flexible is the D&M's model (2002), and it is the most suitable to be employed in a developing country. That is because, according to Petter and McLean [8], the spearheading efforts to diagram IS triumph failed from the perplexing, interdependent and multidimensional scene of information system (IS) measurements.

Few researchers have changed the first DeLone and McLean hypothesis to survey applications including information management (e.g. Kulkarni, Ravindran & Freeze [26, 27] and web-based business [28–30]. When some researchers found effects of IS success on workgroups, industries and societies (e.g. [10, 31], DeLone and McLean replaced individual effect and authoritative contact with net advantages, along these lines representing help at different investigation levels. This idea empowered its application to whatever degree of examination the analyst considered the most extreme significant.

As to date, only a few practical studies pertaining to IS and its achievements in developing nations exist [32, 33]. DeLone and McLean's [11] concept created a vital lens through which to look at the successful implementation of IS. The limited studies about developing regions concerning IS success are a sign of potential to conduct further examinations of the constructs that could propel successful implementation of IS applications and the manner in which those constructs might be correlated. With this in mind, the recognition of the factors that affect IS success might bring about an understanding of what to do insure IS success in those regions.

This research suggests that D&M's theory can be used to look into the possible successful introduction of the technological and infrastructural facilities features that considered imperative in improving the social healthcare procedures of resident's health care. A need exists to address the use of their concepts for evaluating the success of IT in developing regions (like Jordan) and the prospects of developing the model by looking at supplementary aspects (such as technological and infrastructural facilities services quality, data quality and framework system). This would represent the variables that could be included for the examination model. This procedure additionally recognizes the effect of technological and infrastructural facilities, administration esteem, data worth and framework quality on DeLone and Mclean's factors spoke to by individual's well-being fulfilment and expectation of utilization or use as a type of inner free factors. Also, it analyses the net preferred position of IoT as a dependent variable.

3.9 Research Factors

This section presented two (2) types of factor: first type is original factors of IS theory, namely the administration quality, data quality, framework quality, client fulfilment, intention to use and net advantages. Second type of factors is external factors, namely technological and infrastructure facilities factors as following:

3.9.1 Service Quality (SeQu)

Generally, administration quality is derived from the perspective of client attitudes, in which value is characterized as continuing the client's necessities [34, 35]. Effectively satisfying these requirements relies upon an association's ability to identify and meet them [36]. From the organization's perspective, customers can be seen as persons with singular necessities. In case a standard degree of administration quality is set up to fulfil these necessities, associations professing to give great administrations must fulfil clients' prerequisites with the goal that they will create more constructive positive image in the commercial centre over its opponents.

Interestingly, high-quality service does not necessarily translate to decreasing negative quality (poor service and irregularity); however, it can mean expanding positive characteristics like luxury and fun, that lead to the development of significant worth [36]; Grohmann, Hofer and Martin, [37]; Lee et al. [38–40].

Strategic advantage for an institution in the market with respect to products and services can be obtained through measuring quality gaps. This dimension delivers the determination to enable institution to enhance its spot in the marketplace. In any case, earlier examinations dedicated to this topic have demonstrated that estimating quality in a target way of administration portion that is a result of intangible, heterogeneous and inseparable landscape of services [41].

However, Sachdev and Verma [42] assessed the relative significance of value measurements in particular assistance enterprises and featured two (2) perspectives concerning quality measurement: internal and external perspectives. The previous is characterized as zero (0) deformities or conformance to prerequisites while the last reveals an insight into quality estimation with respect to client insights of knowledge, fulfilment, demeanour and delight.

Prior studies have applied many measurement instruments in the hope of contributing to the quality perception literature [43]. In precise, Llusar and Zornoza [43] stated that these tools added to the measurement of technology value and quality studies. Several lessons have attempted to recognize the major facility quality dimensions in the framework of hospitals in which individual collaboration among understudies and Stockholders (staff, nurses, doctor and patients) or lecturers was the principal administration conveyance and correspondence channel.

3.9.2 Information Quality

Data quality refers to the predominance results that data framework creates [9] and often appears as input of feedback. While gauging end-user satisfaction, information quality usually serves as a chief variable; thus, it is normally regarded as part of user satisfaction instead of an independent construct [8].

The strength and validity of the information produced by IS impact users´ satisfaction in applying that information for their purposes. If the information is complicated and not understandable, that information may produce dissatisfaction among users [44]. Concerning its result, few IS researchers have altogether contemplated data quality [45]. Several of the strongest and most vital elements of information quality, as mentioned by Petter and McLean [8], comprise accuracy, wholeness, significance, timeliness and the nature of information.

3.9.3 System Quality Factor

One well-researched component of IS achievement is system framework value. System quality signifies the degree to which the data handling framework itself works and how the equipment and program ready to work together when consolidated. Framework quality has been concentrated through the perspective of assortment factors in the IS space. Nonetheless, the ones that are seen with as progressively important are accommodation of access, adaptability of framework, function efficiency, system integration, reaction time [46] and IS utility perceived [47].

Studies on IS have led to several metrics for gauging system quality, and chief among them are usability and user-friendliness, which are oft-used factors for gauging IS success and user satisfaction. The framework of websites and studies have detected the elements that form system quality features, namely interactivity, navigation, access, hyperlinks and entertaining [48].

3.9.4 User Satisfaction

The possibility of consumer fulfilment was applied to data frameworks (IS) research and assembled in the system identified with client fulfilment. User satisfaction was frequently viewed as a measurement for deciding data framework system achievement [49]. Kotler [50] described consumer gratification as follows: "Satisfaction is an individual's feelings of enjoyment or disappointment arising from gazing at the apparent display of an object equivalent to their wishes". Brown [51] explained consumer satisfaction as: "The condition in which customer needs and expectations are met or exceeded over the entire life of the object or administration, arising in repeated buying, loyalty and good mood".

3.9.5 Intention to Use

Framework practice is identified with the use and correspondence of information system (IS) by individuals, populaces or associations [52, 53]. DeLone and McLean [11] suggested that a substitute estimation of framework use could be the reason to utilize which is a subject of the research framework system. The definition "Use" is a complex perplexing term to comprehend on the grounds that it includes an expansive range of definitions that deliberate, informed or uninformed and effective or ineffective. In some cases, assessing the intention to use (otherwise known as attitude) could be worthy option because gauging intention is linked to behaviour intention [11].

3.9.6 Factor of Net Benefits (NBs)

Net benefits (NBs) are used to be a formed version of the original model structure [9] in which individual elements and organizational impacts were separated into a solitary descriptor of the last achievement variable.

An individual impression alludes such that data from IS have the attitudes of clients with respect to the client's activity [54]. The term includes individual enhancements and the general ramifications for the exhibition of an office or specialty unit according to impacts data from IS have on the executive's choices.

These effects happen when the data are recognized and interpreted by clients and applied to their occupations [9, 52].

3.9.7 Technological Factor

This investigation will consider the mechanical factor that is just four components from the all-inclusive [11] IS achievement model to be specific framework quality, data quality, administration quality and client fulfilment.

The utilization of the patients' online interface was not a priority but rather compulsory to the patients, the build "use" was subsumed in client fulfilment since clients' fulfilment of a data framework must be gone before by its utilization.

Net advantage as a build was dropped since allotting it will be of setting in this investigation. Client fulfilment which incorporates "use" in this setting remains the most feasible proportion of the information system (IS) achievement. This prompts the adjustment of the IS achievement model in accessing user's satisfaction within the context of the research.

3.9.8 Infrastructural Facilities

IS competency refers to how much extend staff has the basic aptitudes and information so as to play out the basic administrations [55]. As indicated by Allen and Boynton [56], IS structure refers to the extent to which the data frameworks are organized or dispersed all through an association. Client support manages the specialized support and help given to clients as far as practical data frameworks in the association [57].

4 Research Methods

This section addresses and explains the methods used in this research. It sheds light on the theoretical framework, research theories, research design, the questionnaire design, gauging scale, population, sampling and data gathering process. To conclude the chapter, a conversation on the statistical methods used to analyse the data is provided.

4.1 Data Collection Method and Framework

An examination analysis approach, wherein a quantitative strategy was utilized to gather the fundamental information, is received in this study. Patients of public and

Table 1 Comparing success theories

Model and criteria	[9]	[10]	[24]	Wang and Liu [12]	[14]	[16]
Well tested and validated	Yes	No	Yes	No	No	No
Simple	Yes	No	Yes	No	Yes	Yes
Captures all factors to DCs	No	No	No	No	No	No
Flexible	No	No	Yes	No	No	No

private hospitals in Jordan are included in the study population through an appropriate sampling technique system. Three hundred thirty-four (700) questionnaires were distributed, and from these, three hundred twenty-five (417) were analysed. The example attributes are then outlined out in Table 1.

4.2 Research Framework and Hypotheses

The research framework—which serves as the foundation of the study problems—illustrates that that all the thoughts, implications and recommendations are connected to the research complications.

This research recommends that, despite the presence of current innovative movements, the DeLone and McLean's information systems (IS) success model gets by as a fundamental reference to the achievement estimation idea that has been generally utilized in the assortment of research since the time it was distributed in 1992 [9] and keeps on being an effective measuring of IS achievement. Starting late, a need to recognize the interest for appraisal procedures that fit the assessment procedure of advances, to be specific, Internet of things for enhancing quality and efficiency during the emergencies of coronavirus has showed up. The recommendation has been made that through coordinating aspects of standard DeLone and McLean's assessment components, a more up-to-date, progressively refined and refreshed version of the DeLone and McLean's IS success model can be utilized in estimating factors affecting the success of Internet of things for enhancing quality and efficiency implementation in hospitals sector in Jordan during the crisis of coronavirus.

Several writers have looked into the aspects (or incorporated variables) that could possibly affect Internet of things for enhancing quality and efficiency implementation in hospitals sector, as well as their success in healthcare sector establishments. This study has acknowledged certain measures, namely the technological and infrastructural facilities factors that considered imperative in improving the social healthcare procedures of resident's health care. Hope that this discovery will convince the administration of hospitals to focus on important viewpoints that impact the utilization of Internet of things (IoT) in healthcare services.

The need to understand the workings of information systems (IS) and their impacts motivated the conception of the first DeLone and McLean IS success model. According to DeLone and McLean [11], this paradigm for the research framework

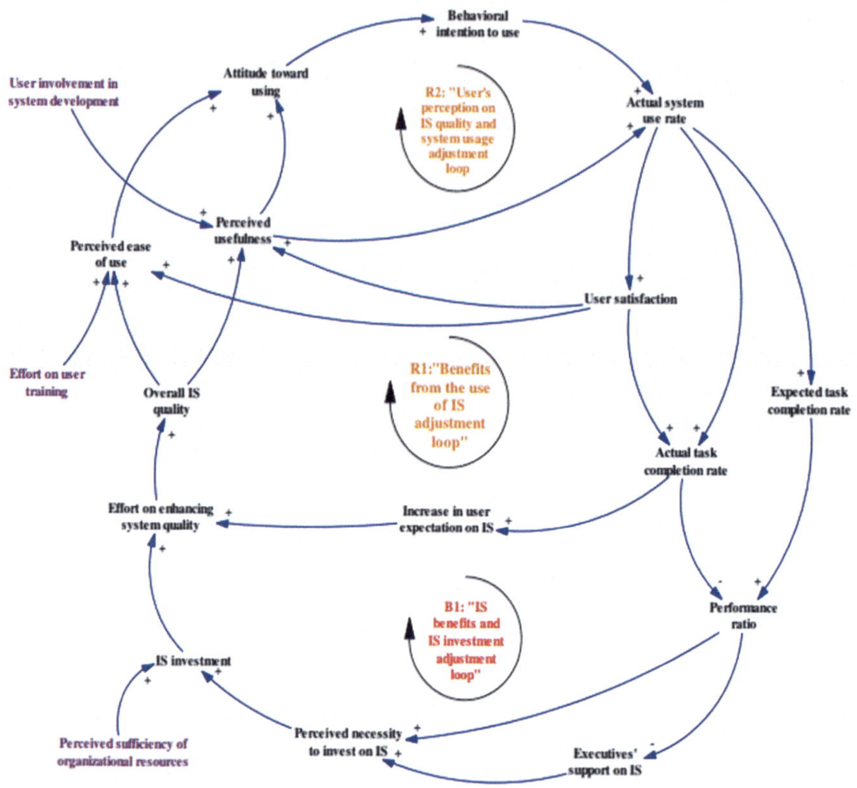

Fig. 3 Wang and Liu system dynamics theory of information system (IS) success *Source* Dynamics theory (2005)

has only three parts: the design of a structure, the use of the structure and the definitions of this model. Every step is appropriate, but not sufficient, for the resulting outcome(s). The concept of the current study sustains the three facets, which are system conception, system use and system significances as illustrated in Fig. 3.

4.3 Instrument Design

A poll of questionnaire survey, that endured face and contents validity, was developed for this study case, for ease of translation from the Likert scale five-point. This survey is separated into two sections: the first part relates to personal information with four (4) items, and the second part relates to the research variables with fifty (50) items. Smart PLS software was applied for the selected partial least square modelling method applied for this study, in such a two-stage approach to structural equation model testing.

5 Reliability of Measuring Instrument

This area presents the consequence of validity and dependability of the information gathered and the instruments. One strategy to make sure that the error of estimation is at a minimum rate is to describe the purity of the measure. The goal of these instument is usually to conduct these tasks assigment in appproraite way. The properties incorporate legitimacy and unwavering quality. To guarantee the legitimacy of the builds, a scientist must lead factor examination; in like manner, to guarantee the unwavering quality of the things, dependability investigation must be performed. This area incorporates the information screening and cleaning, profiles of respondents for real information assortment, validity assessment and reliability assessment.

5.1 Data Screening and Cleaning

The screening and cleaning techniques for information on blunders or exceptions were used before the information was examined.

At that point, the two develops and the constructs in the builds were approved. Factor analysis was performed on the independent and dependent variable items variable things to guarantee the legitimacy of the constructs. Information screening is a procedure that is led to guarantee that there will be no ambiguity in the information qualities that can possibly affect the discoveries. It is basic to do the screening procedure in light of the fact that as often as possible previous advances influence the decisions to be made in the latter steps.

5.2 Profiles of Respondents for Actual Data Collection (N = 417)

By researching the reliability quality, which explicitly refers to interior consistency, united legitimacy just as discriminative validity, the measurement model can be evaluated and assessed, as illustrated in Table 1.

6 Data Analysis

This section presented validity the measures, testing the research model and robustness testing as following.

6.1 Validity the Measures

SPSS software program and smart partial least squares (SPLS) were used to confirm the observations, just as the entire model system was tested. Convergent, discriminating credibility is built upon resulting factors (as seen in Fig. 2). Cronbach's alphas are above 0.80 of all definitions (Table 2). The average variance generated (AVE) square basis of all ideas is above 0.75 (Table diagonal elements.

A specific descriptive analysis of the test set out in Table 3 depicts the overall situation of the hospitals in Middle East. This analysis produces the mean, the normal deviation, maximum and minimum of the concepts. Meanwhile, to make the five-point Likert scale easily construable, three categories are applied in this study as follows: scores less than 2.33 [4/3 + lowest rate (1)] reported to be low; grades of 3.67 [highest value (5)−4/3] were rated as high and referred to as moderate in the middle table.

We have additionally conducted appraisals for normal framework inclination (i.e. change attributed to measurement method as opposed to difference clarified by the investigation's builds). To start with, proof for normal technique inclination exists on

Table 2 Respondents' profiles (N = 417)

Variables	Frequency (%)	Percentage (%)
Gender		
Male	168	40.3
Female	249	59.7
Nationality		
Jordanian	310	74.3
Non Jordanian	107	25.7
Age		
<25	125	30.0
25-35	93	22.3
More than 35	199	47.7
Educational level		
Less than bachelor's degree	184	40.1
Undergraduate degree	97	21.4
Graduation degree	111	23.7
Ph.D degree	61	14.8
Type of treatment received		
Inpatient	182	43.6
Outpatient	83	19.9
Both	152	36.5
Total	417	100%

Table 3 Validity and reliability of measurement

Variables	N	Cronbach's alpha	AVE
Information quality (IQ)	417	0.85	0.93
System quality (SQ)	417	0.88	0.91
Service quality (SerQ)	417	0.87	0.87
Technological (Tech)	417	0.82	0.86
Infrastructural facilities (InFa)	417	0.83	0.85
User Satisfaction (UsSa)	417	0.89	0.83
Use (U)	417	0.86	0.84
Net benefit (NBs)	417	0.79	0.90

the off chance that one principal factor means the greater part of the change clarified [58].

Our essential parts include investigation of full samples that demonstrates the eight (8) builds with eigenvalues predominant than 1.0 record for 78.57% of the fluctuation, while the main develop clarified 19.24% of the change.

Table 4 displays that the most noteworthy link between build association is 0.841, while the predisposition of the basic strategy is generally confirmed by very high connections ($r > .90$)) [59]. These tests show that the propensity of the basic method is definitely not a big problem in this study. The full-example Olkin test ($n = 417$) estimate is 0.978, implying this investigation's example skill [60]. Additionally, collinearity markers (resilience esteems and differential swelling factors) were planned and viewed as not exactly the appropriate cut-off focuses [61], meaning the investigation does not experience the ill effects of multicollinearity problems.

6.2 *Testing the Research Model*

In view of PLS analysis, the basic model and conjectured associations were reviewed by strategies methods for bootstrapping philosophy with 5000 iterations, the quantifiable centrality and the way coefficients were assessed.

For the complete example, we tried the exploration models using the SPLS ($n = 417$). The corroborative angle shown in the SPLS test is appropriate where all loadings exceed 0.71 and are greater than the pass stacking. The results SPLS of the research reviewing the structural model SPLS results are summarized in Fig. 4. In addition to H4 and H5, the proposed research program provided information on the data. In specific, the results show factors: data quality and system quality.

Technological (Tech) and infrastructural facilities (InFa) significantly affect client fulfilment ($b = 0.35, p < 0.01$), ($b = 0.38, p < 0.01$), ($b = 0.33, p < 0.01$), ($b = 0.41, p < 0.01$), along these lines supporting H1, H2, H3 and H4, and the outcomes show that factors in particular: information quality (IQ), service quality (SerQ) technological (Tech), infrastructural facilities (InFa), significantly affects intention to use (ItU) (*b*

Table 4 Result of variables analysis

Variables		Dimensions	Factor loading(FL)	Mean ± SD	(CR)	Cronbach's alpha	(AVE)
Information quality (IQ)	Content usefulness	CU1	0.758	3.755 ± 0.936	0.874	0.717	0.632
		CU2	0.738	3.776 ± 0.834			
		CU3	0.878	3.753 ± 0.723			
		CU4	0.796	3.741 ± 1.083			
		CU5	0.856	3.753 ± 0.723			
	Content adequacy	CA1	0.817	3.761 ± 1.083			
		CA2	0.741	3.728 ± 0.946			
		CA3	0.857	3.736 ± 0.836			
		CA4	0.823	3.723 ± 0.986			
		CA5	0.864	3.766 ± 0.936			
System quality (SQ)	Ease of use	EU1	0.738	3.767 ± 1.071	0.865	0.858	0.653
		EU2	0.753	3.763 ± 1.041			
		EU3	0.738	3.767 ± 1.029			
		EU4	0.726	3.853 ± 0.775			
		EU5	0.871	3.875 ± 0.855			
	Accessibility	Acc1	0.761	3.776 ± 0.834			
		Acc2	0.846	3.753 ± 0.723			
		Acc3	0.874	3.761 ± 1.083			
		Acc4	0.765	3.722 ± 1.064			
	Interactivity	Int1	0.754	3.771 ± 1.071			
		Int2	0.758	3.736 ± 1.077			

(continued)

Table 4 (continued)

Variables		Dimensions	Factor loading(FL)	Mean ± SD	(CR)	Cronbach's alpha	(AVE)
		Int3	0.734	3.741 ± 1.055			
Service quality (SerQ)	Accessibility(Acc)	ACC1	0.753	3.797 ± 1.021	0.768	0766	0.672
		ACC2	0.796	3.752 ± 1.081			
		ACC3	0.874	3.734 ± 1.031			
		ACC4	0.863	3.746 ± 1.062			
	Interface design (IDS)	ID1	0.748	3.733 ± 1.057			
		ID2	0.728	3.783 ± 1.054			
		ID3	0.878	3.871 ± 0.964			
	Reliability and response (R&R)	RR1	0.778	3.824 ± 0.773			
		RR2	0.845	3.831 ± 0.873			
	Content quality(CQ)	CQ1	0.817	3.855 ± 0.883			
		CQ2	0.762	3.657 ± 1.855			
	Personalization (Per)	Per1	0.767	3.784 ± 1.061			
		Per2	0.758	3.739 ± 0.774			
		Per3	0.771	3.744 ± 0.794			
		Per4	0.756	3.872 ± 0.874			
		Per5	0.753	3.738 ± 1.046			
	Privacy and security(P&S)	(P&S)1	0.723	3.731 ± 1.065			
		(P&S) 2	0.739	3.738 ± 1.026			
Technological (Tech)	Availability of human capital (AHC)	AHC1	0.833	3.875 ± 0.981	0.727	0.958	0.841
		AHC2	0.742	3.744 ± 0.764			

(continued)

Table 4 (continued)

Variables		Dimensions	Factor loading(FL)	Mean ± SD	(CR)	Cronbach's alpha	(AVE)
		AHC3	0.776	3.872 ± 0.854			
		AHC4	0.857	3.738 ± 1.026			
	Infrastructure in the field of research and development (IFRD)	IFRD1	0.791	3.731 ± 0.815			
		IFRD2	0.762	3.844 ± 1.042			
		IFRD3	0.847	3.834 ± 0.731			
		IFRD4	0.837	3.825 ± 0.859			
	Cooperation of the private and the public sector (CPPS)	CPPS1	0.749	3.764 ± 0.865			
		CPPS2	0.784	3.827 ± 0.732			
		CPPS3	0.763	3.831 ± 0.875			
Infrastructural facilities (InFaFaci)	Parking facilities	InFaFaci1	0.768	3.854 ± 1.062	0.876	0.853	0.785
	General entrance	InFaFaci 2	0.761	3.834 ± 0.731			
	Emergency entrance	InFaFaci 3	0.857	3.825 ± 0.889			
	Waiting area	InFaFaci 4	0.816	3.734 ± 0.865			
	Seating place	InFaFaci 5	0.823	3.827 ± 0.732			
	Washroom facilities	InFaFaci 6	0.859	3.841 ± 0.875			
	Cleanliness and hygiene	InFaFaci 7	0.871	3.831 ± 0.921			
	Canteen	InFaFaci 8	0.763	3.726 ± 0.882			
	Signboards	InFaFaci 9	0.852	3.724 ± 0.863			
	Technology	InFaFaci 10	0.784	3.843 ± 0.856			
User Satisfaction(UsSa)	UsSa1		0.718	3.821 ± 0.873	0.877	0.862	0.734
	UsSa2		0.715	3.835 ± 0.853			

(continued)

Table 4 (continued)

Variables	Dimensions	Factor loading(FL)	Mean ± SD	(CR)	Cronbach's alpha	(AVE)
	UsSs3	0.829	3.657 ± 1.835			
	UsSa4	0.813	3.764 ± 1.051			
Intention to use (U)	ItN1	0.738	3.739 ± 0.764	0.872	0.846	0.645
	ItN2	0.866	3.724 ± 0.774			
	ItN3	0.754	3.872 ± 0.854			
	ItN4	0.824	3.738 ± 1.034			
	ItN5	0.825	3.721 ± 1.025			
	ItN6	0.876	3.738 ± 1.066			
	ItN7	0.821	3.875 ± 0.961			
Net benefit (NBs)	NB1	0.821	3.754 ± 0.754	0.862	0.858	0.766
	NB2	0.853	3.872 ± 0.874			
	NB3	0.723	3.738 ± 1.026			

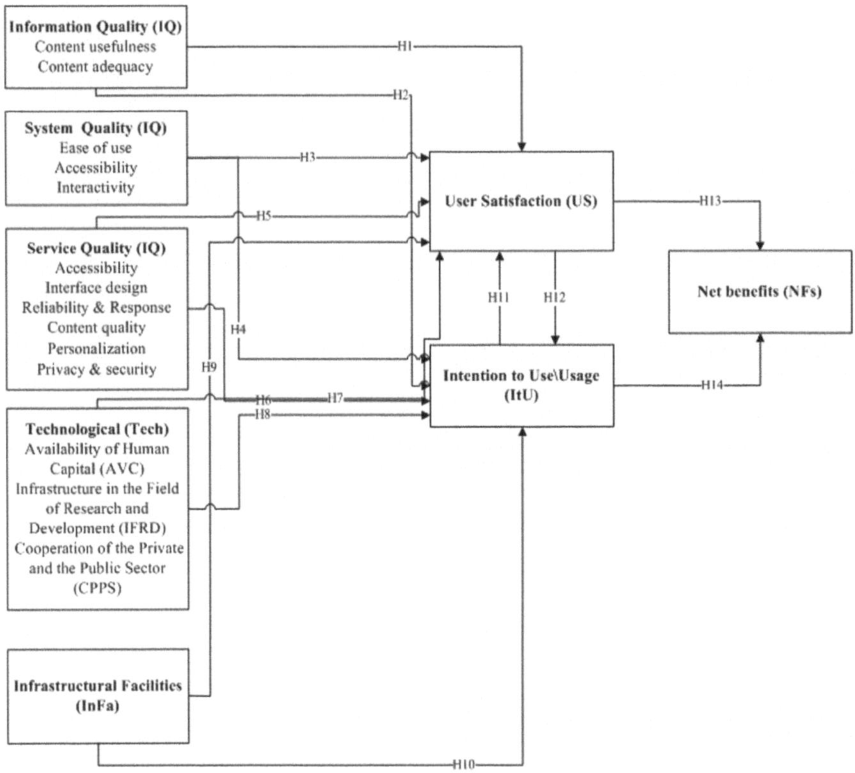

Fig. 4 Research framework and hypotheses

= 0.40, $p < 0.01$), ($b = 0.40$, $p < 0.01$), ($b = 0.59$, $p < 0.01$), ($b = 0.48$, $p < 0.01$), hence supporting H1, H2, H3 and H5.

In any case, we found a substantially negative relationship between the consistency of the system and the intention to use (ItU) ($b = -0.17$, $0.05 < p < 0.10$), dismissing H4 in this manner. It also starts an essentially negative relationship between quality of administration and user satisfaction (UsSa) ($b = -0.12$, $0.05 < p < 0.10$), thereby dismissing H5. The impacts of data quality on both client fulfilment ($b = 0.35$, $p < 0.01$) and use ($b = 0.36$, $p < 0.01$) are both huge, supporting H1 and H2. The connection between technological (Tech) and intention to use ($b = 0.40$, $0.05 < p<0.10$) and intention to use (ItU) ($b = 0.59$, $p < 0.01$) are both critical, supporting H7 and H8. The infrastructure facilities (InFa) and use relationships ($b = 0.41$, $0.05 < p < 0.10$) and intention to use (ItU) ($b = 0.48$, $p < 0.01$) are both noteworthy and support H9 and H10. The findings show that consumer loyalty effectively influences both usage ($b = 0.41$, $p < 0.01$) and net benefits ($b = 0.37$, $p < 0.01$), with support of H12 and H13.

The outcomes show that client fulfilment effectively affects both intention to use ($b = 0.21$, $p < 0.01$) and net benefits ($b = 0.36$, $p < 0.01$), approving H11 and H14.

The clarified fluctuation of net advantages yields 0.43%. The changes clarified by client fulfilment and intention to use (ItU) are 0.56% and 0.36%, separately. Overall, the R^2 results for each needed variable, along with all the AVE, Cronbach's alpha, the unwavering composite quality and the increased factor stacking, provide sufficient decency for the general research model [62].

6.3 Testing Robustness

This same information shows an important serious effect of framework appraisal on intention to use (ItU) and insignificant impact of administration quality on client fulfilment.

So as to inspect whether this result is applicable to discover that impact the accomplishment of Internet of things (IoT) in the implementation of health care from the viewpoint of hospitals in Jordan, we conducted smart PLS analysis with these samples (Figs. 5, 6).

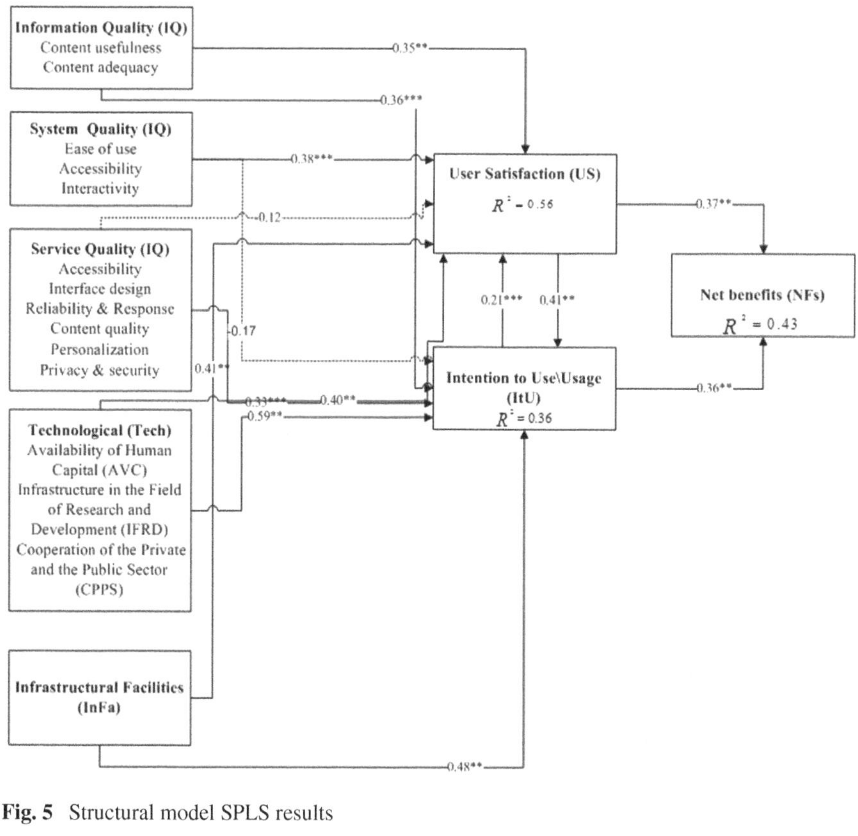

Fig. 5 Structural model SPLS results

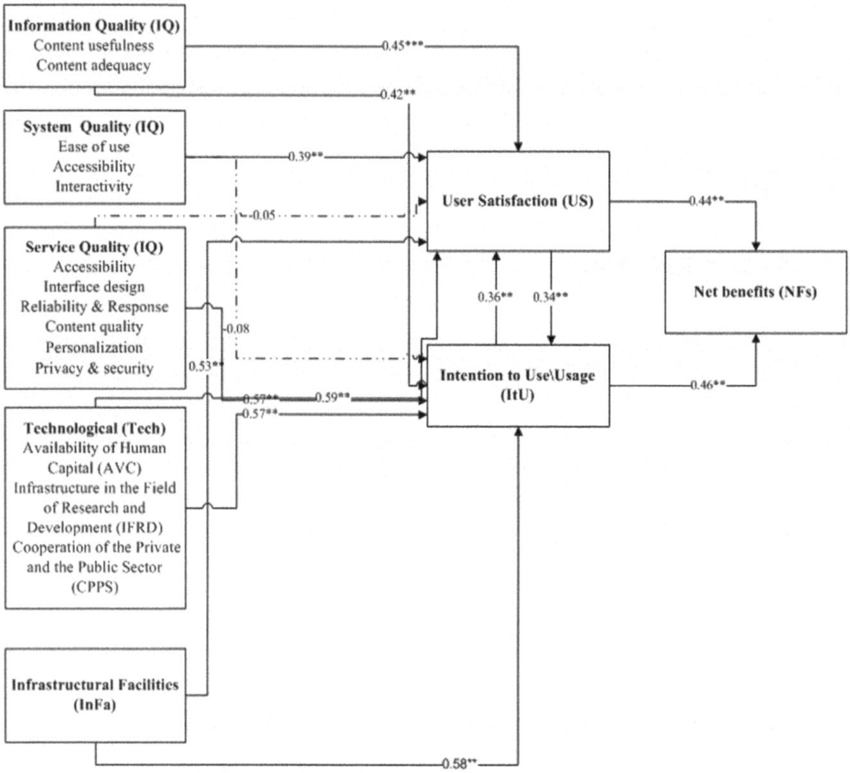

Fig. 6 SPLS results of structural model

The last advance in the PLS-SEM conceptual framework is to test the approximate connections by having to run PLS calculation and modularizing the 2.0 3 M smart PLS algorithm. Despite the fact that coefficients are significant in the analysis of PLS, Hair et al. (2011) confirmed that the earlier theory should be discarded when ways are irrelevant or show signs contrary to the conjectured pathway.

Then again, notable ways of demonstrating the conjectured path support the suggested observational causal relationship. We also conveyed that the hugeness of each coefficient, similar to the loads and loading of the indicators, can be tested using methods for a bootstrapping methodology. Within the past Fig. 4.3, we can observe the loading, path coefficient and R2 values of items clearly.

Utilizing the bootstrapping method in the appraisal of way coefficients includes bootstrap test of 500 and the amount of cases ought to be equivalent to the quantity of perceptions in the original model example (Winnie, Poh-Ming Wong, [63]; Winnie & Ramayah, [64]; Sumo & Regien, [65]; Lorenzo-Romero & Carlota, [66]; Henseler, Jörg, [67]; Monecke & Armin, [68]; Rubel & Mohammad, [69]; Iivari & Juhani, [70]).

In addition, the basic t-values for a two-tailed assessment are 1.64 (with a noteworthiness equivalent of 10%), 1.96 (with an outcome level of 5%) and 2.58 (with an essentials level of 1%).

The specialist set 500 re-examines with an extra number from the bootstrap cases equal to the first number of test (416) so as to create standard blunders and acquire t-statistics. Table 5 contains the path coefficient and the bootstrapping results, where the hypothesized relationships below were tested. (Table 6).

7 Research Contributions

This research makes significant commitments in the system of Internet of things viewpoints for the patients during the Covid-19 crisis in developing nations. This exploration has made subsequent noteworthy contributions.

7.1 Methodological Contribution

- The procedures, speculation, estimation apparatuses set-up in the basic piece of this study give an exceptionally lively viewpoint of the plan and groundwork for this exploration.
  The gathering of the poll study and model structure for this examination have been efficiently and noticeably expressed in this study. This exploration additionally offers legitimization for the choice to utilize the instruments that have been assigned for the fulfilment of this investigation. A basic condition demonstrating (SEM) additionally utilized to 200 approves the structure framework model. This examination adds to the improvement of SEM research in the technology innovation field.
- Firstly, identify and classify the range of IoT solutions and techniques for the patients during the Covid-19 crisis; secondly, identify the technological (Tech) and infrastructural facilities (InFa) issues for these IoT solutions and techniques; thirdly, presenting known technological (Tech), infrastructural facilities (InFa) features for these IoT solutions and techniques; and finally, identifying technological (Tech), infrastructural facilities (InFa) requirements for the IoT applications for the patients during the Covid-19 crisis.

7.2 Theoretical Contribution in Research

(1) The objective of this research involvement relates to how issues affect the level of success of Internet of things for enhancing quality and efficiency implementation in hospitals sector in Jordan during the crises of coronavirus. Furthermore, this

Table 5 Mean, standard deviation (SD), correlations and square root of AVE

Variables	Mean *(N = 417)*	SD *(N = 417)*	*1* *(N = 417)*	2	*3*	*4*	*5*	*6*	7	*8*	α
Information quality (IQ)	3.751	0.9086	***0.78***								0.74
System quality (SQ)	3.773	0.9732	0.64	***0.79***							0.75
Quality of service (SerQ)	3.774	1.0163	0.46	0.42	***0.48***						0.81
Technological (Tech)	3.808	0.8676	0.54	0.60	0.62	***0.96***					0.72
Infrastructural facilities (InFa)	3.804	0.8676	0.42	0.55	0.40	0.61	***0.94***				0.75
User satisfaction (UsSa)	3.769	1.153	0.39	0.59	0.48	0.58	0.46	***0.94***			0.76
Use (U)	3.772	0.9254	0.553	0.342	0.400	0.349	0.306	0.602	***0.86***		0.92
Net benefit (NBs)	3.788	0.8847	0.651	0.414	0.618	.446	0.406	0.310	0.530	***0.85***	0.83

Table 6 Hypothesis testing result

Hypo	Relationship	P coefficient	S. error	*t*-value	Supported	
H1	Information quality (IQ)→ user satisfaction	1.368	0.121	2.971	***	Yes
H2	Information quality (IQ)→Intention to use	0.312	0.094	0.154	**	Yes
H3	System quality (IQ)→User satisfaction	0.595	0.052	01.702	*	Yes
H4	System quality (IQ)→Intention to use	-0.396	0.043	10.334	n.s	No
H5	Service quality (IQ)→User satisfaction	-1.021	0.148	7.011	n.s	No
H6	Service quality (IQ)→Intention to use	0.668	0.115	1.583	***	Yes
H7	Technological (Tech)→User satisfaction	0.522	0.095	5.327	**	Yes
H8	Technological (Tech)→Intention to use	0.063	0.067	0.996	***	Yes
H9	Infrastructural facilities (InFa)→User satisfaction	0.847	0.113	7.853	***	Yes
H10	Infrastructural facilities (InFa)→Intention to use	0.787	0.077	0.558	**	Yes
H11	Intention to use→User satisfaction	0.611	0.061	10.152	***	Yes
H12	User satisfaction →Net benefit	0.204	0.046	5.278	***	Yes
H13	Intention to use→Net benefit	0.771	0.038	20.556	***	Yes
H14	User satisfaction→Intention to use	0.448	0.051	8.842	***	Yes

research highlights the rank of features affecting the context of Internet of things aspects for the patients during the Covid-19 crisis. This thus shows a major job in expanding the standard of success of Internet of things for enhancing quality and efficiency implementation in hospitals sector in developing nations.

(2) This study contemplated the correspondence-related features of Internet of things factors in the framework system of health for smart areas, specifically to know the transmission capacity essential and volume of information generated.

Based on the performance of current business preliminary, it is additionally contemplated and distinguished its qualities and shortcomings as far as Internet of things viewpoints for the patients during the Covid-19 crisis.

As a following stage, the thesis proposed a conceptual model that addressed the disadvantage of existing variables while looking over their qualities. This proposed reasonable model determines the components that impact the accomplishment of Internet of things (IoT) in the implementation of health care from the perspective of hospitals in Jordan for receiving a comprehensive responsiveness of a person's health.

7.3 Practical Contributions

On the basis of the level of observation, analysis and the degree of innovation Internet of things for enhancing quality and efficiency implementation in hospitals sector in Jordan during the emergencies of Covid-19, eight (8) deciding variables have been recognized to determine elements of success of Internet of things. These incorporate the two (2) factors referenced above which have been changed to suit the unit of analysis of this exploration and furthermore includes increasingly factor, which is, technological and infrastructural facilities factors.

These variables impact are accepted to have a significant impact in success of Internet of things within developing nations and along these lines extremely fundamental to this research. The idea of these variables on account of progress of Internet of things is one that mirrors the multilayered values that have been gathered by customers from individual encounters [71].

Lack of trust by patients is progressively influencing the selection of achievement Internet of things; unfortunate cases like hacking has become serious these days and the fear of such can demoralize patients from accomplish enhancing quality and efficiency implementation in hospitals sector in Jordan during the emergencies of Covid-19 [72].

8 Research Implications

This research highlighted the importance of technological and infrastructural facilities factors on success of Internet of things for enhancing quality and efficiency implementation in hospitals level. This outcome is in line through that of [73] who show that it is imperative to emphasis on the enhancing value and efficiency implementation in hospitals sector in Jordan during the crises of coronavirus. These factors are serious issues to be considered when presenting a health for smart regions for the patients during the Covid-19 crisis in developing countries. Internet of things (IoT) providers need to continuously strive to examine the other important factors for smart regions with IoT technology.

This research has revealed that user gratification and intention to use have an important impact on success of net benefits. Then again, notable ways of demonstrating the conjectured path support the suggested observational causal relationship. We also conveyed that the hugeness of each coefficient, similarly to the loads and charging of the indicators, can be tested using techniques for a bootstrapping methodology. Within the past Fig. 4.3, we can notice the loading, path coefficient and R2 values of items clearly and infrastructural facilities (parking facilities, general entrance, emergency entrance, waiting area, seating place, washroom Facilities, cleanliness and hygiene, canteen, signboards and technology).

9 Conclusion

The current present presented a detailed analysis of factors affecting the success of success of Internet of things for enhancing quality and efficiency implementation in hospitals sector in Jordan during the crises of Covid-19 on IS achievement. Most researches are conducted in different settings and IS context. Very little known about the impact of factors related to technological and infrastructural facilities as a determinant of IS success in the context of the success model framework for D&M. Subsequently, this study investigated the relationships between the technological and infrastructural facilities, the service quality, information quality, the system quality, and use of intent and user satisfaction. Additionally, the studies examine the connection between intention to use, in addition to user sense of achievement, user intent and net benefit, customer satisfaction and user intention.

The advantages of investing with technology (human capital availability, research and development infrastructure, and private and public sector cooperation); infrastructural facilities (parking facilities, general entrance, emergency entrance, waiting area, seating place, washroom facilities, cleanliness and hygiene, canteen, signboards and technology); and success of Internet of things for enhancing quality and efficiency implementation in hospitals level were assessed against patients' evaluation of the portal's attributes, in particular quality of framework, quality of data and quality of administration issues. The disclosures of this research can become a sign of the need for administrative hospitals to start taking prompt measures by conveniently supporting and revising the web-based human services framework interface and acknowledging the study's innovative and infrastructure development obstacles.

10 Recommendations for Future Research

This study has assessed effectively the influence of the aspects on satisfaction level and the purpose of using the total advantages of technological and infrastructural facilities factors that considered imperative in improving the social healthcare procedures of resident's health care. Hope that this discovery will convince the administration of hospitals to focus on important viewpoints that impact the utilization of Internet of things (IoT) in healthcare services. Furthermore, this study has emphasized the impact of the user interface and its relationship with the demographic features. However, all the variables affecting the success still need to be inspected of

Internet of things (IoT) in healthcare services. Consequently, this study offers some suggestions for future study as follows:

(1) Other methods could be utilized in future examinations, such as the case study, the contextual investigation, centre gatherings and expert interview to research the connection between segment factors, client fulfilment and expectation to use in the achievement of Internet of things (IoT).
(2) In the future, studies could inspect other features such as empowerment, safety, trust ability and efficiency in accumulation to the issues covered in the study.
(3) The research test was gathered from five hospitals in Jordan, which may not be satisfactory to signify the circumstance across Jordan. Thus, future analysts should be thoughtful when looking to simplify discoveries of this research for the entire nation.

References

1. Worldometers: Current World Population, May-23-[2020] from: https://www.worldometers.info/world-population (2020)
2. Aggelidis, V., Chatzoglou, P.: Hospital information systems: Measuring end user computing satisfaction (EUCS). J. Biomed. Inf. **45**(3), 566–579 (2012)
3. Adeyinka, T., Mutula, S.: A proposed model for evaluating the success of WebCT course content management system. Comput. Hum. Behav. **26**(6), 1795–1805 (2010)
4. Bakıcı, T., Almirall, E., Wareham, J.: A smart city initiative: the case of Barcelona. J. Knowl. Econ. **4**(2), 135–148 (2013)
5. Bai, L., Yang, D., Wang, X., Tong, L., Zhu, X., Bai, C., Powell, C.A.: Chinese experts' consensus on the internet of things-aided diagnosis and treatment of coronavirus disease 2019. Clinical eHealth, (2020)
6. Allam, Z., Jones, D.S.: On the coronavirus (COVID-19) outbreak and the smart city network: universal data sharing standards coupled with artificial intelligence (AI) to benefit urban health monitoring and management. In Healthcare (vol. 8(1)). Multidisciplinary Digital Publishing Institute, Mar 2020, p. 46
7. Irani, Z., Ahmad, N., Amer, N. T., Qutaifan, F., & Alhilali, A. (2013). Technology adoption model and a road map to successful implementation of ITIL. Journal of Enterprise Information Management
8. Petter, S., McLean, E.R.: A meta-analytic assessment of the DeLone and McLean IS success model: An examination of IS success at the individual level. Inf. Manag. **46**(3), 159–166 (2009)
9. DeLone, W.H., McLean, E.R.: Information systems success: the quest for the dependent variable. Inf. Syst. Res. **3**(1), 60–95 (1992)
10. Seddon, P.B., Staples, S., Patnayakuni, R., Bowtell, M.: Dimensions of information systems success. Communications of the AIS, 2(3es), 5, (1999)
11. Delone, W.H., McLean, E.R.: The DeLone and McLean model of information systems success: a ten-year update. J. Manag. Inf. Syst. **19**(4), 9–30 (2003)
12. Wang, W.-T., Liu, C.-Y.: The application of the technology acceptance model: a new way to evaluate information system success. Paper presented at the Proceedings of the 23rd International Conference of the System Dynamics Society. Boston, USA. Retrieved April, (2005)
13. Venkatesh, V., Morris, M., Davis, G., Davis, F.: User acceptance of information technology: toward a unified view. MIS Q. **27**(3), 425–478, (2003)
14. Sabherwal, R., Jeyaraj, A., Chowa, C.: Information system success: individual and organizational determinants. Manag. Sci. **52**(12), 1849–1864 (2006)

15. Rai, A., Lang, S.S., Welker, R.B.: Assessing the validity of IS success models: an empirical test and theoretical analysis. Inf. Syst. Res. **13**(1), 50–69 (2002)
16. Gable, G. G., Sedera, D., & Chan, T. (2008). Re-conceptualizing Information System Success: The IS-Impact Measurement Model. Journal of the Association for Information Systems, 9(7)
17. Ballantine, J., Bonner, M., Levy, M., Martin, A.: The 3-D model of information systems success: the search for the dependent variable continues. Inf. Res. Manag. J. **9**(4), 5 (1996)
18. Seddon, P. B.: A respecification and extension of the DeLone and McLean model of IS success. Inf Sys Res **8**(3), 240–253 (1997)
19. Pitt, L. F., Watson, R. T., & Kavan, C. B. (1995). Service Quality: A Measure of Information Systems Effectiveness. Mis Quarterly, 19(2)
20. Wilkin, C., Hewitt, B.: Quality in a respecification of DeLone and McLean's IS success model. In Proceedings of 1999 IRMA international conference (pp. 663–672, Hershey, PA, Idea Group Inc, (1999)
21. Van Dyke, T. P., Kappelman, L. A., Prybutok, V.R.: Measuring information systems service quality: concerns on the use of the SERVQUAL questionnaire. Mis Quarterly, 195–208, (1997)
22. Hornby, A.S.: Oxford advanced learner's dictionary of current English 6th edn, Oxford University Press, 2002
23. Garrity, E. J., Sanders, G. L. (Eds.).: Information systems success measurement. Igi Global (1998)
24. DeLone, W.H., McLean, E.R.: Information systems success revisited. Proceedings of the 35th annual hawaii international conference on system sciences, IEEE Computer Society, (2002)
25. Mulira, N.: Service systems implementation in volatile networks. (PHD), Delft University of Technology, The Netherlands, (2007)
26. Kulkarni, U.R., Ravindran, S., Freeze, R.: A knowledge management success model: theoretical development and empirical validation. J. Manag. Inf. Syst. **23**(3), 309–347 (2007)
27. Wu, J.-H., Wang, Y.-M.: Measuring KMS success: a respecification of the DeLone and McLean's model. Inf. Manag. **43**(6), 728–739 (2006)
28. Delone, W.H., Mclean, E.R.: Measuring e-commerce success: applying the DeLone & McLean information systems success model. Int. J. Electron. Commer. **9**(1), 31–47 (2004)
29. Molla, A., Licker, P.S.: E-Commerce systems success: an attempt to extend and respecify the delone and maclean model of is success. J. Electron. Commerce Res. **2**(4), 131–141 (2001)
30. Zhu, K., Kraemer, K.L.: Post-adoption variations in usage and value of e-business by organizations: cross-country evidence from the retail industry. Inf. Syst, Res. **16**(1), 61–84 (2005)
31. Myers, B.L., Kappelman, L.A., Prybutok, V.R.: A comprehensive model for assessing the quality and productivity of the information systems function: toward a theory for information systems assessment. Inf, Res. Manag. J. (IRMJ) **10**(1), 6–26 (1997)
32. Avgerou, C.: Information systems in developing countries: a critical research review. J. Inf. Technol. **23**(3), 133–146 (2008)
33. Heeks, R.: Information systems and developing countries: Failure, success, and local improvisations. Inf. Soc. **18**(2), 101–112 (2002)
34. O'Neill, M., Palmer, A., Charters, S., Fitz, F.: Service quality and consumer behavioural intention: An exploratory study from the Australian wine tourism sector. In Conference Proceedings Australian and New Zealand Marketing Academy Conference (pp. 1–5) (2001, December)
35. Welman, C., Kruger, F.: Research methodology for the business & administrative sciences. Oxford University Press (2001)
36. Al-Mushasha, N.F., Hassan, S.: A model for mobile learning service quality in university environment. Int. J. Mobile Comput. Multimedia Commun. **1**(1), 70–91 (2009)
37. Grohmann, G., Hofer, A., Martin, G.: ARIS MOBILE: helping to define the future of mobile learning. In International conference on mobile business (ICMB'05), pp. 213–219. IEEE, July 2005
38. Lee, H., Lee, Y., Yoo, D.: The determinants of perceived service quality and its relationship with satisfaction. J. Serv. Market. **14**(3), 217–231 (2000)

39. Mazur, G.H.: QFD for service industries Proceedings of The Fifth Symposium on QFD, pp. 1–17. Michigan, US, (1993)
40. Yoo, B., Donthu, N.: Developing a scale to measure the perceived quality of an Internet shopping site (SITEQUAL). Q. J. Electron. Commer. **2**(1), 31–45 (2001)
41. Bebko, C.P.: Service intangibility and its impact on consumer expectations of service quality. J. Serv. Mark. **14**(1), 9–26 (2000)
42. Sachdev, S.B., Verma, H.V.: Relative importance of service quality dimensions: a multi-sectoral study. J. Serv. Res. **4**(1), 93–116 (2004)
43. Llusar, J.C.B., Zornoza, C. C.: Validity and reliability in perceived quality measurement models. Int. J. Qual. Reliab. Manag, (2000)
44. Allwood, M.C., Kearney, M.C.: Compatibility and stability of additives in parenteral nutrition admixtures. Nutrition **14**(9), 697–706 (1998)
45. Bharati, P., Berg, D.: Service quality from the other side: information systems management at Duquesne Light. Int. J. Inf. Manag. **25**(4), 367–380 (2005)
46. Belardo, S.K. KR, Wallace, W.A.: DSS component design through field experimentation: an application to emergency management. In Proceedings of the third international conference on information systems (pp. 93–108), (1982)
47. Franz, C.R., Robey, D., Koeblitz, R.R.: User response to an online information system: a field experiment. MIS Q., 29–42 (1986)
48. Santos, J.: E-service quality: a model of virtual service quality dimensions. Manag. Serv. Qual. **13**(3), 233–246 (2003)
49. Khalifa, M., Liu, V.: Satisfaction with internet-based services: the role of expectations and desires. Int. J. Electron. Commer. **7**, 31–50 (2003)
50. Kotler, P.: Gary Armstrong. Am. Prentice-Hall Int. Inc, Principles of Marketing (1997)
51. Brown, S.P.: Effects of advertised customer satisfaction claims on consumer attitudes and purchase intention. J. Adv. Res. (1992)
52. Nielsen, J. (2005). Critical success factors for implementing ERP system. Qualitative case studies on implementation of enterprise wide systems, 211–231
53. Straub, Detmar, Loch, K., Evaristo, R., Karahanna, E., Srite, M.: Toward a theory based definition of culture. J. Glob. Inf. Manag. **10**(1), 13–23 (2002)
54. Santa, R.: An investigation of the alignment between technological innovation effectiveness and operational effectiveness. Central Queensland University, Faculty of Business and Informatics, (2009)
55. Whyte, G., Bytheway, A.: Factors affecting information systems' success. Int. J. Serv. Indust. Manag. (1996)
56. Allen, B.R., Boynton, A.C.: Information architecture: in search of efficient flexibility. MIS Quarterly, 435–445 (1991)
57. Amoroso, D.L.: Organizational issues of end-user computing. ACM Sigmis Database: Database Adv. Inf. Syst. **19**(3–4), 49–58 (1988)
58. Podsakoff, P.M., Organ, D.W.: Self-reports in organizational research: Problems and prospects. J. Manag. **12**(4), 531–544 (1986)
59. Bagozzi, R.P., Yi, Y., Phillips, L.W.: Assessing construct validity in organizational research. Adm. Sci. Q. **36**, 421–458 (1991)
60. Li, J., Rao, H.R.: Twitter as a rapid response news service: an exploration in the context of the 2008 China earthquake. The Electronic Journal of Information Systems in Developing Countries, **42**, (2010)
61. Halawi, L.A., McCarthy, R.V., Aronson, J.E.: An empirical investigation of knowledge management systems' success. J. Comput. Inf. Syst. **48**(2), 121–135 (2008)
62. Leung, Z.C., Cheung, C.F., Chan, K.T., Lo, K.H.: Effectiveness of knowledge management systems in social services: food assistance project as an example. Administration in Social Work **36**(3), 302–313 (2012)
63. Winnie, P. M. W.: The impact of trustworthiness and customer e-loyalty and e-satisfaction. Int J Acad Res Bus Soc Sci **4**(3), 390 (2014)

64. Wong, W. P. M., Lo, M. C., Ramayah, T.: The effects of technology acceptance factors on customer e-loyalty and e-satisfaction in Malaysia. Int J Bus Soc **15**(3), 477 (2014)
65. Sumo, R., van der Valk, W., van Weele, A. J., Bode, C.: Fostering incremental and radical innovation through performance-based contracting in inter-organizational relationships. Johannesburg, South-Africa (2015)
66. Lorenzo-Romero, C., Constantinides, E., Brünink, L. A.: Co-creation: Customer integration in social media based product and service development. Procedia Soc Beh Sci **148**, 383–396 (2014)
67. Henseler, J., Ringle, C.M., Sarstedt, M.: Using partial least squares path modeling in advertising research: basic concepts and recent issues. In Handbook of research on international advertising. Edward Elgar Publishing, (2012)
68. Monecke, A., Leisch, F.: semPLS: Structural equation modeling using partial least squares (2012)
69. Rubel, M.R.B., Kee, D.M.H.: Quality of work life and employee performance: antecedent and outcome of job satisfaction in Partial Least Square (PLS). World Appl. Sci. J. **31**(4), 456–467 (2014)
70. Iivari, J.: An empirical test of the DeLone-McLean model of information system success. ACM SIGMIS Database: The DATABASE for Advances in Information Systems, **36**(2), 8–27 (2005)
71. Lee, S. Y., Petrick, J. F., Crompton, J.: The roles of quality and intermediary constructs in determining festival attendees' behavioral intention. J Travel Res **45**(4), 402–412 (2007)
72. Ratnasingam, P., Pavlou, P.A., Tan, Y.H.: The importance of technology trust for B2B electronic commerce. In 15th Bled Electronic Commerce Conference eReality, Constructing the eEconomy, Bled, Slovenia, June 2002
73. Kopečný, R., Ihnátová, Z.: The use of managing stress strategies in the profession of a media creator, (2014)
74. Amoroso, D.L., Cheney, P.H.: Testing a causal model of end-user application effectiveness. J. Manag. Inf. Syst. **8**(1), 63–89 (1991)
75. Ang, C.L., Davies, M.A., Finlay, P.N.: An empirical model of IT usage in the Malaysian public sector. J. Strateg. Inf. Syst. **10**(2), 159–174 (2001)
76. Bailey, J.E., Pearson, S.W.: Development of a tool for measuring and analyzing computer user satisfaction. Manag. Sci. **29**(5), 530–545 (1983)
77. Brown, T. (2004). The role of m-learning in the future of e-learning in Africa. 21st ICDE World Conference. Retrieved from http://www.tml.tkk.fi/Opinnot/T-110.556/2004/Materiaali/brown03.pdf
78. Chan, T., Sedera, D., Gable, G.G.: Re-conceptualizing information system success: the IS-impact measurement model. J. Assoc. Inf. Syst. **9**(7), 2 (2008)
79. Chin, W.W.: Issues and opinion on structural equation modeling. MIS Q. **22**(1), vii–xvi (1998)
80. Garrity, E., Glasberg, B., Kim, Y.J., Sanders, L., Shin, S.K.: An experimental investigation of web-based information systems success in the context of electronic commerce. Decis. Support Syst. **39**(3), 485–503 (2005)
81. Guimaraes, T., Igbaria, M.: Exploring the relationship between IC success and company performance. Inf. Manag. **26**(3), 133–141 (1994)
82. Hair Jr, J.F., Hult, G.T.M., Ringle, C., Sarstedt, M.: A primer on partial least squares structural equation modeling (PLS-SEM), Sage Publications, 2013
83. Jennex, M.E., Olfman, L.: Organizational memory/knowledge effects on productivity, a longitudinal study. Paper presented at the system sciences, 2002. HICSS. Proceedings of the 35th Annual Hawaii International Conference on, (2002)
84. Kettinger, W.J., Lee, C.C.: Perceived service quality and user satisfaction with the information services function. Decis. Sci. **25**(5–6), 737–766 (1994)
85. Kettinger, W.J., Lee, C.C.: Zones of tolerance: alternative scales for measuring information systems service quality. Mis Quarterly, 607–623 (2005)
86. Khalifa, M., Abidi, R., Limayem, M.: Effects of electronic customer relationship management on online shopping satisfaction. Paper presented at the Pre-ICIS Meeting on French Speaking World IS Research, (2002)

87. Khalifa, M., Shen, N.: Effects of electronic customer relationship management on customer satisfaction: a temporal model. Paper presented at the System Sciences, 2005. HICSS'05. Proceedings of the 38th Annual Hawaii International Conference on, (2005)
88. Kotler, P., Lee, N.R.: Social marketing: influencing behaviors for good, Sage Publications, 2011
89. Leedy, P.D., Ormrod, J.E.: Practical research: Pearson Merrill Prentice Hall Columbus, OH, (2005)
90. Lee-Post, A.: e-Learning success model: an information systems perspective. Electron. J. e-Learning, **7**(1), (2009)
91. Li, Y., Yeh, Y.: Service qualitys impact on mobile satisfaction and intention to use 3G service. Proceedings of the 42nd Hawaii Internatioal Conference on System Sciences, p. 110. Hawaii, US, (2009)
92. Myers, M., Tan, F.: Beyond models of national culture in information systems research. J. Glob. Inf. Manag. **10**(1), 24–32 (2002)
93. Nielsen, J.: Usability metrics: tracking interface improvements. IEEE Softw. **13**(6), 12–13 (1996)
94. Pitt, L. F., Watson, R. T., & Kavan, C. B. (1997). Measuring information systems service quality: concerns for a complete canvas. Mis Quarterly, 209–221
95. Szajna, B.: Empirical evaluation of the revised technology acceptance model. Manag. Sci. **42**(1), 85–92 (1996)
96. Von Dran, G., Zhang, P.: A theoretical model of quality websites: a multi-disciplinary conceptualization. In Decision Sciences Institute 2002 Proceedings pp. 645–650, (2002)

IoMT-Based Smart Diagnostic/Therapeutic Kit for Pandemic Patients

M. Parimala Devi, G. Boopathi Raja, V. Gowrishankar, and T. Sathya

Abstract In the present situation, most of the patients suffered from pandemic diseases such as COVID-19, Ebola, etc. The infected people might have an incubation period of 1–14 days before creating any symptoms. The most widely recognized symptoms of coronavirus illness are high fever, breathing problem, and dry cough. Most of the patients (about 80%) recover from the illness without developing any major symptoms. This disease may be complicated rarely since it is more critical for aged people and even become fatal. The people with other major health problems, for example, asthma, diabetes, obesity, or heart disease might be progressively helpless against getting seriously sick. They lost their life before diagnosing specific medical problems. Since it requires huge investment in maintenance, diagnosis as well as treatment, and also it consumes time to provide a test as well as to investigate the patients' past clinical history. Numerous researches were undergone all over the world to smart kit the patients' past clinical records were stored in IoT cloud database. The security and privacy medical record of the patients is protected. This cloud access database provides the past medical history to the healthcare professionals to rescue the patient from a serious illness. Also, the current health status of the pandemic patients is continuously monitored through wireless telemetry technique Message Queue Telemetry Transport Protocol (MQTT). Based on the patient's live status, the health specialists suggest the medicine and/or recommend the precaution steps and provide the treatment effectively without direct contact with them.

M. Parimala Devi (✉) · G. B. Raja · V. Gowrishankar · T. Sathya
Department of Electronics and Communication Engineering, Velalar College of Engineering and Technlology, Erode, Tamil Nadu, India
e-mail: parimaladevi.vlsi@gmail.com

G. B. Raja
e-mail: g.boopathiraja14@gmail.com

V. Gowrishankar
e-mail: shankargow@gmail.com

T. Sathya
e-mail: sathyamce@gmail.com

© The Editor(s) (if applicable) and The Author(s), under exclusive license to Springer Nature Singapore Pte Ltd. 2020

C. Chakraborty et al. (eds.), *Internet of Medical Things for Smart Healthcare*, Studies in Big Data 80, https://doi.org/10.1007/978-981-15-8097-0_6

Keywords COVID-19 · Smart kit · IoMT · Pandemic · MQTT

1 Introduction

Tragically, the elder aged population and the patients with constant health ailment is setting critical strain on present day patients' health monitoring frameworks [1, 2] and increasing demand rapidly on the assets and/or resources from patients' clinic beds to specialists and medical caretakers [3]. Rapidly increasing demand on healthcare frameworks may be reduced with the suitable way that gives highest consideration to the highly risk patients.

The Internet of medical things (IoMT) has been perceived as the most appreciable way to minimize the demand on healthcare monitoring frameworks [4–8]. A lot of this exploration takes more concentration in the monitoring of patients' health with most explicit conditions such as diabetes [6] or Parkinson's illness [7]. Further research would like to fill express needs, for instance, supporting recovery (aiding rehabilitation) through consistent checking of a patient's progression [8]. Crisis medicinal services administrations have furthermore been perceived as an opportunity by related works [9, 10], anyway has not yet been for the most part investigated.

A few similar existing works have recently introduced explicit zones and the modern advancements identified and studied with Internet of things (IoT) health care. A major research review has been introduced in [11, 12], which mainly focuses on commercially accessible frameworks, potential applications, and other associated issues. Each and every concept is considered individually, instead of as a feature of an overall design framework. Several sensor types such as pulse, temperature, pressure, and humidity are available in practice and are compared in [13], with some emphasis on communication. Finally, in [10], sensing the physical quantity and big data handling management is identified as the most essential for any network that supports communication.

In this way, this report makes a unique responsibility in that it recognizes every key components of end-to-end IoT healthcare monitoring framework and proposes a traditional model that could be applied to all IoT-based healthcare monitoring systems. This is most essential as there are still no known end-to-end IoT frameworks for constant remote monitoring of patients' health.

This work further gives a broad review of the cutting edge progressions that fall inside the proposed model. The primary objective is determined to sensors for monitoring distinctive clinical parameters, short-and-long-range communication measures, and cloud procedures. This work isolates itself from the past critical audit duties by considering every fundamental and essential part of an IoT-based healthcare monitoring system both separately and as a system.

Further, the significant commitment is made by setting target around low-power wide-area networks (LPWANs), including their intriguing suitability for use with regards to IoT structures. The upcoming approved band measures, for instance, narrowband IoT, are differentiated and the battling unlicensed-band standards, with explicit excitement for appropriateness to social insurance applications [14].

The remaining outline of this chapter is structured as follows. Section 1 explored the Internet of things (IoT) field in healthcare system and analyze the various concepts and techniques existing in the field of IoMT. Section 2 discusses the various pandemic diseases along with symptoms that arise in the world. Section 3 reviews the attractive features of existing healthcare systems available in market and also discuss the problem associated with it. Section 4 highlights the various types of telemetry techniques. Section 5 enhances the functionalities of proposed system in healthcare services and provides recommendations to enhance this research. Section 6 concludes the work, summarizing the important innovations and highlight the outline of IoMT areas where further research is needed.

2 Pandemic Diseases—Symptoms and Treatments

An outbreak is the case at which an ailment occurs in startling high numbers. It might remain in one zone or broaden all the more generally. An outbreak can occur within few days or it may take several days or sometimes years. In such case, specialists think about a solitary instance of an infectious disease to be an outbreak. This might be valid if it's an obscure illness, if it's new to a network, or if it's been missing from a populace for quite a while.

An epidemic is the situation at which an irresistible sickness spreads quickly to a greater number of people than pros would envision. It influences a greater zone than an outbreak.

A pandemic is a severe disease outbreak that spreads across several nations, probably entire world. It affects a larger number of peoples rapidly in a dense area and takes a greater number of lives than an epidemic. The World Health Organization (WHO) announced COVID-19 to be a pandemic when it turned out to be uncertain that the disease was serious and that it was spreading rapidly over a wide territory.

Figure 1 shows the different stage of disease outbreak along with their impact on economy and possibility of occurrences annually.

Figure 2 shows the comparison table of various pandemic outbreaks occurred in the world along with their mortality rate.

The WHO's pandemic prepared system ranges from Stage 1 (a for the most part protected) to Stage 6 (a full pandemic):

- **Stage 1**: An infection disease has caused to people with unknown infection from animals.
- **Stage 2**: The infection from animals has made people to sick.
- **Stage 3**: There is large number of affected patients from the infection. If the infection is spreading from human to human, it's not extensive enough to cause network level flare-up.

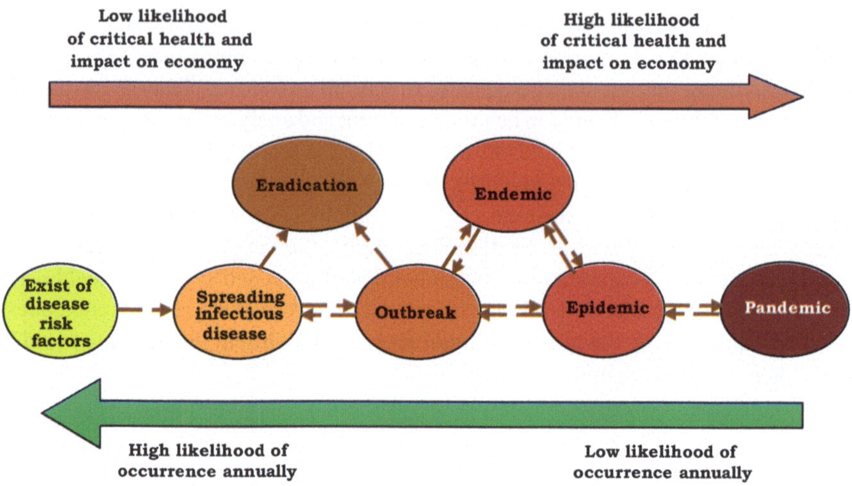

Fig. 1 Different stages of disease outbreak

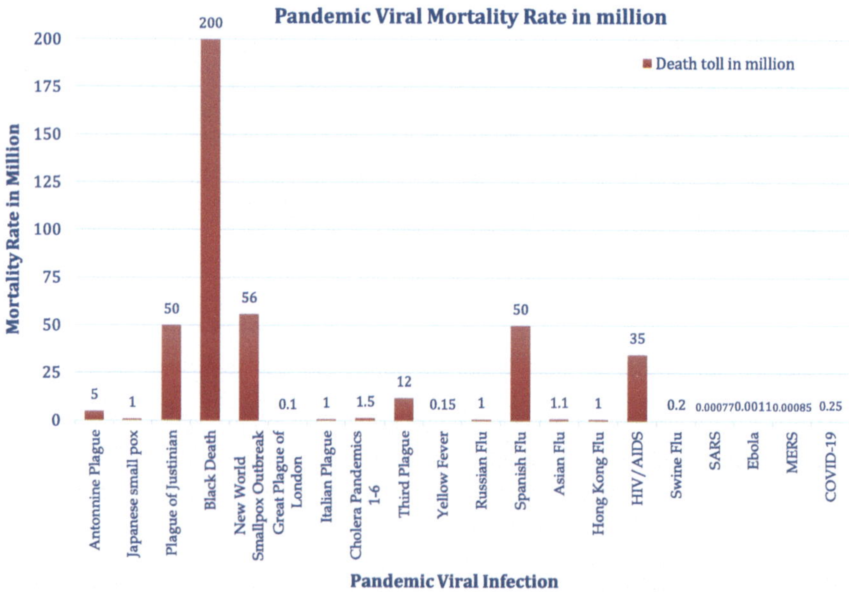

Fig. 2 Comparison of various pandemics with mortality rate

- **Stage 4**: The infection disease is effectively spreading from affected person to healthy person with affirmed flare-up which influences community level.
- **Stage 5**: The infectious disease is growing exponentially among people in more than one country.

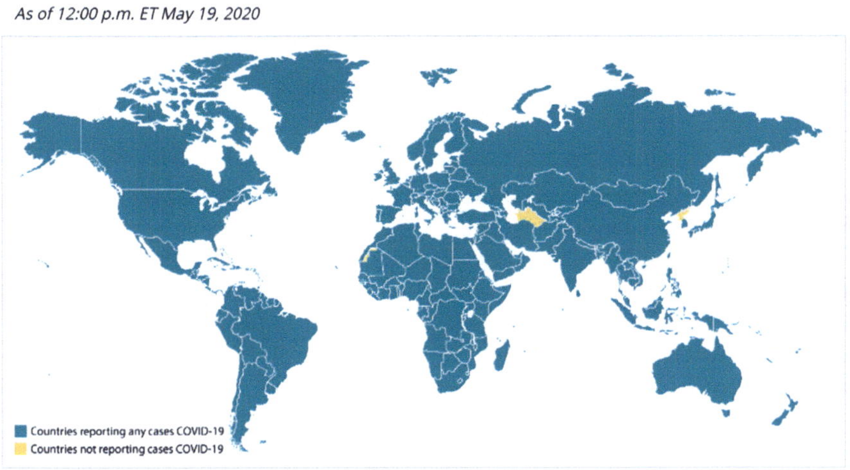

Fig. 3 Global case numbers reported by WHO and CDC (*data obtained from www.cdc.gov) [15]

- **Stage 6**: At least one more nation, in a substitute zone from Stage 5, has a community level outbreak.

2.1 Coronavirus Disease 2019 (COVID-19)

The region of corona affected and unaffected regions in the world are shown in Fig. 3. This global case number data can be reported by WHO and taken from official CDC Web site [15].

2.2 COVID Symptoms

Patients with corona infection may have mild symptoms to severe health illness. Elder peoples and adults who have extreme health ailments like heart or lung infection or diabetes appear to be at higher risk for COVID-19 illness.

The COVID-19 patients have larger possibilities of side effects detailed—going from mild indications to severe illness.

The symptoms may be noted visibly in the coronavirus affected patients even from second day and/or sometimes it takes up to 14 days after the corona infection. The most commonly observed side effects of COVID-19 patients are listed as follows, [16]:

- Dry cough
- Severe fever
- Shortness of breathing or breathing difficulty

- Body/muscle pain
- Chillness
- Lack of taste or smell
- Sore throat.

This is not all potential indications of corona patients. In few cases, some other different side effects have been observed including gastrointestinal side effects like nausea, vomiting, or diarrhea.

The Indian Council of Medical Research gave guidelines to begin fast antibody-based blood tests for COVID-19 in certain control zones and in enormous gathering center. Figure 4 shows the different phases of COVID-19 treatment.

The testing convention is portrayed in a given Fig. 5. That is, the individuals who have suspected for flu-like diseases could, after 14 days of being isolated, could be tested for an antibody-based test. If the test is negative, a hereditary test could be done to confirm or they could be isolated for 14 days more before another antibody-based test.

Serological tests can play an essential role during a lockdown since they can be utilized to recognize the individuals who do and don't have immunity to the new coronavirus. For instance, all health personnel as well as workers who perform essential functions (including police and fire-fighters) could be tested to allow those with immunity to get back to the frontlines.

The tests can distinguish forthcoming blood-plasma donors. Plasma is the one which is left over after separating the various cells in blood which contains antibodies and coagulant factors. The researchers identified and concluded that plasma from infected people containing neutralizing antibodies could improve the clinical illness of COVID-19 patients.

3 Application of IoT in Health care

Several efficient systems are available in practice nowadays in order to diagnosis and/or to provide treatment for pandemic patients [17]. Some of them are explained as below.

3.1 IoT-Based PCR for the Identification of Pandemic Disease

The block diagram of IoT-based PCR framework for pandemic disease detection is shown in Fig. 6 [18]. When the sample possibly containing the DENV is handled at focal point area, the results of diagnostic techniques as well as GPS directions of the patients' area are consequently moved by means of the client's cell phone interface through a worldwide system to a control community. The recovered information can

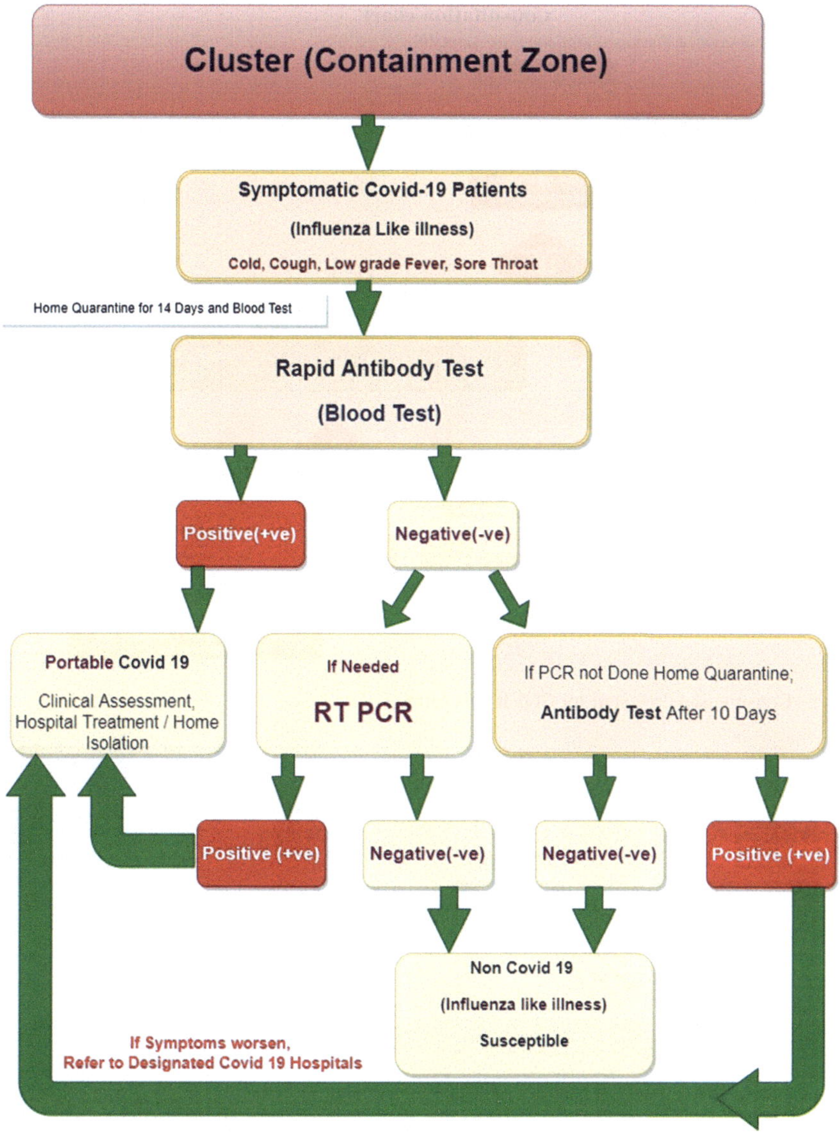

Fig. 4 Different phases of COVID-19 treatment

be prepared and put away in cloud. In light of this gathered data, infection flare-up guide can be created by indicating the illness episode zone and carry out regular monitoring.

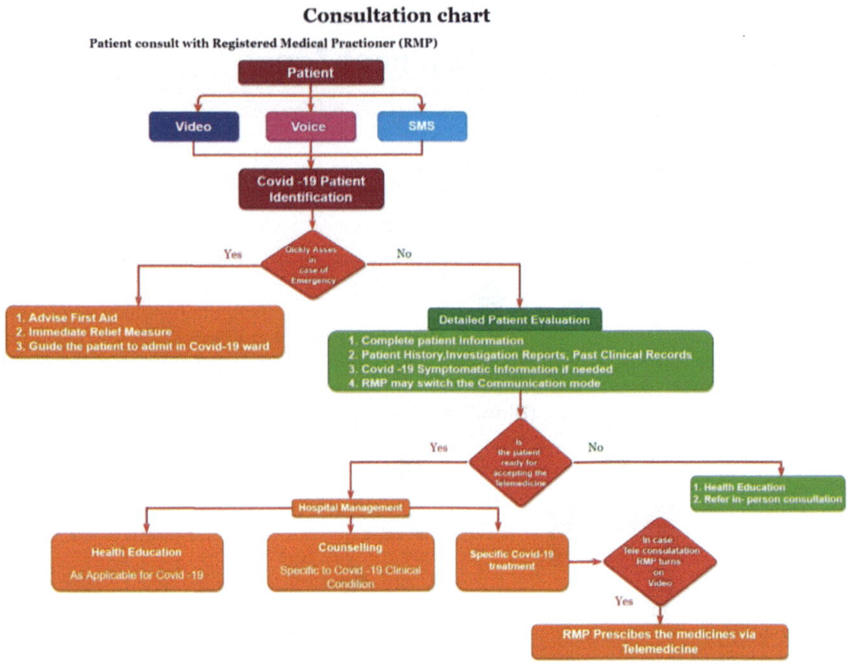

Fig. 5 Consultation flowchart for COVID-19 patients

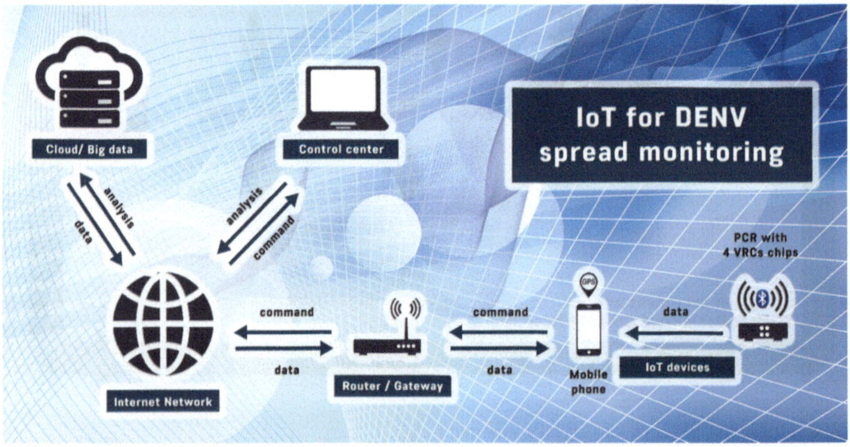

Fig. 6 Schematic diagram illustrates the IoT framework for the DENV spread monitoring [18]

3.2 IoT for Smart Health care

Figure 7 shows the concept of IoT-based smart healthcare setup for patient monitoring, [1]. The essential parameters such as respiratory rate, pulse rate, and body temperature are captured through sensors, processed and stored in the cloud as a patient database. Whenever need arises, these data can be accessed by specialist or other technicians effectively.

(1) Central node and wearable sensor

Wearable sensor nodes are only a devices or gadgets that can quantify physiological conditions. The recommended sensors are those that measure the imperative symptoms, for example, respiratory rate, pulse rate, and body temperature level. The each and every single sensor hubs gathers physiological information independently and moves altogether to the central node. It performs procedure on this information, in view of this, it might take some choice and afterward moves this data to an external environment.

(2) Communication over short-range

For sensors to communicate with the central node, this short-range communication technique is required. There are a couple of noteworthy necessities to consider while selecting a short-range communication standard, in view of the impacts on the human body, security, and latency.

(3) Communication for long-range

The sensed data collected by the central node is not valuable except if something should be conceivable with it. This data should be sent to a database where applicable gatherings, (for example, guardians or specialists) can safely access it. Also, there are a couple of considerations since quite a while ago run correspondences standard

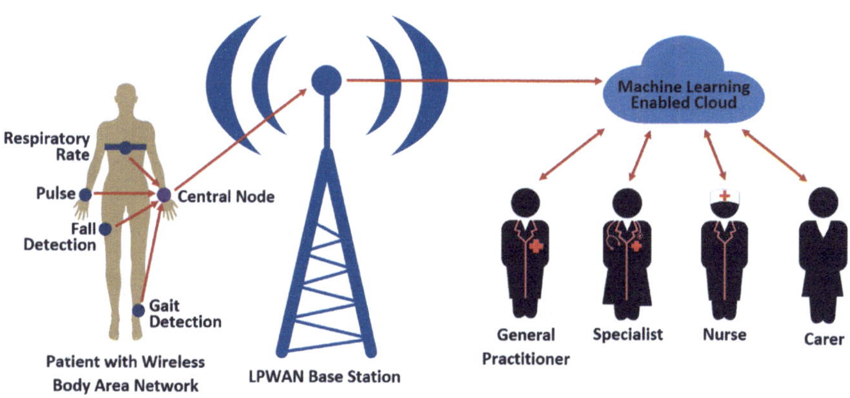

Fig. 7 Smart healthcare model for patient monitoring using IoT [1]

for use in a healthcare systems, including data security, error detecting and correcting capabilities, robustness, lower delay, latency and higher data accessibility. The error correcting capabilities and robustness are considered as more important in long-range communication against noise interference, as these guarantee that the data sent is equivalent to the data received.

(4) Secured architecture for cloud storage

The medical record and clinical data procured from patients must be taken care of securely for sometime later. Social insurance specialists benefit by knowing a patient's clinical history, machine learning (ML) and deep learning (DL) fruitful with the exception of if tremendous databases of information are available to it. The distributed cloud storage is the most useful practical method for putting away immense huge data. In any case, giving availability to social insurance experts without trading-off security is a key worry that ought to be tended to by specialists creating healthcare IoT devices. ML offers the likelihood to perceive inclines in clinical information that were beforehand dark, give treatment plans and diagnostics, and offer best proposals to social protection specialists that are express to individual patients.

3.3 *IoT-Based Wearable Smart Health Monitoring System*

Figure 8 describes the block diagram of smart health monitoring system with wearable sensors based on IoT concepts to monitor the status of patients' health, [19]. In this system, Arduino Pro Mini is utilized as microcontroller and the communication module is preferred as HC-06 Bluetooth module. Mostly, the physiological parameters can be measured by using pulse sensor and the body temperature can be continuously sensed with the help of smart thermometer or temperature sensor. The

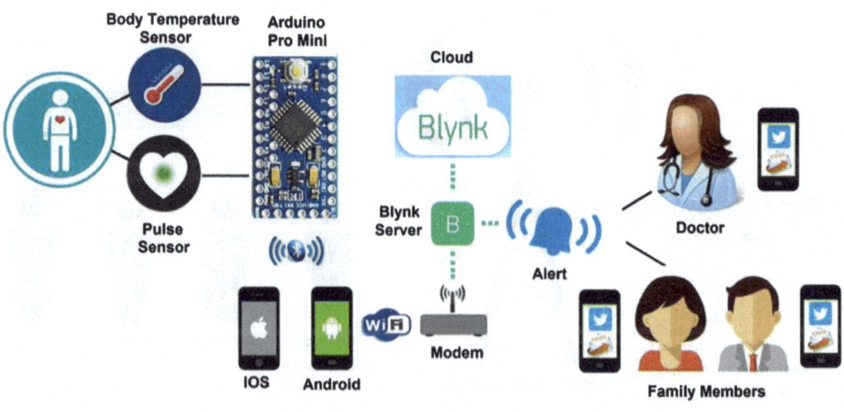

Fig. 8 IoT-based wearable smart health monitoring system [19]

basic idea of this efficient health monitoring system is shown in figure. This system consists of Arduino board (especially Arduino Pro Mini), Bluetooth module (HC-06), physiological sensors, and Blynk application with Wi-Fi/Internet connectivity.

4 Telemetry Principles

Telemetry is defined as the technique that collects measured parameters or other information at inaccessible or remote points and it allows sharing the sensed information to the desired persons/control unit or receiver for continuous monitoring, [20]. The word telemetry is arises from Greek word, where ‘tele’ means remote and ‘metry’ means measure.

A telemeter is a device used to measure any physical parameter remotely. It comprises of a sensor/actuator, a transmitting channel and a display unit, recording, or controlling gadget. Telemeters are the physical component utilized in telemetry. Telemetry techniques utilize several electronic gadgets and can be accessed remotely or hard-wired, it may be simple or computerized.

4.1 Wireless Radio Telemetry

Radio telemetry allows to analyze the physiological information of human under critical emergency conditions and in normal environmental factors with no inconvenience or deterrent to the individual or creature under scrutiny [20]. Elements impacting sound and wiped out people during the presentation of their every day errands may in this way be effortlessly perceived and assessed. Remote bio-telemetry has made conceivable the investigation of dynamic subjects under conditions that so far disallowed estimations. It is, along these lines, an imperative strategy in circumstances where no link association is plausible.

By bio-telemetry, the physiological signs can be acquired from swimmers, riders, competitors, pilots, or unskilled workers. Telemetric reconnaissance is generally helpful during transportation inside the medical clinic territory also for the consistent observing of patients sent to different wards or facilities for registration or treatment.

5 IoMT Framework for Pandemic Patients

The objective of the IoMT framework is to remotely monitoring the COVID-19 suspected and confirmed patients with primary symptoms and also those patients are allowed This framework not only monitor the key clinical data’s who are kept at self-quarantine safely in the home environment with least complications and with necessary safety guidelines and forward the time stamped sensor value of the patient

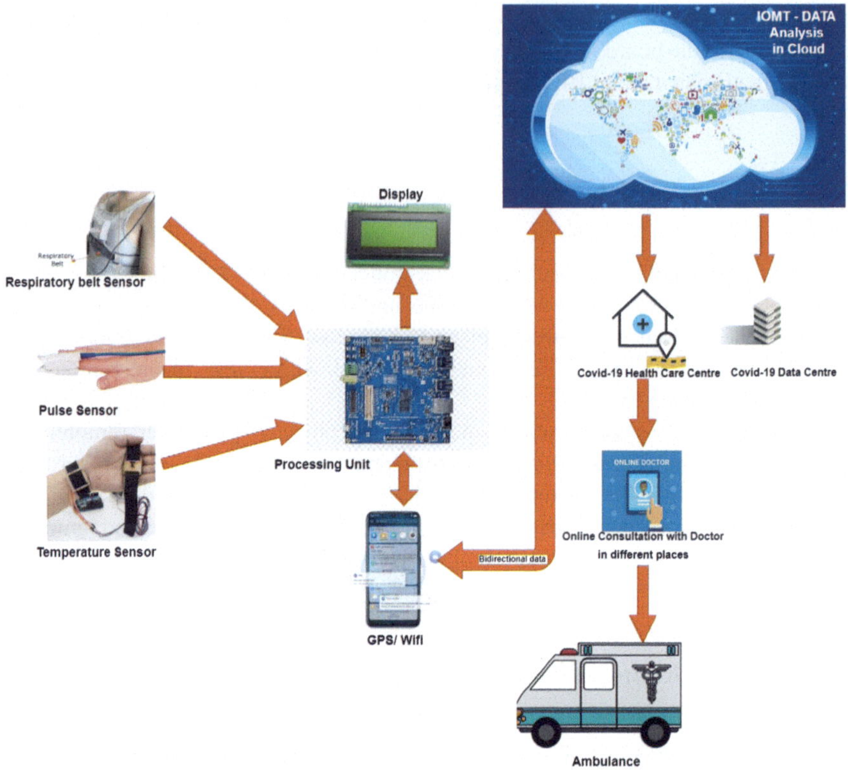

Fig. 9 Overall system architecture and communication

to IoT platform for data analysis and visualization. The patients' aggregate data is forward to healthcare center and alerts would be triggered based on the individual patient readings. Figure 9 shows overall IoMT framework for pandemic patients.

Because of implementing the proposed assisting and monitoring system, there exists a harmonious environment which is created between the family and friends of COVID-patients.

This kit helps the doctors and healthcare professionals to prefer the proper decision in due course. This system also helps the healthcare workers to monitor the clinical data of the COVID-19 patients with ease of time and the data of patients are collected without being contacted from the patients. These systems have four sensors to periodically get the patient data, mobile phones for monitoring and connectivity, IoT which enables cloud services and software to establish a connectivity.

Figure 10 shows the architecture of the smart healthcare kit for COVID-19 patients. The smart kit consists of different precision sensors to monitor breathing rate, fever, and heartbeat rate of a patient through data acquired by the processing unit which is connected to the patient mobile phones through inbuilt Wi-Fi. The patient data are post or published to IoT cloud platform using HTTP or MQTT protocol

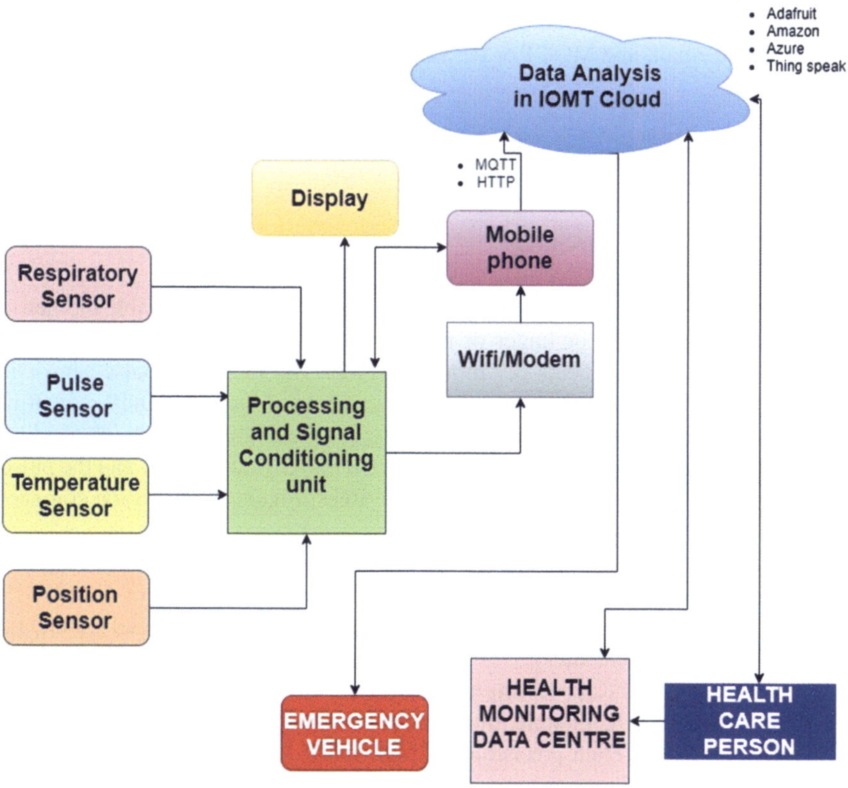

Fig. 10 Architecture of smart healthcare kit

for data analysis and management. The smart kit monitors COVID-19 patients in real time in the prescribed time stamp interval. The efficiency of this monitoring kit can be improved effectively by the data from the various sensors interfaced particularly with that system and the obtained data are stored in the cloud. The proposed healthcare system is providing highly reliable and it is convenient for the COVID-19 patients who are kept at quarantine and recommended to stay away for about 14 days to 28 days as mentioned by the guidelines of World Health Organization (WHO). These kits also help the suspected COVID-19 patients who wish follow the self-quarantine and also helps the patients and healthcare providers to monitor many patients at a time and improve the improve healthcare system of the country in the medical emergency period.

The vital importance of the proposed smart kits is not only monitored health status collected from patient's data through the IoMT frameworks but also allows the pandemic data center to save the critical illness of the patient continuously. The cloud storage of the patient's record helps the clinical data by authorized healthcare personals and doctors at any time across the country or world. The live status of the patients can be send to the family members through any of the services webhook, Twitter, SMS, email, and MQTT or REST-based mobile app.

5.1 Components in the Smart Kit Design

5.1.1 Heartbeat Measurement

The heartbeat rate of the individual patient can be measured by wearable biometric pulse sensor in the wrist or finger of the patient. This compact biometric sensor measures the number of beats per minute (BPM). The biometric pulse sensor is connected to processing unit to read out the heart rate of the COVID-19 patient in quarantine center or hospital. The analogously detected value changes, depending on the pulse beat. The analog values are converted into digital by ADC and the pulse is measured on the basis of the last measured values. Figure 11 shows the compact wrist pulse sensor for pandemic patients.

A small module which is connected to the processing unit Raspberry Pi, the pulse sensor will measures pulse of the patient and the health condition of COVID-19 patients is monitored. This sensor consumes low-power consumption and it could be operated by lithium–ion battery.

The Raspberry Pi the processing unit can read only digital information as they do not have inbuilt ADC module, thus an analog-to-digital converter is needed for taking measurements. High precision and high speed ADC module are needed for effective performance.

In order to convert the analog data of the pulse sensor 10 bit MCP3008 ADC is utilized. Figure 11 shows Raspberry Pi and heart rate monitor—connection setup. The positive pin of the biometric pulse sensor is connected to supply pin of the Raspberry Pi and negative is connected to ground. The signal which is to be measured is connected to Channel 0 of the ADC. The processing units aggregate the collected

Fig. 11 Wrist pulse sensor for patient

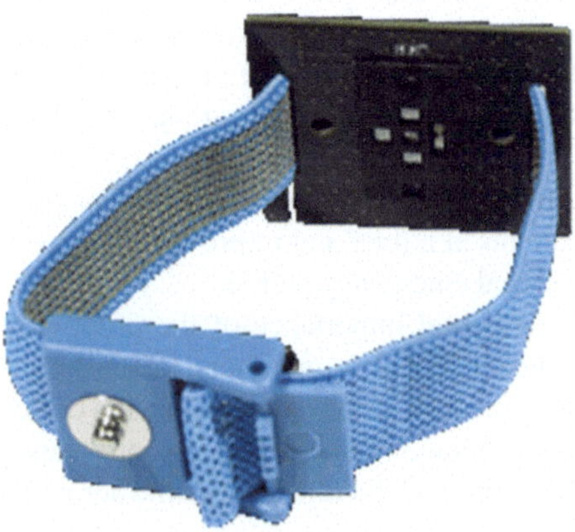

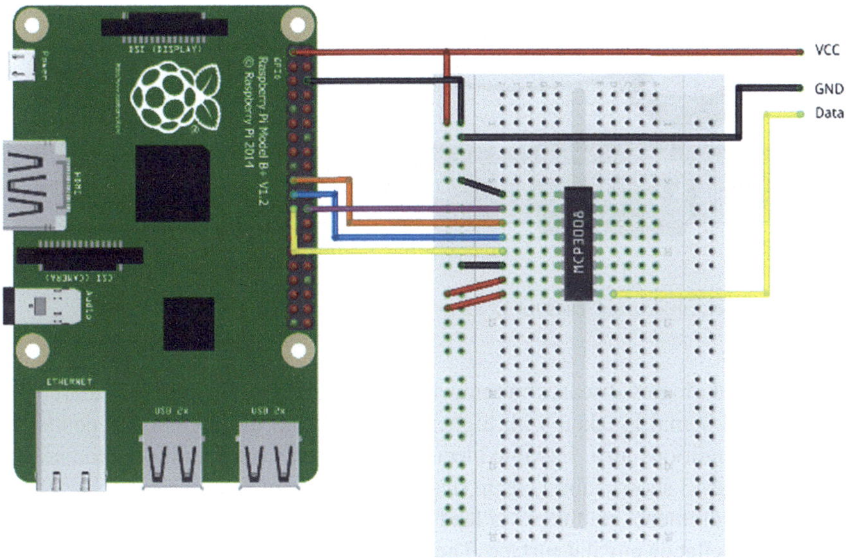

Fig. 12 Raspberry Pi and heart rate monitor—connection setup

data and publish it to the IoT cloud. The module would provide unobstructed heart health condition for individuals (Fig. 12).

Breathing Rate Sensor

For COVID-19 patient's serious symptoms is difficult in breathing and chest pain. It is very important to measure the breathing rate with heterogeneous wearable respiration belt sensor and ECG monitoring for COVID-19 patients with least patient contact. By precisely tracking respiratory rate, the abnormality can be detected in earlier stage without any indication of deterioration. This helps to identify the abnormalities due to COVID-19 for the suspected cases clearly.

From the literature survey, respiratory rate and ECG sensor technologies have evolved many different types for medical applications and use wide parameters to arrive at accurate readings.

The two sensors connected inside of a soft, flexible, and washable belt of the patient are ECG sensor and breathing sensor. The belt is strapped around the chest. When the chest of the patient expands and contracts regularly because of breathing the air in and out lungs. The analog signal received from the sensor is converted into digital by using appropriate ADC.

The on-body electrocardiogram (ECG) is diagnostic tool which is used to measure the bioelectrical and muscular functionality of the human heart. Hence, ECG biosignal is recorded at regular interval for COVID-19 patients who are under quarantine and those who are suspected. The ECG is recorded to analyze and identify the myriad

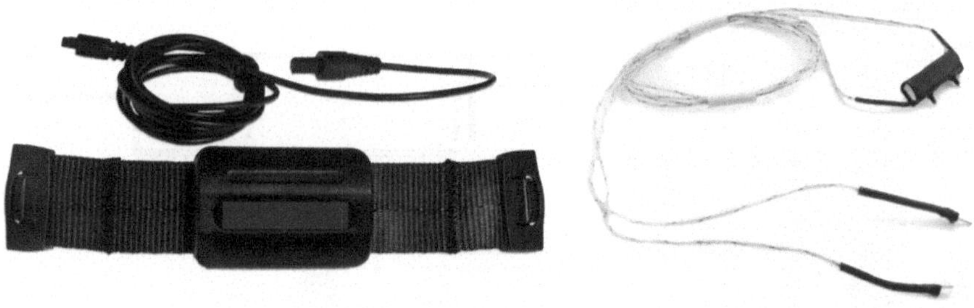

Fig. 13 Fabric electrodes and leads for ECG monitoring

of cardiac pathologies diseases ranging from myocardial ischemia and infarction. The bio-ECG signal is taken with highest accuracy and the accuracy depends on the testing conditions also. Flexible electrodes are to measure multiple biomedical signals. Figure 13 shows fabric electrodes and leads for ECG monitoring.

ECG measurements are taken via leads that are placed on the patient body while the patient lies flat on any flat surface. The graph or a regular pattern of PQRST wave shows the abnormal electric activity if there are any abnormal cardiac rhythmic activities. The underlying heart beat and abnormal rhythm mechanism of the heart are measured effectively and passed to IoT cloud platform for further processing.

Mobile App

The mobile app using MQTT protocol subscribes the individual patient health status. Figure 14 shows the snapshot of the patient or healthcare professional mobile application. The application has feature to view individual sensor value and its graph.

GLCD

Figure 15 shows wrist GLCD displaying the ECG graph which had been sent by the processing unit of the smart kit.

Figure 16 shows the Microsoft Azure IoT dashboard with live ECG wave.

5.1.2 Respiration Rate Sensor

The essential and foremost symptoms of SARS are abnormal respiratory rate. The COVID-19 patients are severely affected by respiratory troubles and hence it is very important to measure the respiratory rate at the earliest as soon as possible. But it is not an easy thing to measure respiratory rate during critical stage as it is an indicator of patient live status. Respiration rate module not only can provide an early warning of breathing problem and tiredness but also the critical illness due to COVID-19.

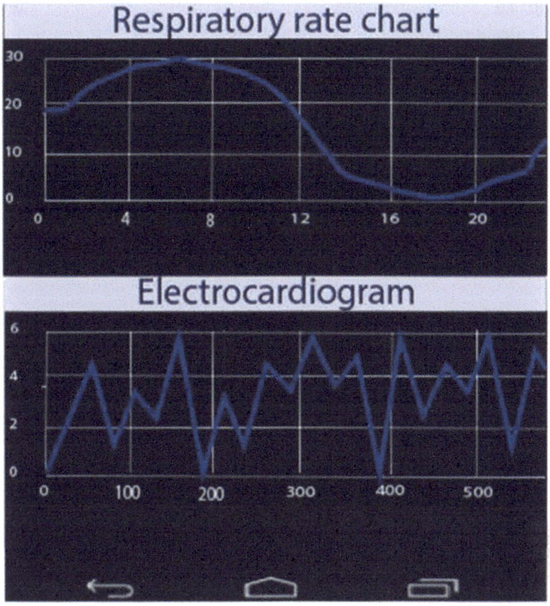

Fig. 14 Mobile app respiration and ECG status of the patient

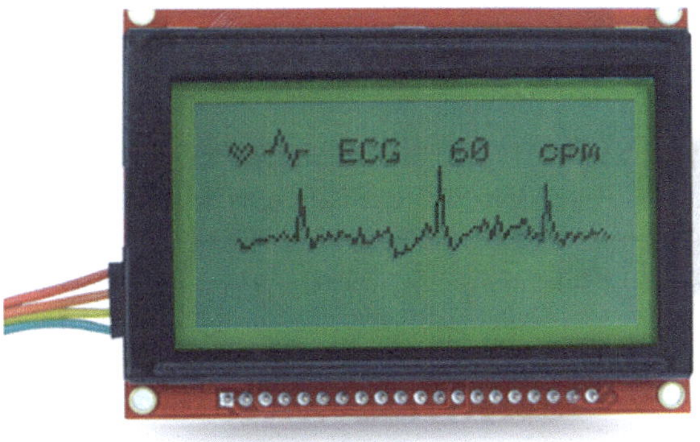

Fig. 15 Wrist GLCD ECG waveform of the patient

Nostril type sensor measures the breathing rate of the patient under critical condition and it indicates the abnormalities in continuous interval. This sensor module has a flexible hose which placed behind the ears, and a set of prongs which are placed under the human nostrils. Breathing rate is measured by these prong sensor module.

The thermocouple is placed in the compact small holder that allows the placement adjustment of sensor in the required position to accurately measure the airflow changes as well as the nasal air temperature. This sensor module is an easy to install and use. The healthy human has a breathing rate of 15–30 breaths per minute.

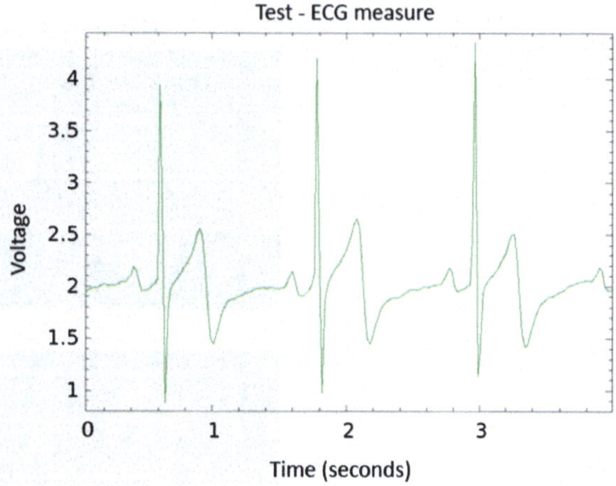

Fig. 16 Microsoft Azure IoT dashboard ECG measured graph

Figure 17 shows the mobile app showing the waveform of respiratory rate and electrocardiogram of the pandemic patients (Fig. 18).

Figure 19 shows the wrist GLCD of the pandemic patients connected to the processing unit. The live data is shown in patient wrist band.

Figure 20 shows the Microsoft Azure IoT dashboard respiration measured graph.

5.1.3 Temperature Sensor

The important symptom of pandemic disease COVID-19 is prolonged high fever. To measure temperature in different places of human body, the very high accurate thermometer sensor is utilized in the smart kit. More than one sensor unit is placed in different parts of the human body. The measured temperature would help the healthcare personals to identify the level illness of the patients in the quarantine. Figure 21 shows the body contact type thermometer module for Raspberry Pi.

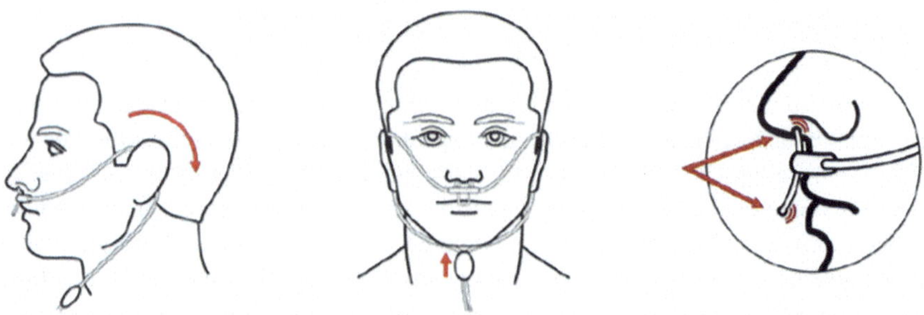

Fig. 17 Respiration measurement

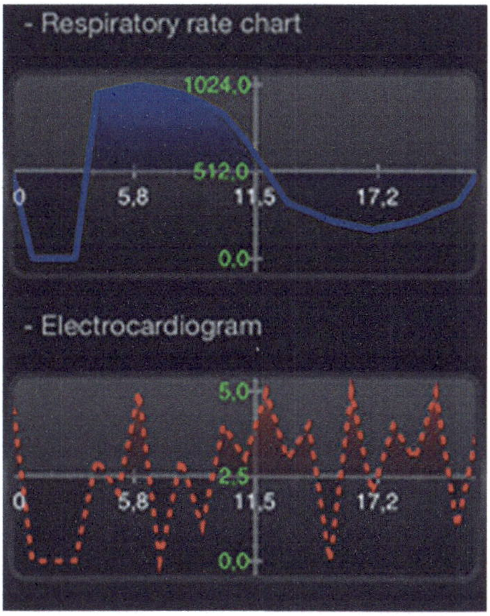

Fig. 18 Respiration live time stamp graph on mobile app

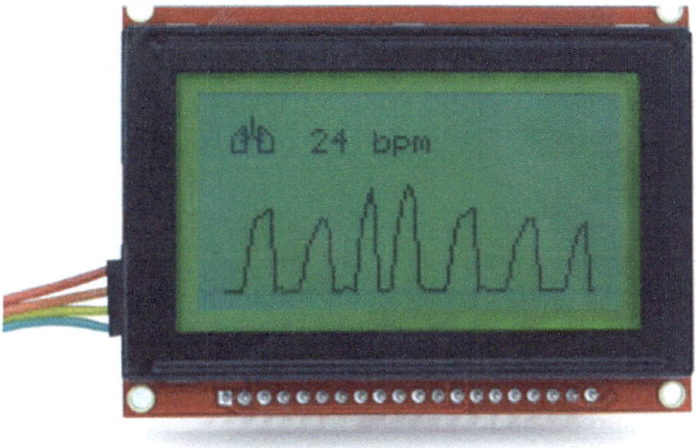

Fig. 19 Wrist GLCD respiration waveform of the patient

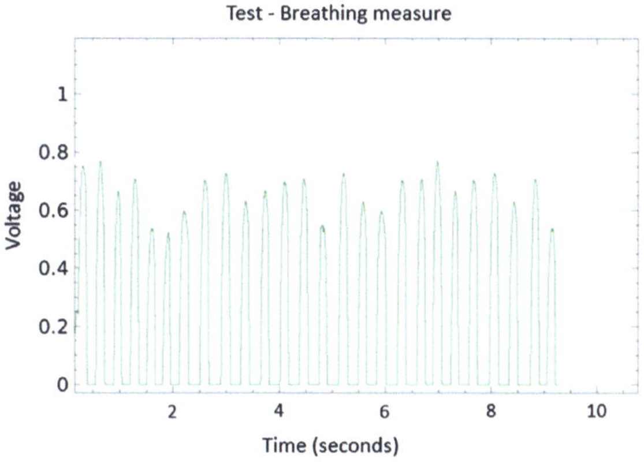

Fig. 20 Microsoft Azure IoT dashboard respiration measured graph

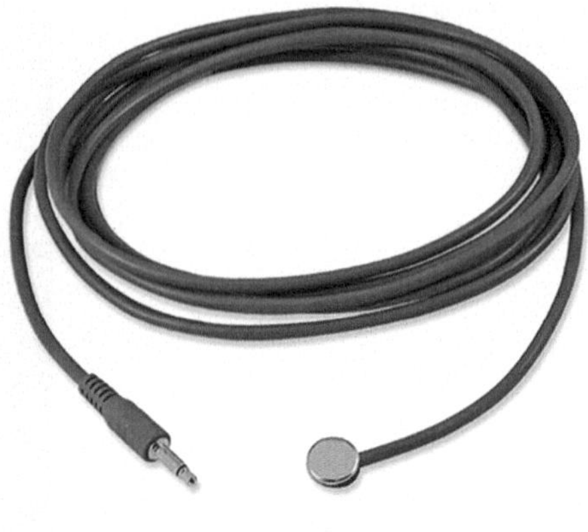

Fig. 21 Body contact type thermometer

A normal body temperature of a non-affected person is 37.0°C (98.6°F). The normal temperature of the adults may vary about 0.9°F in a day, and hence the continuous monitoring is needed.

Most of the pandemic diseases symptoms are fever that can be continuously monitored by the IoT cloud platform with thermometer sensor module attached to human body and the efficiency of evaluation and treatment done by the physician improves largely by this continuous monitoring technique. The smart kit utilizes the body contact type thermometer instead of contact-less infrared type as they could be easily sanitized after the use by the patient. Table 1 shows temperature range for various pandemic diseases.

For taking measures of temperature, the sensor is connected and there should be a contact between the metallic strip and skin of the human whose body temperature is to be monitored. Figure 22 shows thermometer connection with processing unit. Using adhesive tape or the wrist belt type sensor, it may be attached to the skin without causing inconvenience to the patient. After the patient recovers, the smart kit would be sanitized easily.

Table 1 Temperature range for various pandemic diseases

Disease	Temperature in °F
Hypothermia	< 95.0 °F
Normal	97.7–99.5 °F
Fever or hyperthermia	99.5–100.9 °F
Hyperpyrexia	104–106.8 °F

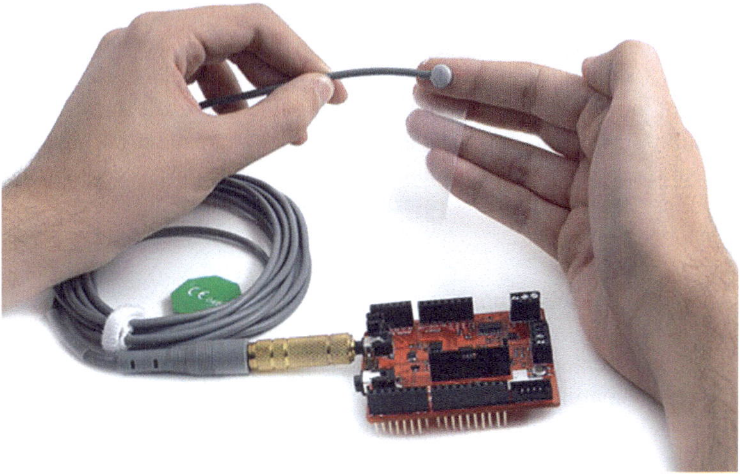

Fig. 22 Thermometer connection with processing unit

5.2 *Processing Unit*

The kit has processing unit for gathering, processing data from the sensor module. The various function of the unit is power management for sensors and communication between the IoT hub and kit. The processing unit has to be compact, low-power consumption, and high speed operation. The microcontroller or minicomputer is mostly used processing unit. The proposed smart kit utilizes Raspberry Pi minicomputer as it has inbuilt Wi-Fi and LAN capabilities. The Pi has interacts with 4G module and capabilities to utilize the full bandwidth.

5.2.1 Internet of Medical Things Platform

The IoT platform is responsible for integration of smart healthcare kit with healthcare professionals. The IoT platforms need to be configured based on the user requirement. They provide sensor data storage, analysis, visualization, and event processing of the pandemic patient. The IoT platforms also have to support 24 × 7 availability, scalability, and security. Today's market is flooded with lot of IoT middleware platforms. The most popular platforms are Amazon Web service IoT, Google Cloud Platform, Microsoft Azure IoT, and IBM Watson IoT. The designed IoMT framework utilize Microsoft Azure IoT platform as this hybrid services platform and able manage billions of the devices. Azure IoT supports large number of smart kits. They can analysis real-time stamp with patients past history of disease. The autonomous IoT framework for each district or hotspot can be created using Microsoft Azure. The healthcare professional, patient family, and district magistrate could subscribe the live health status. The patient kits connection and failure status could easily tracked by Azure IoT hub. The azure stream analytics would run live data analysis and evaluation on the stream of big data coming from kits in the district and automatically post the transformed set of information to healthcare center and pandemic crisis management center of the government. Figure 5.14 shows the Microsoft Azure monitor for patient health visualization. Based on the data analytics of patient's health, the azure IoT hub notify/alert if it detects any abnormal condition in the patients by email and webhook (Fig. 23).

Health Monitoring Mobile App

Figure 24 shows the android mobile app designed for pandemic patients and their doctors. The app continuously subscribe the pandemic patient health status through MQTT protocol from the IoT cloud database and trigger the alert through SMS and

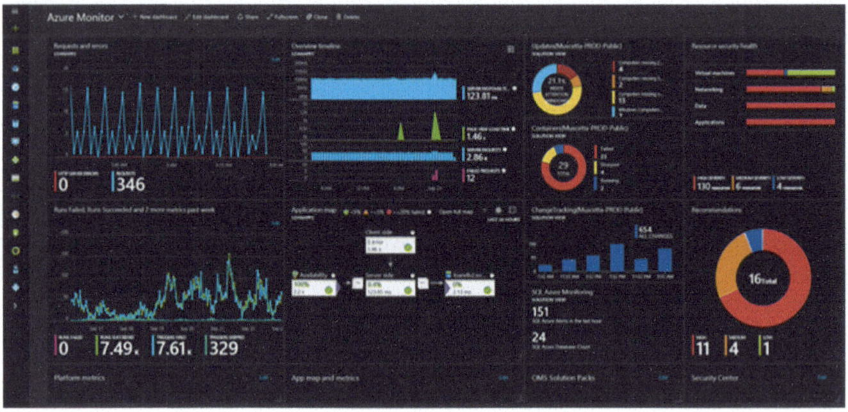

Fig. 23 Microsoft Azure monitor for patient health visualization

Fig. 24 Health monitoring mobile app

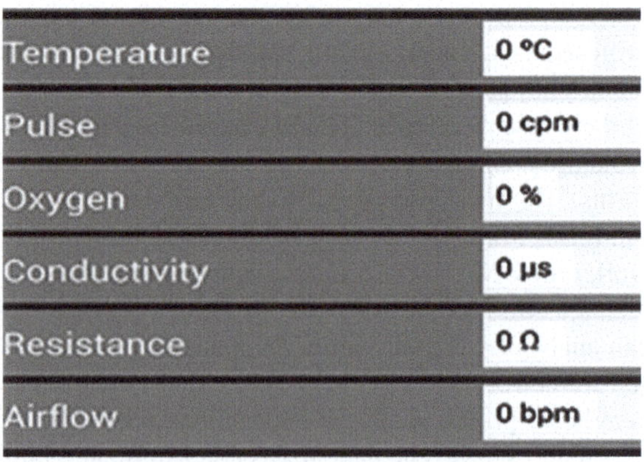

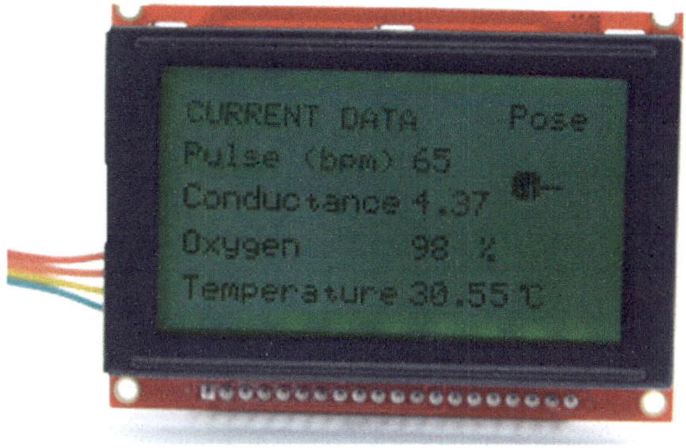

Fig. 25 GLCD for smart wrist band

email. The individual patients vital sign information are displayed in mobile app and also can be viewed through Web browser using webhook technique.

GLCD for the Wrist Band

The individual patient can know their current health status through GLCD of the smart wrist band. The wrist band alerts the patient if any vital signs are abnormal. Figure 25 shows the GLCD used in the kit prototype design and current sensors data information gathered by the kit processing unit.

6 Conclusion and Future Work

Today, numerous administrations can be reached with advancement in new technology and the quantity of utilizations that utilization this innovation is continually expanding. IoT innovation is extending step by step to incorporate various applications domains like smart cities, smart farming, and smart grid. The IoT-based smart health monitoring kits is one of them and this smart kits offers way to improve public health infrastructure of emerging countries like India. The consistent monitoring of pandemic patients in the emergency clinic condition is exceptionally troublesome with the current healthcare infrastructure and strategies. Patients under monitoring in medical clinics are in isolation ward and affect the mental health status. Numerous medical issues require early diagnose for better treatment since they cannot be treated effectively in later stages of the disease. The early testing is staggeringly significant for patients with coronary illness.

In this investigation, IoMT-based smart diagnostic/therapeutic kit for a patient monitoring system permits patients to be versatile in their quarantine zones. The created IoMT framework consistently gauges vital signs the pulse rate, fever, and rate of breathing of the pandemic patients and gives checking and following alerts various services like mobile app, SMS, email, and webhook. At the point, when the patient's essential information arrives at a foreordained cutoff esteem, the portable application cautions the patient and the individuals in the region. In the rare cases that there is no one in the hotspot region for the pandemic patient who can support him, the patient's pulse, heat level, and coordination data are sent to relatives and the healthcare professional as notices through the IoMT cloud platform. The primary motivation behind the smart kit is to make give that they get clinical guide as quickly as time permits, in the event of a potential inconvenience for heart sicknesses.

Our future work includes improving the trust in IoMT by providing the efficient security and privacy solution for the stakeholders (pandemic patients, healthcare professionals). The compactness of the smart kit can be enhanced by evolving sensor technologies and data processing techniques.

References

1. Baker, S. Xiang, W., Atkinson, I.: Internet of things for smart healthcare: technologies, challenges, and opportunities. IEEE Access. pp. 1–25 (2017)
2. Australian Institute of Health and Welfare, "Australia's Health," (2014). [Online]. Available: http://www.aihw.gov.au/WorkArea/DownloadAsset.aspx-?id=60129548150
3. Perrier, E.: Positive Disruption: Healthcare, Ageing & Participation in the Age of Technology. The McKell Institute, Australia (2015)
4. Gope, P., Hwang, T.: BSN-care: a secure iot based modern healthcare system using body sensor network. IEEE Sens. J. **16**(5), 1368–1376 (2016)
5. Zhu, N., Diethe, T., Camplani, M., Tao, L., Burrows, A., Twomey, N., Kaleshi, D., Mirmehdi, M., Flach, P., Craddock, I.: Bridging e-health and the internet of things: the sphere project. IEEE Intell. Syst. **30**(4), 39–46 (2015)
6. Chang, S.H., Chiang, R.D., Wu, S.J., Chang, W.T.: A context-aware, interactive m-health system for diabetics. IT Prof. **18**(3), 14–22 (2016)
7. Pasluosta, C.F., Gassner, H., Winkler, J., Klucken, J., Eskofier, B.M.: An emerging era in the management of Parkinson's disease: Wearable technologies and the internet of things. IEEE J. Biomed. Health Inform. **19**(6), 1873–1881 (2015)
8. Fan, Y.J., Yin, Y.H., Xu, L.D., Zeng, Y., Wu, F.: IoT based smart rehabilitation system. IEEE Trans. Indus. Inform. **10**(2), 1568–1577 (2014)
9. Sarkar, S., Misra, S.: From micro to nano: the evolution of wireless sensor-based health care. IEEE Pulse **7**(1), 21–25 (2016)
10. Yin, Y., Zeng, Y., Chen, X., Fan, Y.: The internet of things in healthcare: an overview. J. Indus. Inf. Integr. **1**, 3–13, 3–2016
11. Islam, S.M.R., Kwak, D., Kabir, H., Hossain, M., Kwak, K.-S.: The internet of things for health care: a comprehensive survey. IEEE Access **3**, 678–708 (2015)
12. Dimitrov, D.V.: Medical internet of things and big data in healthcare. Healthc. Inform. Res. **22**(3), pp. 156–163 (July 2016)
13. Poon, C.C.Y., Lo, B.P.L., Yuce, M.R., Alomainy, A., Hao, Y.: Body sensor networks: in the era of big data and beyond. IEEE Rev. Biomed. Eng. **8**, 4–16 (2015)
14. Tamboli, A.: Build your own IoT platform. Springer publication, (2019)
15. www.cdc.gov
16. www.webmd.com
17. Zhu, H., Podesva, P., Liu, X., Zhang, H., Teply, T., Xu, Y., Chang, H., Qian, A., Lei, Y., Li, Y., Niculescu, A., Li, Y., Iliescu, C., Neuzil, P.: IoT PCR for pandemic disease detection and its spread monitoring. Sens. Actuators: B. Chem. **303**, 127098 (2020)

18. Zhua, H., Podesvaa, P., Liua, X., Zhanga, H., Teplyb, T., Xua, Y., Changa, H., Qiang, A., Leic, Y., Lig, Y., Niculescud, A., Iliescue, C., Neuzila, P.: IoT PCR for pandemic disease detection and its spread monitoring. Sens. Actuators: B. Chem. **303**, Elsevier, (2020)
19. Taştan, Mehmet: IoT based wearable smart health monitoring system. Celal Bayar Univ. J. Sci. **14**(3), 343–350 (2018)
20. Khandpur, R.S.: Handbook of biomedical instrumentation. Tata McGraw Hill, 2nd edn, (2003)

Dr. M. Parimala Devi received B.E. (Electronics and Communication) from Bharathiyar University, Coimbatore, M.E. (VLSI Design) from Anna University, Chennai, M.B.A. (Human Resource Management) from Anna University and Ph.D. (Information and Communication Engineering) from Anna University, Chennai. Currently, she is an Assistant Professor in the Velalar College of Engineering and Technology, Erode. She has published 25 papers in national and international journals and conferences. She has been the reviewer for many SCOPUS indexed journals and received the best paper awards at international conferences. She has published a book named "Advanced Microprocessors and Microcontrollers" with University Science Press, New Delhi. She is a lifetime member of IETE. Her research interests include VLSI & SoC, IoT, Microprocessor-based system design, and Nanoelectronics.

Mr. G. Boopathi Raja received B.E. (Electronics and Communication Engineering) from Anna University of Technology, Coimbatore, M.E. (Applied Electronics) from Anna University, Chennai. Currently, he is an Assistant Professor in the Velalar College of Engineering and Technology, Erode. He has published 10 papers in national and international journals and conferences. He is a lifetime member of IETE. His research interests include VLSI design, Medical Electronics and Signal Processing.

V. Gowrishankar received bachelor degree (B.E) in Electronics and communication engineering from Anna university, Chennai and postgraduate degree (M.E) in VLSI Design from Anna University, Chennai in 2008 and 2010, respectively. He completed Ph.D. from Anna University, Chennai in 2020. He is currently an Assistant Professor at the department of Electronics and Communication Engineering, Velalar college of Engineering and Technology, Erode since 2010. His research areas of interest are low-power embedded devices, open source hardware, Internet of things, wireless sensor networks, low-power system on chip, and optimization of analog-to-digital conversion in deep-submicron technologies. He has authored or co-authored more than 30 publications in journals (mostly Scopus indexed journal) and conference proceedings. He is lifetime member of IETE and ISTE society.

Ms. T. Sathya received B.E. (Electronics and Instrumentation Engineering) from Anna university, Chennai, M.E. (Applied Electronics) from Anna university, Chennai. Currently, she is an Assistant Professor (Sr. Gr) in Dept. of ECE, Velalar College of Engineering and Technology, Erode. She has published six papers in national and international journals and conferences. She received the best paper awards at international conferences. She is a lifetime member of ISSE. She published a book titled Fundamentals of Electric Circuits and Electronic Devices in the year 2018. Her area of interest includes Circuit theory, Signal and image Processing and Sensor Measurements and Instrumentation.

The Prediction Analysis of COVID-19 Cases Using ARIMA and KALMAN Filter Models: A Case of Comparative Study

Murali Krishna Iyyanki and Jayanthi Prisilla

Abstract The time series technique in machine learning is one of the important spaces for analysis and prediction. It includes many approaches to predict that involves time component. In the chapter, two approaches, i.e., autoregressive integrated moving average (ARIMA) and KALMAN filter models were demonstrated on the corona data (India) that was obtained from Ministry of Health and Family Welfare Web site. On modeling, it was found that ARIMA model gave better performance model over the KALMAN filter model. ARIMA (1, 1, 0) gave the approximate value of 35,303 for May 1, 2020 with sigma equal to 199.32, whereas the state-space model and error model of KALMAN filter generated the value of 33,116 and variance equal to 1356.18. The key purpose of the study is to understand and estimate the number of hospital beds and nursing care beds for the COVID-19 (CV-19) patients and make the indispensable arrangement for the patient treatment and avoid delay in action. In recovery cases, the highest value of difference is observed as 1153 on April 27, 2020, whereas the increases in reported cases are 2082 on April 28, 2020. More number of cases are reported with the peak in Maharashtra of 9915 (confirmed) and 1593 (recovery) on April 30, 2020. COVID-19 data visualization was carried out geographical information system with red color referring to the danger or more number of COVID-19 affected areas/state. Green color refers to normal and blue color refers to safe zone with no or single digit cases reported.

M. K. Iyyanki (✉)
Defence Research Development Organization, Hyderabad, India
e-mail: iyyanki@gmail.com

J. Prisilla
Technical Support Engineering, The Airports Authority of India Ltd, Hyderabad, India
e-mail: prisillaj28@gmail.com

© The Editor(s) (if applicable) and The Author(s), under exclusive license to Springer Nature Singapore Pte Ltd. 2020

C. Chakraborty et al. (eds.), *Internet of Medical Things for Smart Healthcare*, Studies in Big Data 80, https://doi.org/10.1007/978-981-15-8097-0_7

1 Introduction

In machine learning, the analysis of time series is found to be very popular and standard that is performed using various models. The experimental data analysis was observed at various points in time leads to new and unique complications in statistical modeling and inference [1]. In this chapter, ARIMA and KALMAN filter models are discussed for predicting COVID-19 cases. The prediction approach of events through a time sequence is referred as time series forecasting. By analyzing the historical trends of the past, assumption is favored for future trends. Time series (TS) are used in every field from medicine to finance, business, inventory planning, and dynamic system theory. The modern application of TS forecasting uses computer technologies that include machine learning, artificial neural networks, support vector machines, and so on. It is well-quoted by a data scientist that "time series forecasting is something of a dark horse in data science." On the other hand, according to Tealab [2] time series is a general problem solution of great practical interest in various disciplines. TS have evidence about the predictor variables of any system which determines dynamically. It is a sequence of values over the time of a system $y(t)$ which registers a sequence of experimental values given as $y\ (t_1)$, $y\ (t_2)$, $y\ (t_3)$,..., $y\ (t_n)$ for certain interval $t = n$ where $t_0 < t_1 < \ldots < t_n$. The aim of the study is to have the count of hospital beds and nursing beds made available on the prediction made to avoid delays and rushing. This would help the healthcare centers to arrange and be vigilant.

2 Predictive Modeling

Predictive modeling (PM) is a practice that uses data and mathematics to predict outcomes with data models. On the other hand, machine learning (ML) algorithms build the mathematical model based on the training data for prediction; ML algorithms uses statistical techniques to allow a computer to construct PMs. Predictive model stirs relations between ML, pattern recognition, and data mining. PM includes much more than the tools and techniques for unveiling patterns within data. PM training defines the development of a model process in a way that can understand and quantify the model's prediction accuracy on future, yet-to-be-seen data. The prime aim of PM is to produce accurate predictions and next is to interpret the model and understand how it works. But unfortunate reality/certainty is that as the model is pushed toward higher accuracy, models become more complex and their interpretability becomes more difficult [3]. PM performs curve and surface fitting, TS regression, or/and ML methods. One such example of TS regression; where the key convention of regression methods is that the patterns in the past data will be repeated in the future [4]. In this work, time series approach is carried out using ARIMA and KALMAN filter approach, the predictive results of CV-19 were analyzed to find that the ARIMA model gave the nearest results of the confirmed cases in India. The objective of this prediction study is to understand the need of hospital beds and nursing care beds for CV-19 patients. This study helps to make the necessary arrangements for number of patient in-advance and to be cared for.

3 Time Series Using COVID-19 Datasets

A time series (TS) is a set of series of data points listed in the time order. A sequence that is successive equal spread out in points with time. The analysis encompasses methods for analyzing TS data to extract meaningful statistics and other data characteristics. The forecasting model of TS uses future values based on previously observed values for prediction. The time series data components are trend, seasonal variation, cyclical variation, and other irregular fluctuations.

Elmousalami [5] in their case study of CV-19 of analysis and modeling performed single exponential smoothing (SES) on the datasets of international confirmed cases. Figure 1 shows the graph of SES obtained and the Eq. 1 of SES is given as

$$F_{t+1} = (1 - \alpha)F_t + \alpha\, D_t \tag{1}$$

The results in Table 1 show that SES has the most accurate model for forecasting recovered cases of CV-19 with 517.54, 523335.16, 723.42, and 16.38% for mean absolute deviation (MAD), mean square error (MSE), root mean square

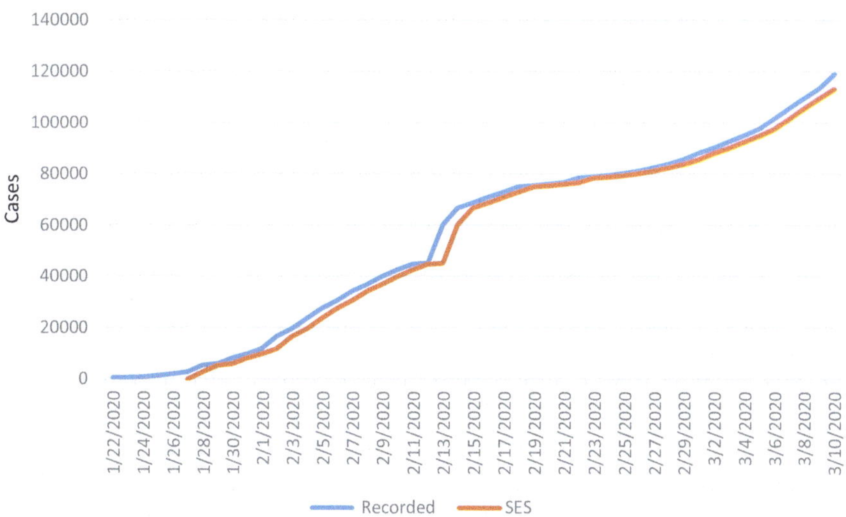

Fig. 1 SES for predicting the confirmed cases (international) [5]

Table 1 Forecasting models for international confirmed cases [5]

Model/Criteria	MAD	MSE	RMSE	MAPE
MA				
5 weeks ahead	7602.60	77470882.22	8801.75	21.42%
10 weeks ahead	18039.43	242692414.14	15578.59	28.18%
WMA	4614.96	32413677.85	5693.30	11.16%
SES	3385.65	20050014.56	4477.72	9.68%

error (RMSE), mean absolute percentage error (MAPE), respectively, against moving average (MA) and weighted moving average WMA.

Siedner [6] in their study of CV-19 in USA suggests that the due to social distancing, there is a lot of reduction in mean daily growth rate of CV-19 cases. The study involved a cumulative epidemic size of 4,171 cases (USA) where the reduction in growth rate estimated corresponds with a reduction in total cases from 26,356 to 23,266 at 7 days, and from 156,360 to 88,105 at 14 days after implementation. In brief, the uninterrupted TS model suggests that social distancing reduced the total number of CV-19 cases by nearly about 3,090 cases in 7 days after implementation and by 68,255 cases in 14 days. Table 2 displays the outcome of regression model for the growth rate daily wise after the social distancing was implemented.

In this study of CV-19 with dataset of different states of India, TS graph was implemented to understand the visualization of reported and recovery cases at a time. The data was obtained from https://www.mohfw.gov.in/ and the analysis is carried out on STATA-12 software.

The graph displays the different states confirmed (Fig. 2) and recovery (Fig. 3), in both the graphs Maharashtra is at the peak with 9915 (confirmed) and 1593 recovery cases on April 30, 2020.

Table 2 Linear regress for daily growth rate before versus after implementation of the first state-wide social distancing measure and state-wide restrictions on the internal movement [6]

	First state-wide social distancing measure			State-wide restriction on internal movement		
	Coef.	95% CI	P-value	Coef.	95% CI	P-value
Const	0.306	0.286 to 0.327	<0.001	0.209	0.190 to 0.229	<0.001
Time	−0.002	−0.007 to 0.004	0.53	−0.009	−0.011 to −0.006	<0.001
Post-intervention period	0.002	−0.032 to 0.035	0.92	−0.039	−0.138 to 0.06	0.44
Time x post-intervention period	−0.008	−0.014 to −0.002	0.008	0.003	−0.014 to 0.020	0.72

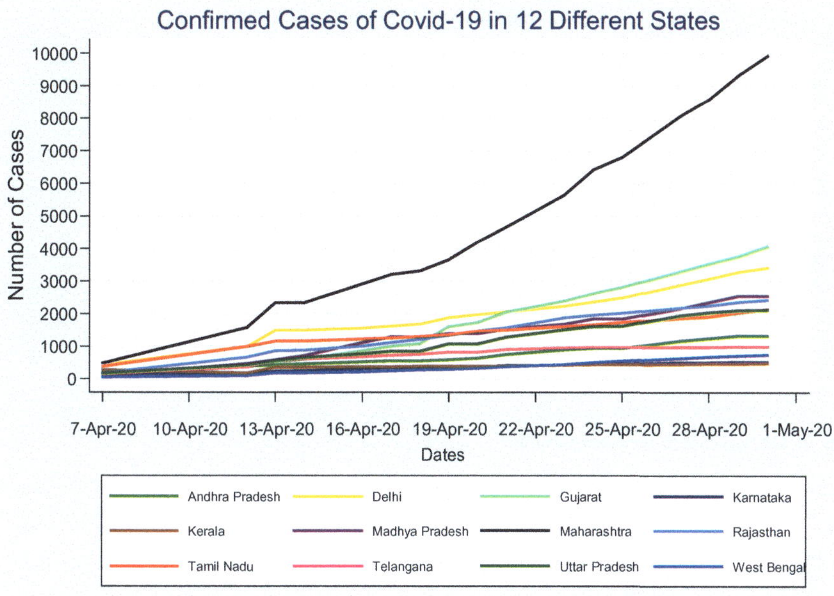

Fig. 2 Reported cases of different Indian states affected due to COVID-19

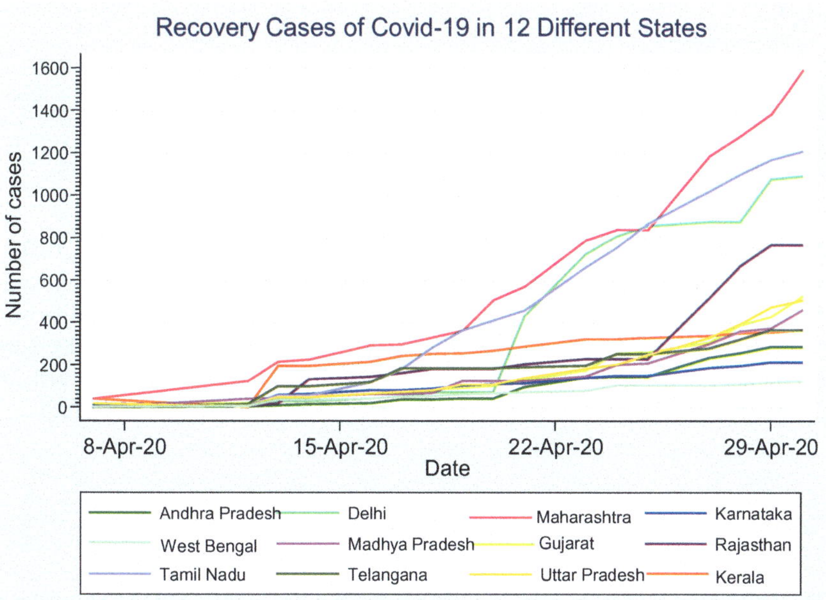

Fig. 3 Recovery cases in different states of India

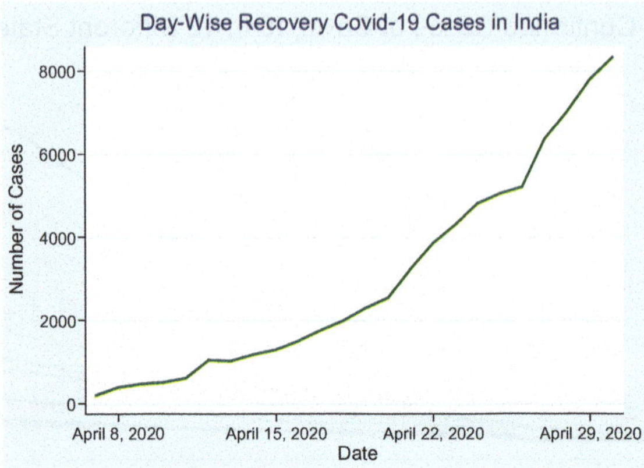

Fig. 4 Day-wise recovery cases graph

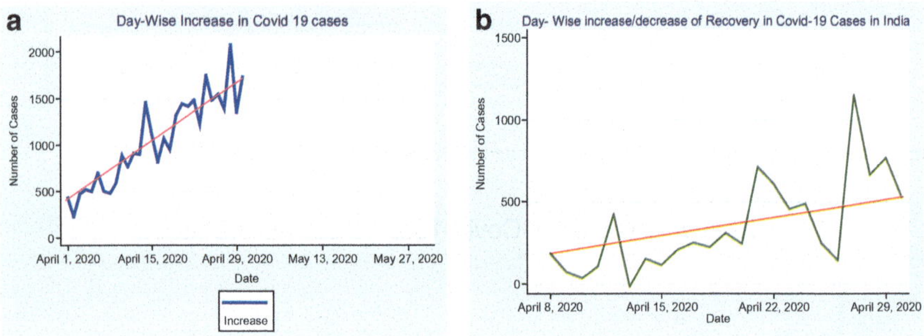

Fig. 5 **a** Day-wise increase in confirm cases, **b** increase/decrease graph for recovery cases

Figure 4 shows the recovery cases of CV-19 in India from March 14, 2020 to April 30, 2020. The graph represents slight decrease on April 13, 2020 giving April 14 on subtracting from April 12, 2020 recovery data. Figure 5 shows the comparison of two—reported cases (Fig. 5a) and recovery cases (Fig. 5b) with increase/decrease in the number of cases. The peak value in recovery difference is 1153 on April 27, 2020, whereas the highest increase in confirmed case is 2082 on April 28, 2020.

4 ARIMA

In TS exploration, an autoregressive integrated moving average (ARIMA) model is a generalization of an autoregressive moving average (ARMA) model. ARIMA (ARM) models are the best models for the statistical models for analyzing and forecasting TS data. An ARM model is a filter that separates the data from the noise, and the data is then extrapolated to obtain forecasts. The forecasting equation of ARM for stationary TS is a linear (regress) equation in which the predictors include of lags of the response variable and/or lags of the forecast errors. Predicted value (Y) is calculated with a constant and/or a weighted sum of one or more current values of Y and/or a weighted sum of one or more current values of the errors.

ARM models complex data pattern; and uses the export modeler for outlier detection, and produces for the drive of eXtended Markup Language (XML) files for prediction modeling of future data.

4.1 The Notation of ARIMA (P, D, Q)

The ARM model consists of autoregressive (AR), moving average (MA), and seasonal autoregressive integrated moving average (SARIMA) models [7]. The autoregressive terms are lags of the stationaries series in the forecasting equation; moving average are lags of the forecast errors, and a TS which needs to be differenced to be made stationary is integrated of a stationary series.

A non-seasonal ARM model is written as an ARIMA (p, d, q) model where p is the sum of autoregressive terms, d is the sum of integrated differences order, and q is the sum of moving average (lagged forecast errors) in the prediction equation.

Hence, the forecasting Eqs. 2, 3, and 4 is built as follows [8, 9].

$$\left(1 - \Phi_1 B - \ldots - \Phi_p B^p\right)\left(1 - \Phi_1 B^s - \ldots - \Phi_p B^{\text{ps}}\right)(1 - B)^d \tag{2}$$

$$\left(1 - B^s\right)^D y_t = \left(1 + \theta_1 B + \ldots + \theta_q B^q\right)\left(1 + \ominus_1 B^s + \ldots + \ominus_Q B^{QS}\right) \in_t \tag{3}$$

where B represents the backshift operator that is defined by the following operation:

$$B^m y_t = y_t - m \tag{4}$$

whenever the parameter has a value of 0 is used; it represents that not to use that element of the model.

4.2 ARIMA in COVID-19 Cases—Datasets

In a case study of ARIMA model, [10] used the model for predicting the electricity prices. The two ARIMA models −1 and 2 were used predicted hourly prices in the electricity markets of Spain and California. The model of Spanish requires 5 h to predict future prices, as opposed to the 2 h needed by the Californian model. The

spot markets and long-term contracts, price forecasts are essential for developing bid strategies or negotiation skills.

Model 1 is given as

$$\begin{aligned}&\left(1-\Phi_1 B^1-\Phi_2 B^2-\Phi_3 B^3-\Phi_4 B^4-\Phi_5 B^5\right)\\&\times\left(1-\Phi_{23} B^{23}-\Phi_{24} B^{24}-\Phi_{47} B^{47}\right.\\&\left.-\Phi_{48} B^{48}-\Phi_{72} B^{72}-\Phi_{96} B^{96}-\Phi_{120} B^{120}-\Phi_{144} B^{144}\right)\\&\times\left(1-\Phi_{168} B^{168}-\Phi_{336} B^{336}-\Phi_{504} B^{504}\right)\log p_t=c\\&+\left(1-\theta_1 B^1-\theta_2 B^2\right)\left(1-\theta_{24} B^{24}\right)\\&\times\left(1-\theta_{168} B^{168}-\theta_{336} B^{336}-\theta_{504} B^{504}\right)\varepsilon_t\end{aligned} \tag{5}$$

Model 2 is given as

$$\begin{aligned}&\left(1-\Phi_1 B^1-\Phi_2 B^2\right)\times\left(1-\Phi_{23} B^{23}-\Phi_{24} B^{24}-\Phi_{47} B^{47}-\Phi_{48} B^{48}\right.\\&\left.-\Phi_{72} B^{72}-\Phi_{96} B^{96}-\Phi_{120} B^{120}-\Phi_{144} B^{144}\right)\\&\times\left(1-\Phi_{167} B^{167}-\Phi_{169} B^{169}-\Phi_{192} B^{192}\right)\times(1-B)\left(1-B^{24}\right)\left(1-B^{168}\right)\\&\log p_t=c+\left(1-\theta_1 B^1-\theta_2 B^2\right)\left(1-\theta_{24} B^{24}-\theta_{48} B^{48}-\theta_{72} B^{72}-\theta_{96} B^{96}\right)\\&\times\left(1-\theta_{144} B^{144}\right)\times\left(1-\theta_{168} B^{168}-\theta_{336} B^{336}-\theta_{504} B^{504}\right)\varepsilon_t\end{aligned} \tag{6}$$

Tables 3 and 4 are the statistical values of forecast mean square of errors (FMSE) was obtained on application of model 1 and 2. Table 5 displays the estimated and parameter values of two countries models.

Table 3 Statistical without explanatory variables [10]

	MWE (%)	$\bar{s}_R$	$\sqrt{FMSE}$
January (Spain)	12.06	0.106	71.98
February (Spain)	8.05	0.106	36.77
March (Spain)	11.28	0.104	71.75
April (Spain)	19.37	0.104	61.51
May (Spain)	4.99	0.083	19.91
June (Spain)	9.97	0.061	81.14
July (Spain)	9.39	0.067	42.59
August (Spain)	8.17	0.092	48.13
September (Spain)	12.01	0.097	70.82
October (Spain)	13.63	0.097	80.33
November (Spain)	7.32	0.098	47.51
April (California)	5.01	0.060	21.19
August (California)	15.65	0.121	469.85
November (California)	13.6	0.074	393.23

Table 4 Statistical with explanatory variables [10]

	MWE (%)	$\bar{s}_{\mathbf{R}}$	$\sqrt{FMSE}$
January (Spain)	9.97	0.106	64.72
February (Spain)	8.13	0.107	45.10
March (Spain)	10.5	0.105	71.57
April (Spain)	14.68	0.102	45.24
May (Spain)	7.75	0.082	33.35
June (Spain)	10.8	0.061	80.99
July (Spain)	8.83	0.066	41.80
August (Spain)	9.39	0.092	49.35
September (Spain)	10.72	0.097	65.50
October (Spain)	13.69	0.094	77.57
November (Spain)	9.88	0.098	73.73
April (California)	5.21	0.060	21.82
August (California)	21.03	0.123	674.58
November (California)	13.68	0.074	397.27

Noureen [9] in a case study of ARIMA in forecasting is a small-scale agricultural load. For the TS data, ARIMA method was applied on the stationary TS data. As seasonal variations make a TS nonstationary, this study presented an analyses on testing stationarity and transforming non-stationarity into stationarity. The model was developed with a specific order selection for autoregressive terms, moving average terms, differencing and seasonality and the forecasting performance has been tested and compared with the actual value. After the plotting of ACF and PACF, augmented Dickey fuller (ADF) test is performed for hypothesis testing to confirm stationarity of TS. ADF is also known as unit root test. The model for the ADF test is shown in Eq. (7):

$$\partial Y_t = \mu + \beta t + \rho Y_{t-1} + \partial Y_{t-1} + \ldots + \partial_p Y_{t-p} + e_t \tag{7}$$

The seasonal ARIMA model is implemented to forecast the agricultural loads for the last one year of the three-year data. The mean absolute error (MAE) of our forecast is calculated to be 13.23%.

Benvenuto [7] implemented ARIMA on a dataset consisting of 22 number determinations. The overall prevalence of CV-19 presented an increasing trend that reached the epidemic plateau as shown in Fig. 6 and Table 6 gives the predicted values for the two days. The difference between cases of a day and cases of the previous day Δ(Xn-Xn-1) showed a non-constant increase in the number of confirmed cases. Figure 7 displays the correlogram and ARIMA forecast graph for the 2019-nCoV incidence.

Table 5 Estimated parameter values of the Spanish and Californian ARIMA models [10]

Spanish market		Californian market	
Parameters	Estimate	Parameters	Estimate
c	−0.0052	c	−0.00015
Φ_1	0.5432	Φ_1	0.447
Φ_2	0.8373	Φ_2	0.206
Φ_3	−0.4174	Φ_{23}	0.0625
Φ_4	−0.0271	Φ_{24}	−0.0193
Φ_5	0.0243	Φ_{47}	−0.0095
Φ_{23}	0.0384	Φ_{48}	−0.3013
Φ_{24}	0.4165	Φ_{72}	−0.021
Φ_{47}	0.0532	Φ_{96}	−0.0581
Φ_{48}	0.004	Φ_{120}	−0.0698
Φ_{72}	0.0196	Φ_{144}	−0.2739
Φ_{96}	0.019	Φ_{167}	0.0222
Φ_{120}	−0.003	Φ_{168}	−0.5922
Φ_{144}	0.1474	Φ_{169}	0.0595
Φ_{168}	0.3342	Φ_{192}	−0.0681
Φ_{336}	0.2873	θ_1	0.9326
Φ_{504}	0.2661	θ_2	0.0291
θ_1	−0.0941	θ_{24}	0.7752
θ_2	0.6998	θ_{48}	−0.2376
θ_{24}	0.1607	θ_{72}	0.2386
θ_{168}	0.2304	θ_{96}	−0.0053
θ_{336}	0.1726	θ_{144}	−0.2713
θ_{504}	0.2232	θ_{168}	0.0248
		θ_{336}	0.5082
		θ_{504}	0.0007

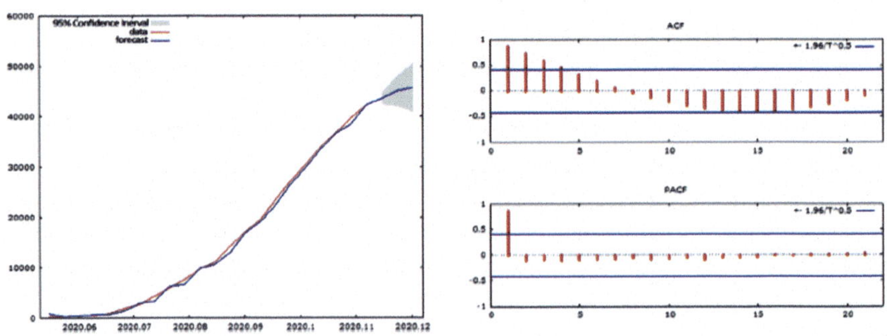

Fig. 6 Correlogram and ARIMA forecast graph for the 2019-nCoV prevalence [7]

Table 6 Forecast value for two days after the analysis for the prevalence and for the incidence of the CV-19 [7]

	Date	Forecast	95% CI
Prevalence	February 11, 20	43599.71	42347.53–44851.9
	February 12, 20	45151.45	42084.88–48218.02
Incidence	February 11, 20	2070.66	1305.23–2836.09
	February 12, 20	2418.47	1534.43–3302.51

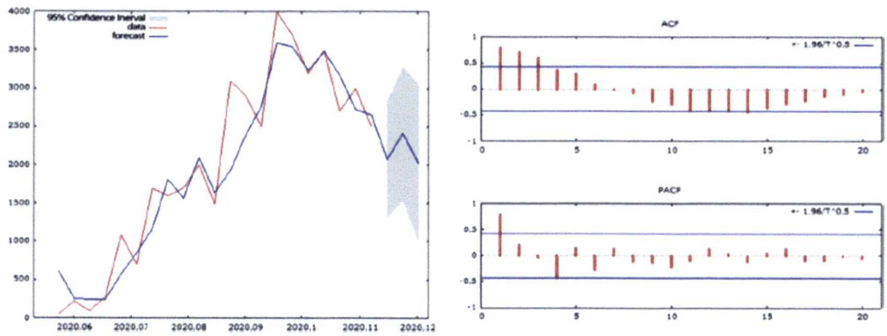

Fig. 7 Correlogram and ARIMA forecast graph for the 2019-nCoV incidence [7]

4.3 *ARIMA Model on COVID-19—India Dataset*

In this case study of COVID-19 (India), ARIMA (ARM) model was built using STATA software. Here, the comparative study on the prediction results obtained from the two models state that ARIMA (1,1,0) model gives much better accurate results over the KF predicted values. The number of cases reported is shown in Table 7 and ARIMA (1,1,0) was modeled to obtain Table 8 with log likelihood value of −316.86; and the predicted value of both the models is shown in Table 15.

Using ARM model, when the parameters of the model were given as $p = 1$, $d = 1$, and $q = 0$; then the p-value = 0 and the predicted values were to the nearest data values. The z-test statistic for the predictor (ConfirmCases) is 823.3/554.8 = 1.48. Coefficient of ARMA(ar) = 0.96; wald chi2(1) is wald chi-square statistic. It is mainly used for hypothesis test where at least one of the predictors' regression coefficients is not equal to zero. Here, in this case, 1 refers to the number of degrees of freedom of the chi-square distribution used to test the wald chi-square statistic and is distinct by the number of predictors (1)./sigma is the estimated standard error of the ARM regression with 199.32 value.

Correlograms/autocorrelation function (ACF) and partial correlograms/partial autocorrelation function (PACF) are shown in Fig. 8, with confidence interval (CI) of −0.9–0.9 in ACF and in PACF, CI is −0.03–0.03. The x-axis denotes the lag and y-axis represents the first-order differential of cases. The blue dot represents the autocorrelation between the lag variable and unlag variable of cases in this study. The

Table 7 Number of cases reported

Date	Number of cases reported
March 14, 2020	84
March 15, 2020	110
March 16, 2020	114
March 17, 2020	137
March 18, 2020	151
March 19, 2020	173
March 20, 2020	223
March 21, 2020	315
March 22, 2020	360
March 23, 2020	468
March 24, 2020	519
March 25, 2020	606
March 26, 2020	694
March 27, 2020	834
March 28, 2020	918
March 29, 2020	1,024
March 30, 2020	1,251
March 31, 2020	1,397
April 1, 2020	1,834
April 2, 2020	2,069
April 3, 2020	2,547
April 4, 2020	3,072
April 5, 2020	3,577
April 6, 2020	4,281
April 7, 2020	4,789
April 8, 2020	5,274
April 9, 2020	5,865
April 10, 2020	6,761
April 11, 2020	7,529
April 12, 2020	8,447
April 13, 2020	9,352
April 14, 2020	10,815
April 15, 2020	11,933
April 16, 2020	12,759
April 17, 2020	13,835
April 18, 2020	14,792
April 19, 2020	16,116

(continued)

Table 7 (continued)

Date	Number of cases reported
April 20, 2020	17,565
April 21, 2020	18,985
April 22, 2020	20,471
April 23, 2020	21,700
April 24, 2020	23,452
April 25, 2020	24,942
April 26, 2020	26,496
April 27, 2020	28,380
April 28, 2020	29,974
April 29, 2020	31,787
April 30, 2020	33,610

dots which are well-outside the interval are known to be large and will be least equal

Table 8 ARIMA model—ARIMA(1,1,0)

Arima Confirm_Cases1, arima (1,1,0)					
ARIMA regress					
Sample: March 15, 2020–April 30, 2020			Num. of obs = 47		
			Wald chi2(1) = 256.04		
LL = − 316.86			Prob > chi2 = 0.0000		
D.ConfirmCases1	Coef.	OPG SE.	z	P > |z|	[95% CI]
ConfirmCases1_con	823.3	554.8	1.48	0.138	−264.07 to 1910.74
ARMA ar.L1	0.96	0.60	16.00	0.000	0.84 to 1.08
/sigma	199.32	19.02	10.48	0.000	162.04 to 236.60

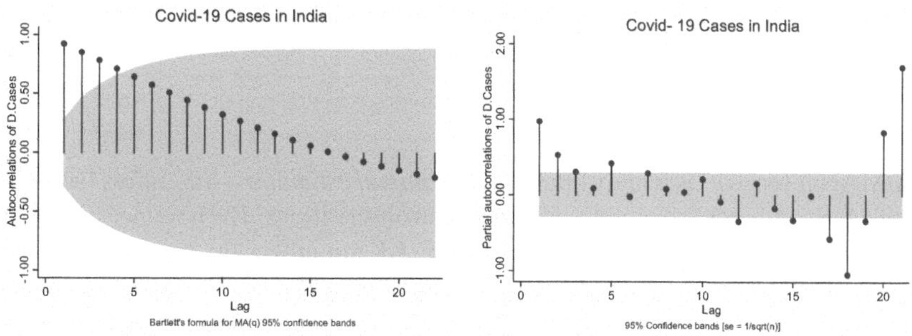

Fig. 8 ACF and PACF graph of COVID cases

Table 9 ACF and PACF values

Correlogram Confirm_Cases1, lags(20)					−1 0 1	−1 0 1
LAG	AC	PAC	Q	Prob > Q	[Autocorrelation]	[Partial autocor]
1	0.9176	1.0686	39.629	0.0000		
2	0.8364	−0.5011	73.34	0.0000		
3	0.7564	−0.3528	101.58	0.0000		
4	0.6801	−0.1634	124.99	0.0000		
5	0.6042	−0.1479	143.93	0.0000		
6	0.5309	−0.4203	158.95	0.0000		
7	0.4605	0.0746	170.54	0.0000		
8	0.3936	−0.3604	179.25	0.0000		
9	0.3298	−0.2024	185.54	0.0000		
10	0.2670	−0.2052	189.79	0.0000		
11	0.2063	−0.3993	192.4	0.0000		
12	0.1462	−0.4029	193.75	0.0000		
13	0.0893	0.4218	194.27	0.0000		
14	0.0389	0.5808	194.37	0.0000		
15	−0.0088	−1.0014	194.38	0.0000		
16	−0.0533	0.9417	194.58	0.0000		
17	−0.0949	0.5621	195.26	0.0000		
18	−0.1325	2.0889	196.63	0.0000		
19	−0.1674	1.5300	198.89	0.0000		
20	−0.2005	2.5197	202.28	0.0000		

to 1, i.e., $p = 1$. Each spike that rises above or falls below the CI range is considered to be statistically significant. ACF and PACF table is mentioned in Table 9.

The analysis procedures include ACF and PACF that are used to calculate correlation in the data [11].

5 KALMAN Filter

KALMAN filter (KF) is widely known as an *optimal estimator*—i.e., infers factors of interest from indirect, inaccurate, and uncertain observations. The new measurements are processed by the recursive property of KF. KF minimizes the mean square error of the estimated parameters, if the noise is Gaussian; and it is a best linear estimator, given the mean and standard deviation of the noise. The technique of finding the best estimate from noisy data amounts to filter out the noise is referred as filtering; and this practice is carried out by KF (Kleeman). KF is a two-step process, namely prediction and update steps. For the likelihood, one has to find f ($y_t|Y_{t-1}$) [12]. The two steps are given in Eqs. 8 and 9. (prediction) and Eqs. 10, 11, and 12 (update).

1. Prediction equation

$$\hat{\mathbf{x}}_k^- = A\,\hat{\mathbf{x}}_{k-1}^- + BU_k \tag{8}$$

$$\mathbf{P}_k^- = A\,\mathbf{P}_{k-1}^- + A^T + \mathbf{Q} \tag{9.}$$

2. Updating equation

$$\mathbf{K}_k = \mathbf{P}_k\mathbf{C}^T\left(\mathbf{C}\mathbf{P}_k^-\mathbf{C}^T + \mathbf{R}\right)^{-1} \tag{10}$$

$$\hat{\mathbf{x}}_k = \hat{\mathbf{x}}_k^- + \mathbf{K}_k\left(\mathbf{Y}_k - \mathbf{C}\hat{\mathbf{x}}_k^-\right) \tag{11}$$

$$P_k = (1 - K_k C)P_k^- \tag{12}$$

The state-space model consists of covariance and error forms; both the forms follow two equations first one is state Eq. 13 and observation Eq. 14. The notation of a state-space model is as follows:

$$y_t = Z_t\alpha_t + S_t\xi_t \tag{13}$$

$$\alpha_t = T_t\alpha_{t-1} + R_t\eta_t \tag{14}$$

with $\begin{pmatrix}\eta_t\\ \xi_t\end{pmatrix}$ ~ iid N $\left(0, \begin{bmatrix} Q & 0\\ 0 & H\end{bmatrix}\right)$ and the initial observation is given as $y_1 \sim N(y_{1|0}, F_1)$.

5.1 *KALMAN Filter—for Prediction in Different Studies*

Rhudy [13] in their work of KF using MATLAB gives an illustration of a simple object in freefall presuming that there is no air resistance. The purpose of filter is to determine the location of the object based on uncertain information about the starting location of the object as well as measurements of the location provided by a laser rangefinder. The acceleration of the given object will be the same to the acceleration due to gravity. In their study, the measurement system has a standard deviation of error of 2 m, and variance of 4 m^2. In the measurement noise, uncertainty in the initial state is considered. The starting point is known to be 105 m before the ball is dropped, while the actual starting point is 100 m as shown in Fig. 9. The initial guess

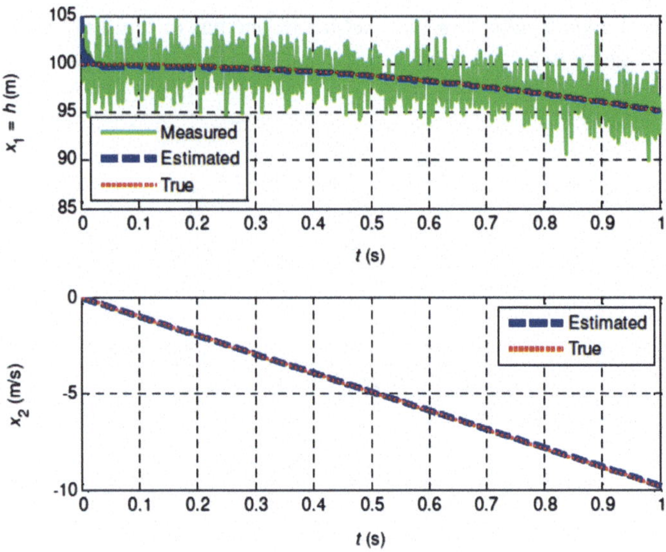

Fig. 9 Example of KF estimated and true states [13]

was roughly determined and has a relatively high corresponding initial covariance. The error of 10 m^2 for the initial position is assumed as the object starts from rest; a smaller uncertainty value of 0.01 m^2/s^2 is obtained as shown in Fig. 10.

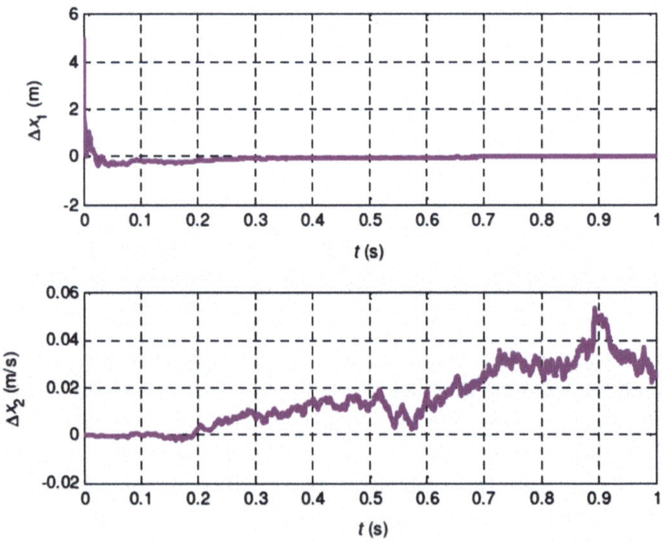

Fig. 10 Example of KF using estimation errors [13]

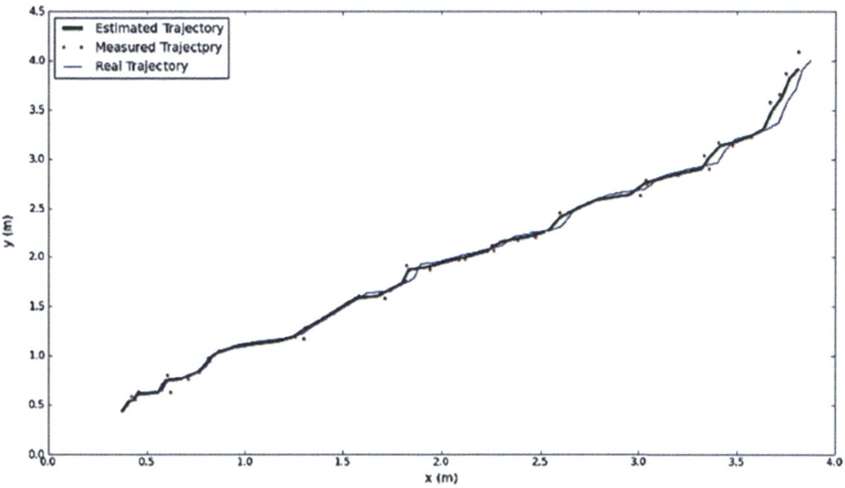

Fig. 11 KF applied to ToA-based localization [14]

Laaraiedh [14] in a case study of KF in telecommunications used on the mobile tracking user connected to a wireless network. A simple tracking algorithm was implemented using Python language by a mobile user who is moving in a room and connected to at least three wireless antennas. The estimated position of the mobile using a trilateration algorithm is indicated by matrix of measurement Y with at least three values of time of arrival (ToA) at time step k as shown in Fig. 11. The values are computed using ranging procedures between the mobile and the three antennas. Initialization of different matrices and using the updated matrices for each step and iteration; estimated, and the real trajectory of the mobile user, and the measurements are performed by the least square-based trilateration. KF enhances the tracking accuracy compared to the static least square-based estimation.

Rankin [15] in their case study of KF for the market price application was based on yearly, quarterly, monthly, weekly, and daily prices. A study was also carried out on open, high, low, and close prices. The use of averages (e.g., weekly or monthly) or stock indexes may alter the results of a study. Table 10 shows the comparison of expenses for the consumer strategy. The first sample (DJT#1) consisted of 1036 hourly readings from February 22, 1985 to September 23, 1985. The second (DJT#2) was of 896 hourly readings from January to June, 1984. The third sample (DJT#3) was gathered from July through December, 1983 and consisted of 896 samples from the 128 day period. KF program produced N-step ahead forecasts for TS. MSE of the forecast errors are calculated to measure model accuracy.

Malleswari [16] in a case study of KF in the error modeling (like ionospheric delays, atmospheric delays, tropospheric delays, and so on) affecting the GPS signals as they travel from satellite to the user who is on earth. In this methodology, it showed that the variations in the signal related to WGS—84 data can be smoothened using KF with the studies made and the analysis yielded better accuracies as shown in

Table 10 Expense comparison for consumer strategy [15]

Strategy	DJT#1	DJT#2	DJT#3
1-Day Period Open Close KF	\$51,772 \$51,785 \$51,697	\$57,576 \$57,459 \$57,429	\$65,559 \$65,585 \$65,506
2-Day Period Open Close KF	\$26,220 \$26,230 \$26,128	\$28,832 \$28,718 \$27,670	\$32,747 \$32,782 \$32,699
3-Day Period Open Close KF	\$18,141 \$18,145 \$18,047	\$19,788 \$19,665 \$19,642	\$22,401 \$22,433 \$22,342
4-Day Period Open Close KF	\$13,439 \$13,443 \$13,542	\$14,754 \$14,622 \$14,607	\$16,642 \$16,679 \$16,587
5-Day Period Open Close KF	\$10,748 \$10,741 \$10,678	\$12,231 \$12,088 \$12,061	\$13,765 \$13,806 \$13,705

*DJT = Dow Jones Transportation

Tables 11 and 12 that Φkf—the latitude in degrees on KF application is 0.004221766 for Gandipet and 0.00003667424 for Hussain Sagar. Similarly, λkf—longitude in degrees on KF application KF is 0.03084715 for Gandipet and 0.0006331302 for Hussain Sagar.

Table 11 Comparison of longitude for Gandipet (left) and Hussain Sagar (right) [16]

Longitude	Variance	Longitude	Variance
λ**rx**—Longitude in degrees (Receiver)	27.0337204	λ**rx**—Longitude in degrees (Receiver)	13.39910013
λ_{prg}—Longitude in degrees before applying KALMAN filter	27.0337194	λ_{prg}—Longitude in degrees before applying KALMAN filter	0.001264126
λ_{kf}—Longitude in degrees after applying KALMAN filter	0.03084715	λ_{kf}—Longitude in degrees after applying KALMAN filter	0.0006331302
$\lambda_{s/w}$—Longitude in degrees after applying Web soft	6.904284042	$\lambda_{s/w}$—Longitude in degrees after applying Web soft	0.00355667

Table 12 Comparison of latitude for Gandipet (left) and Hussain Sagar (right) [16]

Latitude	Variance	Latitude	Variance
Φrx—Latitude in degrees (Receiver)	6.89938593	Φrx—Latitude in degrees (Receiver)	0.020659696
Φ_{prg}—Latitude in degrees before applying KALMAN filter	7.3488	Φ_{prg}—Latitude in degrees before applying KALMAN filter	0.000292464
Φ_{kf}—Latitude in degrees after applying KALMAN filter	0.004221766	Φ_{kf}—Latitude in degrees after applying KALMAN filter	0.00003667424
$\Phi_{s/w}$—Latitude in degrees after applying Web soft	0.011725697	$\Phi_{s/w}$—Latitude in degrees after applying Web soft	0.000198005

5.2 KALMAN Filter—for COVID-19 Prediction—India Dataset

There are two forms in state-space model, namely covariance and error form models. There are shown in Tables 13 and 14, respectively.

Table 13 State-space model—covariance

Space (CC L4.Datee, state) (Confirm_Cases1 L4.Datee) in 34/44					
State-space model					
Sample: April 16, 2020—April 26, 2020			Num. of obs = 11		
			Wald chi2(1) = 2923.86		
LL = − 77.19			Prob > chi2 = 0.0000		
ConfirmCases1	Coef.	OIM SE.	z	P > |z|	[95% CI]
CC Date L4. _cons	−0.468 0.301	– –	– –	– –	– –
Confirm_Cases1 Date L4. _cons	1392.43 −3.06e + 07	25.75 567088.4	54.07 −54.04	0.000 0.000	1341.96 to 1442.89 −3.18e + 07 to −2.95e + 07
Var. CC Confirm_Cases1	1356.18 73018.58	31135.21	2.35	0.010	11994.69 to 134042.5

*LL = Log Likelihood, I0 to I8 = Iteration 0 to 9, SE = standard error

Table 14 State-space model—error form

Space (CCE L4.Datee, state) (Confirm_Cases1 L4.Datee) in 34/44					
State-space model					
Sample: April 16, 2020—April 26, 2020				Num of obs = 11	
				Wald chi2(1) = 2923.86	
LL = − 77.19				Prob > chi2 = 0.0000	
ConfirmCases1	Coef.	OIM SE.	z	P > |z|	[95% CI]
CCE Date L4. _cons	−0.468 0.301	– –	– –	– –	– –
Confirm_Cases1 Date L4. _cons	1392.43 −3.06e + 07	25.75 567088.4	54.07 −54.04	0.000 0.000	1341.96–1442.89 −3.18e + 07 to −2.95e + 07
Var CCE Confirm_Cases1	1356.18 73018.58	−31135.21	– 2.35	– 0.010	– 11994.69–134042.5

5.2.1 Covariance

See Table 13.

5.2.2 Error Form

In Fig. 12, the dotted lines show the prediction of CV-19 data obtained using ARIMA and KF model. The solid blue line indicates cases of training data. The results of KF model—covariance and error model are shown in Tables 13 and 14, respectively. The log likelihood in refine estimates is −77.19, wald chi2(1) is 2923.86. Z-test

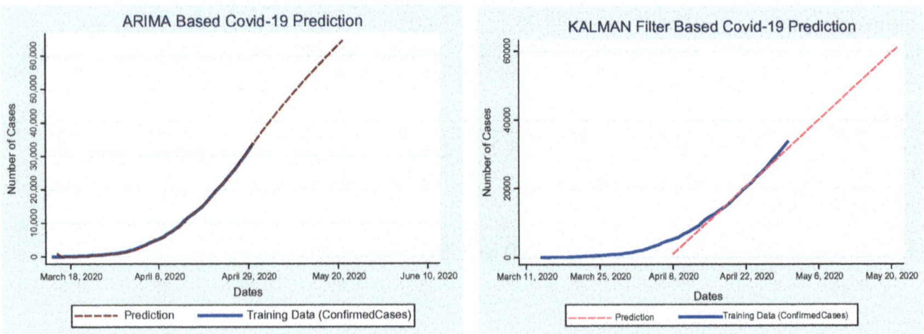

Fig. 12 Comparison of ARIMA and KALMAN filter prediction graphs

of predictor (Confirm_Cases1) is 73018.58/31135.21 = 2.35 and z-test of date is 1392.43/25.75 = 54.07. The variance is given as 1356.18. Two models are best fit model; as all of the *p*-values are very significant with $p < 0.001$ and $p < 0.05$.

Table 15 shows the ARM and KF predicted value from May 1, 2020 and the data. The prediction was calculated from May 1, 2020 up to May 20, 2020. The predicted values are thus compared with the data to check if it lies within the nearest range. Figure 13 describes the prediction of ARM and KF along with data in a single graph and on comparison one can see the predictive curve of ARM increases accurately with the dates, whereas the KF would not give accurate predicted values.

6 Geographic Information Systems—Visualization and Prediction—COVID-19 Datasets

Geographic information systems (GIS) are a computer-based tool that examines spatial relationships, patterns, and trends. This through connecting geography with data, GIS better understands data using a geographic context. It stores, analyze, and visualize data for geographic positions on earth's surface. The four main characteristics of GIS *create* geographic data, *manage* it in a database, *analyze* and find patterns, and *visualize* it on a global map. In viewing and analyzing data on maps gives better understanding of data, and one can make better decisions. It helps in understanding what is where. Spatial-temporal GIS, or 4D GIS, has become necessary in areas where GIS is needed for predicting dimensions across time. GIS is increasingly needed with a real-time platform that offers not just monitoring of events but can take input and predict what could happen as a type of forecasting tool. Figure 14 shows the GIS visualization of CV-19 in different states of India. The color red in Maharashtra indicates that the numbers of reported cases (confirmed cases) are more in number and is known as red zone. The less brightness of red indicates the little less than Maharashtra state. The green color indicates normal with less number of CV-19 cases. The color blue refers to safe zone where no or single digit confirmed cases are reported. In red and green zone states, one find lockdown implemented to overcome the increase in the number of cases. If no lockdown was implemented in India, one would find more number of cases as in aboard along with death cases.

7 Conclusions

In a comparative study of two predictive models of TS, ARIMA, and KALMAN filter in this chapter predicts day-wise cases in COVID-19 of India. Both the models are used on the stationary TS datasets. But, it was found that ARIMA model gave better results over KALMAN filter model for the COVID-19 dataset.

Table 15 Predicted values using ARIMA and KALMAN filter from April 27, 2020 to May 20, 2020

Date	ARIMA predicted values	KALMAN filter projected values	Number of cases reported	Remarks
March 14, 2020			84	
March 15, 2020	907		110	
March 16, 2020	166		114	
March 17, 2020	149		137	
March 18, 2020	190		151	
March 19, 2020	195		173	
March 20, 2020	225		223	
March 21, 2020	302		315	
March 22, 2020	434		360	
March 23, 2020	434		468	
March 24, 2020	603		519	
March 25, 2020	599		606	
March 26, 2020	721		694	
March 27, 2020	810		834	
March 28, 2020	1,000		918	
March 29, 2020	1,030		1,024	
March 30, 2020	1,157		1,251	
March 31, 2020	1,500		1,397	
April 1, 2020	1,568		1,834	
April 2, 2020	2,286		2,069	
April 3, 2020	2,326		2,547	
April 4, 2020	3,038		3,072	
April 5, 2020	3,608		3,577	
April 6, 2020	4,094		4,281	
April 7, 2020	4,989		4,789	
April 8, 2020	5,309	1,091	5,274	
April 9, 2020	5,772	2,483	5,865	
April 10, 2020	6,465	3,875	6,761	
April 11, 2020	7,654	5,268	7,529	
April 12, 2020	8,299	6,660	8,447	
April 13, 2020	9,361	8,053	9,352	
April 14, 2020	10,254	9,445	10,815	
April 15, 2020	12,254	10,838	11,933	
April 16, 2020	13,040	12,230	12,759	
April 17, 2020	13,585	13,622	13,835	

(continued)

Table 15 (continued)

Date	ARIMA predicted values	KALMAN filter projected values	Number of cases reported	Remarks
April 18, 2020	14,902	15,015	14,792	
April 19, 2020	15,744	16,407	16,116	
April 20, 2020	17,421	17,800	17,565	
April 21, 2020	18,991	19,192	18,985	
April 22, 2020	20,383	20,585	20,471	
April 23, 2020	21,932	21,977	21,700	
April 24, 2020	22,914	23,369	23,452	
April 25, 2020	25,169	24,762	24,942	
April 26, 2020	26,407	26,154	26,496	
April 27, 2020	28,023	27,547	28,380	
April 28, 2020	30,224	28,939	29,974	
April 29, 2020	31,539	30,332	31,787	
April 30, 2020	33,563	31,724	33,610	
May 1, 2020	35,303	33,116		
May 2, 2020	37,009	34,509		
May 3, 2020	38,681	35,901		
May 4, 2020	40,322	37,294		
May 5, 2020	41,932	38,686		
May 6, 2020	43,512	40,079		
May 7, 2020	45,064	41,471		
May 8, 2020	46,589	42,863		
May 9, 2020	48,087	44,256		
May 10, 2020	49,560	45,648		
May 11, 2020	51,008	47,041		
May 12, 2020	52,433	48,433		
May 13, 2020	53,836	49,825		
May 14, 2020	55,217	51,218		
May 15, 2020	56,576	52,610		
May 16, 2020	57,916	54,003		
May 17, 2020	59,236	55,395		
May 18, 2020	60,538	56,788		
May 19, 2020	61,822	58,180		
May 20, 2020	63,088	59,572		

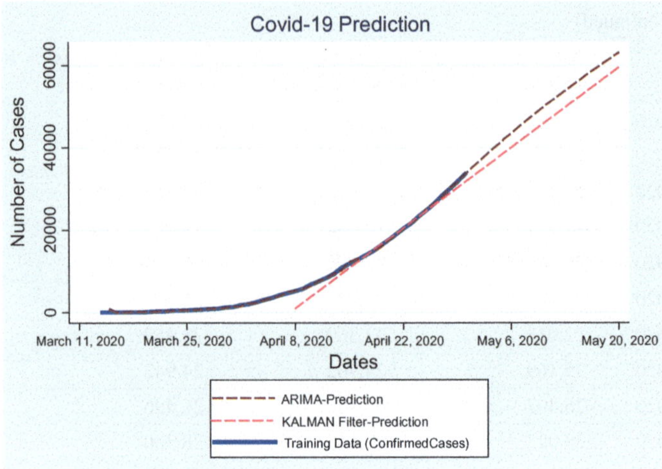

Fig. 13 Two models prediction graph of COVID-19 India cases

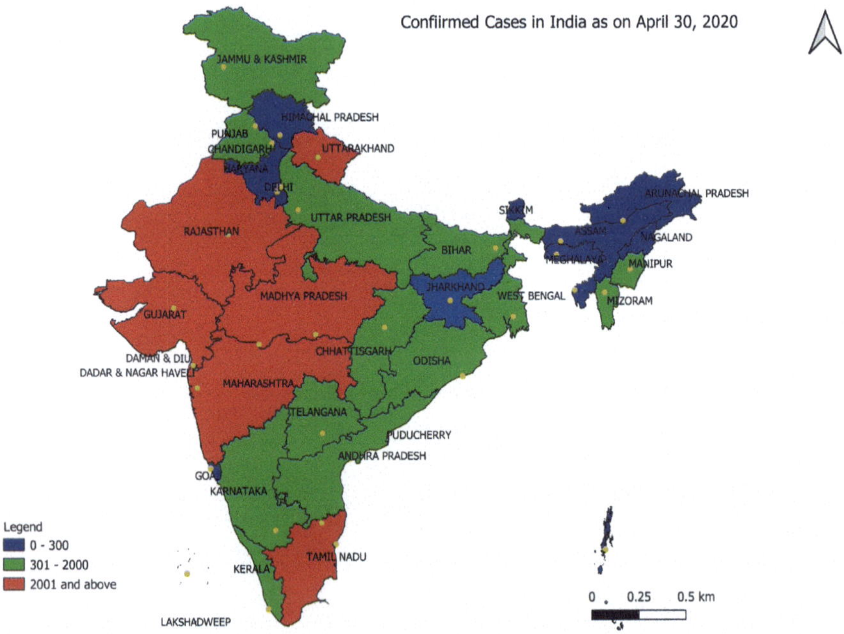

Fig. 14 GIS visualization on COVID-19 in different states on India

Conflict of Interest The authors declare that they have no known conflict of interests.

References

1. Shumway, R. H., & Stoffer, D. S. (2006) Characteristics of Time Series. In: Time Series Analysis and Its Applications. Springer Texts in Statistics. Springer, New York, NY
2. Tealab, A.: Time series forecasting using artificial neural networks methodologies: a systematic review. Faculty of Computers and Information Technology, Future University in Egypt. Elsevier B. V. Future Computing and Informatics Journal. **3**, 334e340 (2018). https://doi.org/10.1016/j.fcij.2018.10.003. 2314-7288/
3. Kuhn, M., Johnson, K.: Measuring performance in classification models. Appl. Predictive Model. doi 10.1007/978-1-4614-6849-3 11,© Springer Science and Business Media, New York, 2013, p. 247
4. Pavlyshenko, B.M.: Machine-learning models for sales timeseries forecasting. Data. **4**, 15 (2019). https://doi.org/10.3390/data4010015 www.mdpi.com/journal/data
5. Elmousalami, H.H., Hassanien, A.E.: Day level forecasting for coronavirus disease (COVID-19) spread: analysis, modeling and recommendations. (2020). arXiv:2003.07778
6. Siedner, M.J., Harling, G., Reynolds, Z., Gilbert, R., Venkataramani, A.S., Tsai, A.C.: Social distancing to slow the U.S. COVID-19 epidemic: interrupted time-series analysis. (2020). medRxiv preprint doi:https://doi.org/10.1101/2020.04.03.20052373
7. Benvenuto, D., Giovanetti, M., Vassallo, L., Angeletti, S., Ciccozzi, M.: Application of the ARIMA model on the COVID-2019 epidemic dataset, 2352–3409/© 2020 The Authors. Published by Elsevier Inc. (2019). https://doi.org/10.1016/j.dib.2020.105340
8. Cleophas, T.J., Zwinderman, A.H.: Autoregressive models for longitudinal data (120 mean monthly population records). Machine Learning in Medicine- a Complete Overview. (2015). ISBN 978-3-319-15194-6, https://doi.org/10.1007/978-3-319-15195-3
9. Noureen, S., Atique, S., Roy, V., Bayne, S.: Analysis and application of seasonal ARIMA model in energy demand forecasting: a case study of small scale agricultural load. (2019). 978-1-7281-2788-0/19/$31.00 ©2019 IEEE
10. Contreras, J., Espínola, R., Nogales, F.J., Conejo, A.J.: ARIMA models to predict next-day electricity prices. IEEE Trans. Power Syst. **18**(3), (Aug 2003)
11. Martin, R.D., Victor J.Y.: Influence functionals for time series. Ann. Stat. **14**(3), 781–818 (1986). Accessed September 8, 2020. http://www.jstor.org/stable/3035535
12. Mikusheva, A.: Filtering. State space models. Kalman Filter.course materials for 14.384 TimeSeries Analysis. MITOpenCourseWare (http://ocw.mit.edu), Massachusetts Institute of Technology. (2007)
13. Rhudy, M.B, Salguero, R.A., Holappa, K.: A kalman filtering tutorial for undergraduate students. Int. J. Comput. Sci. Eng. Surv. (IJCSES). **8**(1), (Feb 2017). https://doi.org/10.5121/ijcses.2017.8101
14. Laaraiedh, M.: Implementation of Kalman filter with Python language, (2012). https://arxiv.org/pdf/1204.0375
15. Rankin, J.M.: Kalman filtering approach to market price forecasting. Retrospective Theses and Dissertations. 8291, (1986). https://lib.dr.iastate.edu/rtd/8291
16. Malleswari, B.L. MuraliKrishna, I.V., Lalkishore, K., Seetha, M., Hegde, N.P.: The role of kalman filter in the modelling of GPS errors. J. Theor. Appl. Inform. Technol. (2009). www.jatit.org
17. Kleeman, L.: Understanding and applying kalman filtering, https://www.cs.cmu.edu/
18. Ramirez-Amaro, K., Chimal-Eguia, J.C.: Machine learning tools to time series forecasting. IEEE Xplore. (2007). https://doi.org/10.1109/micai.2007.42

Exploration of Cough Recognition Technologies Grounded on Sensors and Artificial Intelligence

S. R. Preethi, A. R. Revathi, and M. Murugan

Abstract Artificial intelligence is ruling all industrial sectors and has its hand on the medical and healthcare field too. Cough is a symptom of divergent respiratory disorder diseases from a common cold to the current coronavirus disease. Cough is not only extant in humans, but it similarly found to be existing in numerous animals primarily in pigs [1]. Cough is generally a good self-reaction of the body to prevent secretions and its blockages in the upper airway. The frequency, sequence and pattern of the cough reveal the disease along with its severity. Thus, sensing platform and artificial intelligence are used intensively for cough analysis. This chapter is to explore about cough detection and throws light on the various cough detection methodologies, the artificial intelligence algorithms implemented, features involved in cough detection and constraint existent in implementation. In architectural analysis of cough detection; divergent types of the sensors, auxiliary equipment and neural network sustenance instruments deployed are entailed. Cough detection is enacted by voluminous machine and deep learning algorithms using classifiers such as random forest, decision tree, logistic regression, support vector machine, feed forward artificial neural network, convolutional neural network hidden Markov model, multiclass classifier with multilayer perceptron model, and validation is achieved through K-cross validation. The chapter also articulates about the dataset availability of various patterns of cough, the visualizing of sound pattern in frequency and time domain.

S. R. Preethi (✉) · M. Murugan
Department of Electronics and Communication Engineering, SRM Valliammai Engineering College, Kattankulathur, Chengalpatu, Tamil Nadu, India
e-mail: srpreethi31090@gmail.com

M. Murugan
e-mail: vp@valliammai.co.in

A. R. Revathi
Department of Information Technology, SRM Valliammai Engineering College, Kattankulathur, Chengalpatu, Tamil Nadu, India
e-mail: revathiar.it@valliammai.co.in

© The Editor(s) (if applicable) and The Author(s), under exclusive license to Springer Nature Singapore Pte Ltd. 2020

C. Chakraborty et al. (eds.), *Internet of Medical Things for Smart Healthcare*, Studies in Big Data 80, https://doi.org/10.1007/978-981-15-8097-0_8

Further cough is found to have two set of features namely superordinate and subordinate sound features. Superordinate features include Mel-frequency cepstral significant, non-Gaussianity score, Shannon entropy, energy, zero intersection ratio, spectral centroid, spectral bandwidth and spectral roll-off. Subordinate feature covers cough sequence type and duration, bouts occurred in a sequence, cough sequence number in prescribed interval time. The chapter also includes extensive analysis of above feature sets of cough sound. Hence, cough detection using artificial intelligence helps doctors to diagnose early and at ease. At times, it also overcomes the misdiagnosis of the disorders. The chapter also discusses in detail about the various datasets used for cough detection. Finally, includes the constraint of deployment of cough detection that covers the challenges in computational cost, size, budget and ease of deployment with ubiquitous computing.

Keywords Cough detection · Sensors · Machine learning · Deep learning algorithms · Classifiers · Superordinate features · Subordinate features

1 Introduction to Sick Sound—COUGH

One of the most important sickness indicating sounds is cough. Cough occurs due to the presence of disturbance in respiratory track. Based on the presence of liquid, airway passages and lasting time period, the cough can be classified on types, patterns and endurance. The cough along with its acoustic quality sound can be as wet or dry cough types. Wet cough is due to the presence of the disturbance at times due to occurrence of secretions such as mucus and pus. Dry cough is due to inflammations without any fluid secretions [2].

Cough occurring pattern may be obstructive and restrictive based on the nature of airway [3, 4]. In obstructive pattern, airway is widened or narrowed than the normal size. In restrictive pattern, fluid occupied air sacs are present. At time, there is a presence of combined pattern including both the patterns of obstructive and restrictive [5]. Endurance of the cough denotes the time period of existence of the cough as acute, subacute and chronic [6]. Acute coughs are durable for maximum three weeks, and subacute exists more than three weeks up to eight weeks. Chronic cough is serious infections lasting for a longer time period than 8 weeks. In terms of sound signal, the cough possesses two sorts namely airflow and acoustic signal. The airflow signal is plotted as graph between flow in L/sec and time period in second measured in patients mouth. Acoustic cough signal represents sound graph between amplitude and time in seconds generally tested at sternal manubrium. The taxonomy of cough based on types, pattern and endurance is given in Fig. 1 and Table 1.

Cough is a symptom of respiratory medical, non-respiratory medical and environment condition as described in Fig. 2. In case of respiratory medical condition, the reason could be upper respiratory tract infection, lower respiratory tract infect, pneumonia, bronchitis, influenza, asthma, whooping cough, post nasal drip, tuberculosis and corona.

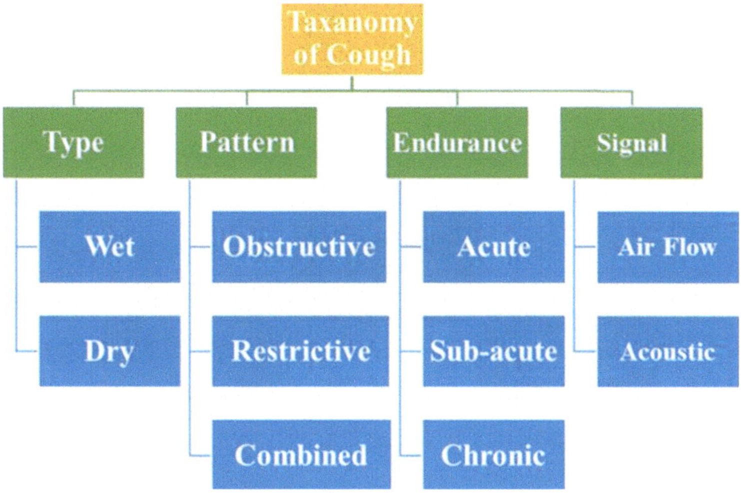

Fig. 1 Taxanomy of cough

Table 1 Details of cough taxanomy

Authors and year	Cough taxonomy	Subclassification	Indications
Mannino David M et al. 2003	Type	Wet	With the presence of acoustic sounds
		Dry	No presence of acoustic sounds
Jaclyn A Smith et al. 2006	Pattern	Obstructive	Widened or narrowed airways
Swarankar Vinayak et al. 2013		Restrictive	Air sacs filled with fluid
Gowrisree Rudraraju et al. 2020		Combined	Together forms of obstructive and restrictive
De Blasio et al. 2011	Endurance	Acute	Enduring less than 21 days
		Subacute	Existing for 3–8 weeks
		Chronic	More than 8 weeks existence
Yan Shi et al. 2018	Signal	Airflow	Represents air movement through mouth
		Acoustic	Denotes tussis echo

Non-respiratory medical conditions are gastroesophageal reflux, heart failure and tumors. Environment conditions like cooking fumes, smoking, air pollutants cause cough.

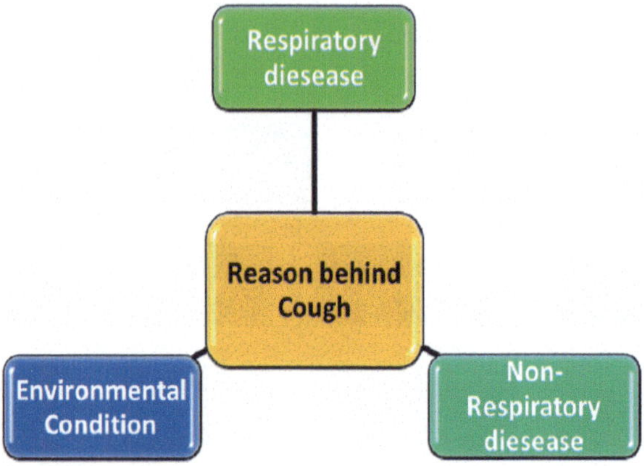

Fig. 2 Cough causing conditions

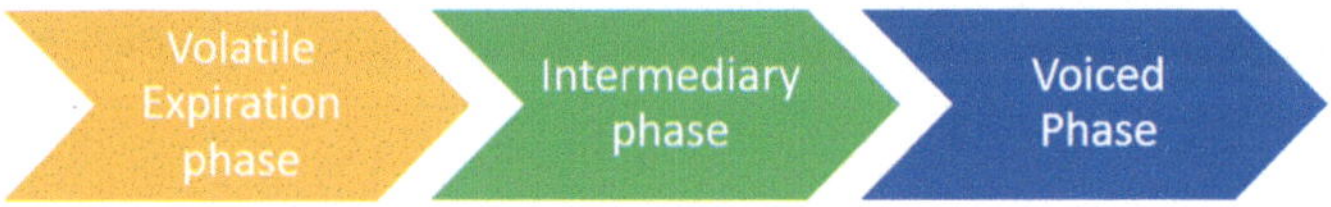

Fig. 3 Phases of cough

2 Cough Pattern Phases

Cough pattern has three phases as shown in Fig. 3, namely volatile expiration, intermediary and voiced phase [7]. At times, the cough possesses only two phases intermediary and voiced phase due to the nature of disease that causes cough.

3 Features of Cough

Generally, in case of clinical trials, cough has found to consist of many features such as Mel-frequency cepstral significant, explosive cough sounds, cough seconds, cough breaths, cough epochs, cough intensity, cough pattern, zero intersection ratio, spectral centroid, spectral bandwidth, and spectral roll-off as shown in Fig. 4 and Table 2.

Mel-frequency cepstral significant (MFCS) feature enables to recognize characteristics of human auditory [8], and hence, it is used in large scale for cough detection [9–11]. A 13 dimensional MFCS obtained through the Mel filter is processed through amplitude and zero crossed coupled first-order and second-order differentiator to enhance to 41 dimensional MFCS [12]. Along with cough frequency; explosiveness of cough sounds, the duration seconds, respiration rate inclusive of least cough and number of repeated cough sounds with less interval (epochs) are also important

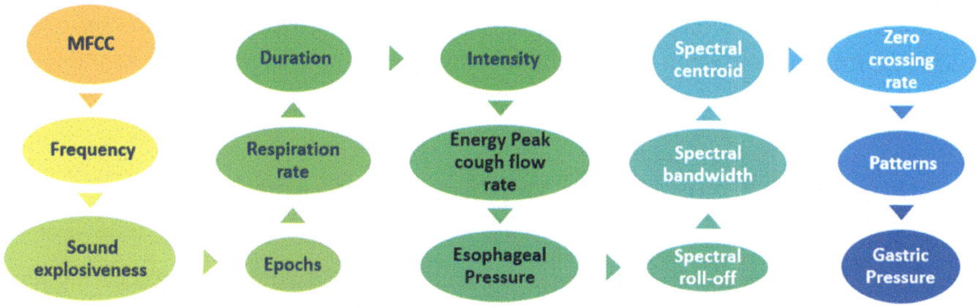

Fig. 4 Vital cough features

Table 2 Details of cough features

Author	Year	Feature
V. Tiwari et al.	2010	Mel-frequency cepstral significant
D. Parker et al.	2013	
Y. Yin et al.	2012	
Y. Chung et al.	2013	
Bowen Dua et al.	2017	
Y. Shi et al.	2016	Cough frequency
		Cough sound impulsiveness
		Cough duration
		Cough respiration rate
		Epochs
L. Pavesi et al.	2001	Cough intensity
K. K. Lee et al.	2012	
G. J. Gibson et al.	2002	Energy peak cough flow rate, Esophageal pressure, Gastric pressure
Y. Shi et al.	2017	
A. A. Abaza et al.	2009	Cough patterns
Gowrisree Rudraraju et al.	2020	Zero intersection ratio, Spectral centroid, Spectral bandwidth, Spectral roll-off

features [13]. Cough intensity is also taken into account by considering peak and mean energy [14, 15]. Along with energy peak cough flow rate, esophageal pressure and gastric pressure are also thrown light for voluntary, induced and spontaneous cough [16, 17]. Cough patterns also form an important end point for disease identification [18]. Zero intersection ratio indirectly implies the frequency of the cough sound generated. Spectral centroid is used to characterize the spectrum, and further, the extent of spectrum data is provided by spectral bandwidth. Spectral roll-off is used to distinguish between voice-related sounds with nonvoice-related sounds [5].

4 Methods and Algorithms Deployed for Cough Detection

Cough detection is performed by many researchers using two main methods namely instinctive cough segmentation and instinctive cough classification as shown in Fig. 5. In instinctive cough segmentation method, the cough-related audio sounds are riven into fragments to identify the features of interest for cough detection.

In case of instinctive cough classification, classifiers are used to analyze and detect the cough sounds. In Instinctive cough segmentation, the fragmenting is done automatically, whereas in instinctive cough classification, manual segmentation is performed before the classification [19].

Many algorithms are deployed by researchers for cough detection animal houses, cough-related diseases and up to detection of COVID-19 through cough. A cough device for recording the ambulatory cough with help of electromyography (EMG), electrocardiogram (ECG) and microphone was devised [20]. A Holter monitor with EMG and audio signal for based ambulatory cough meter [21].

Semi-automated device utilizes audio and EMG signal for cough detection in children [22]. Automated tagging of EMG and audio signal for objective cough monitoring in infants [23]. Accelerometer portable device with no programmed examination software for nocturnal cough and to study the sleep patterns for children with cough [24]. Lifeshirt [25] is programmed scrutiny of an amalgamation of EMG, ECG and plethysmography for quantification of cough frequency in chronic disorder patients.

A spontaneous instrument, hull instinctive cough summer [26], is devised using linear predictive coding significant and predictable neural Web. Hidden Markov model (HMM) is deployed for MFCS characteristic avulsion [27]. Device performing audio recording and physical totaling of sound of interest was performed in chronic obstructive pulmonary disease [28]. Decision tree-based discriminator is used to

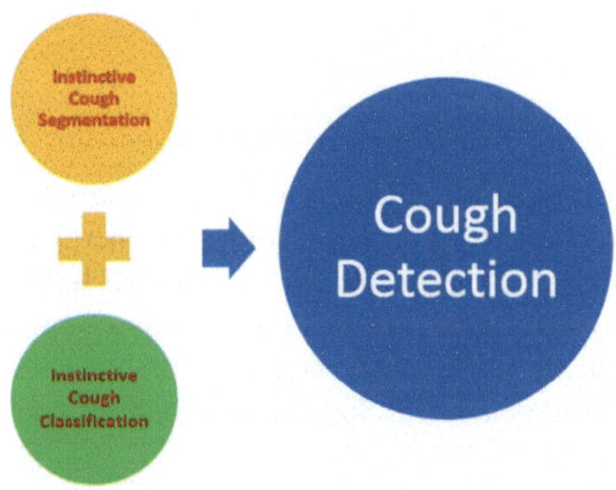

Fig. 5 Methods of cough detection

segment intended coughs and dialogue to extract rate of recurrence and entropy features [29].

Leicester cough monitor (LCM) [30] built using HMM also depends on audio recordings to pre-fragment probable cough events. Cough monitor [31] to observe chronic cough delivers evaluation of respirational sickness. An amalgamation of artificial neural network (ANN) and support vector machine (SVM) classifiers to monitor cough detection of tuberculosis patients by extracting MFCS [32]. Random forest classification [33] identifies cough segments in audio recordings with capability to reconstruct the cough sounds. Simple threshold method [34] differentiates numerous phases of dry and wet coughs and found that dry coughs posed low energy.

VITALOJAK—a cough observing structure [35] applied semi-automated recognition by means of physical corroboration. An aural introverted structure [36] based on Artificial Neural Network (ANN) for recognition of cough. Neural network [37] intended for cough recognition with sorts such as MFCS, formant rate of recurrence, kurtosis and B score. Support vector machine (SVM) with Gammatone cepstral coefficient (GMCC) feature for cough signal recognition [38].

Differentiation of wet and dry coughs in pediatric patients with logistic regression model (LRM) classifier with features such as MFCS, formant frequencies, kurtosis, zero crossing and B score. First cough classification for pertussis uses three classifiers namely ANN, random forest and K-nearest neighbor algorithm (KNN) with MFCS feature and energy level extraction. The tool significance for automatic cough detection was reported in 2013 [39].

Voluntary cough detection [40] was achieved with fast Fourier transform (FFT) coefficient using KNN. Automatic childhood pneumonia detection [41] uses LRM classifier with interest on features such as MFCS, wavelet and non-Gaussian. Non-contact pediatric ward cough segmentation deployed with ANN [42].

The acquired data exploited with ANN supporting accurate cough duration and cough detection with mutual information from sensors [43]. Mobi Cough [44] amalgamates Gaussian mixture model and universal background model (GMM-UBM) for forecasting cough sounds. Smart watch [45] records sounds and performs conformal prediction analysis to detect cough or sneezing events. HMM grounded on cough revealing [46] using univariate and multivariate time series cough data. Convolutional neural network (CNN) is deployed for cough detection [47] with mathematical model for sound analysis.

Asthma cough sound detection [48] through GMM-UBM deals with features such as MFCS and constant-Q cepstral coefficients. WheezeD [49] perceives respiration stage and installs CNN with acoustic in 2D spectro temporal image for breathless recognition. Power spectral density of cough sounds in different air quality conditions is tested by recognition algorithm deployed with principal component analysis (PCA) and SVM [50].

AI4COVID-19 [51] is artificial intelligence (AI) deployed for COVID-19 initial symptoms recognition with novel multipronged mediator centered risk averse architecture. FluSense [52] is innovative edge computing technology for crowd behavior and influenza indicators—cough. The exhaustive detail explaining the methods and their purpose is tabulated in Table 3, and important algorithms are highlighted in Fig. 6.

Table 3 Methods deployed for cough recognition at a glance

Author	Year	Methods deployed
Munyard et al.	1994	Ambulatory cough footage mechanism with assistance of EMG, ECG pulses
Chang et al.	1997	Holter observer-based tussis observer
Hamutcu et al.	2002	Cough monitoring with EMG and audio signal in children with cystic fibrosis
Corrigan et al.	2003	Automated tagging of EMG and audio signal for objective cough monitoring in infants
Paul et al.	2004	Accelerometer portable device with no programmed examination software
Coyle et al.	2005	Lifeshirt [25] is programmed scrutiny of a amalgamation of EMG, ECG and plethysmography
Barry et al.	2006	Hull instinctive cough summer using linear predictive coding significant and predictable neural Web
Matos et al.	2006	HMM for MFCS
Smith et al.	2006	Physical totaling of sound of interest was performed in chronic obstructive pulmonary disease
Martinek J et al.	2008	Intentional cough and speech discriminator based on decision tree
Birring S et al.	2008	Leicester cough monitor using HMM
Smith, J et al.	2010	Cough observer to observe chronic cough
Tracey et al.	2011	An amalgamation of artificial neural network (ANN) and support vector machine (SVM) classifiers for tuberculosis patients
Larson et al.	2011	Random forest classification cough identification
Chatrzarrin et al.	2011	Simple threshold to differentiate phases of coughs
McGuinness K. et al.	2012	VITALOJAK—a cough monitoring system
Drugman T et al.	2012	ANN based on acoustic solitary system
Swarnkar et al.	2013	Neural network-based cough detection
Liu et al.	2013	SVM for cough recognition
Swarnkar et al.	2013	LRM classifier for pediatric patients
Parker et al.	2013	Pertussis cough classification using ANN, random forest and KNN
Drugman T et al.	2013	Automatic cough detection tool significance
Lucio et al.	2014	Voluntary cough detection using KNN
Kosasih et al.	2014	Pneumonia detection with LRM classifier
Amrulloh et al.	2015	ANN automatic cough segmentation
Drugman T et al.	2016	ANN with accurate cough duration and detection
Pham C. et al.	2016	Mobi cough using Gaussian mixture model

(continued)

Table 3 (continued)

Author	Year	Methods deployed
Nguyen et al.	2018	Smart watch with Android app and conformal prediction analysis
Teyhouee et al.	2019	HMM grounded on cough revealing
Kvapilova et al.	2019	Cough detection using CNN
Hwan Ing Hee	2019	GMM-UBM asthma cough detection
Soujanya Chatterjee et al.	2019	WheezeD—CNN-based wheezing detection
Wang et al.	2019	PCA and SVM for cough recognition
Imran et al.	2020	AI4COVID-19—AI-based COVID-19 initial diagnosis.
Hossain et al.	2020	FluSense based on edge computing

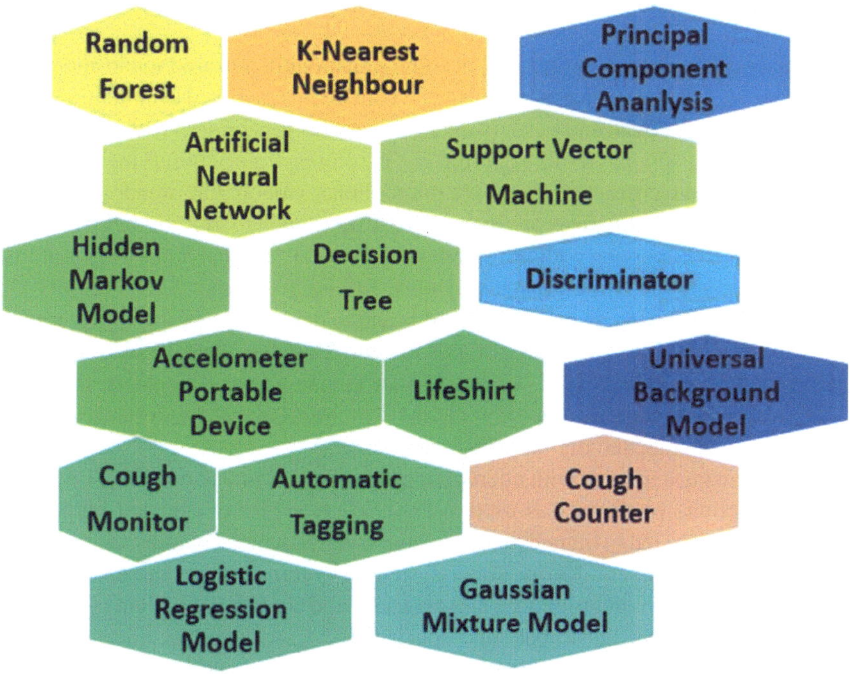

Fig. 6 Highlighted procedures of cough revealing

5 Instruments Organized in Cough Detection

In deploying, Internet of things six building blocks such as deployment types, sensor time, sensor types, architecture, application types and data requirements are considered [53]. Generally, IoT is used for automation of various devices for specific applications such as light controls and video surveillance [53, 54]. In this section, the instruments utilized for cough detection is discussed.

Multiparametric cough monitoring system [20] monitors cough along with activity and heart rates. Accelerometer, electrodes and microphone are deployed to record ECG, ECG and cough signal, respectively. Cough monitor [21] achieved with deployment of Holter monitor, a computer-based cough processor with selected filters and tape recorders used overnight. Cystic fibrosis-based cough is monitored with Logan Research (LR) 100 cough recording device. In addition, conventional tape recorder is used in first or second day of hospitalization for the duration of chest physiotherapy period.

Infant cough monitor was through LR100 cough monitor, infrared sound and video recorder [23]. Accelerometer portable device with no programmed examination software for nocturnal cough and to study the sleep patterns for children with cough [24]. Lifeshirt [25] was prepared of a A peripatetic cardiorespiratory observing structure, adapted unimaneuvering, touching base microphone, videoing in pseudo organized circumstance. Hull instinctive cough summer [26] is simulated by a computing device with MATLAB 6.1 version with LS_Toolbox version 2.1.1, signal processing toolbox version 5.1, neural network toolbox version 4.0.1 and Voicebox.

HMM for cough signals in audio recordings [27] deployed digital sound recorder and microphone placed in chest of the patient. Portable digital voice recorder with miniature omnidirectional condenser microphone wrapped in plastic foam for distinction of voluntary coughs [29]. LCM was inserted with unrestricted arena necklace microphone and digital sound recorder [30].

Cough sensing deployed with microphone present in mobile phone [33], T-Mobile G1 mobile phone platform was used. VITALOJAK [35] implemented with lapel microphone connected to trained manual cough counter, which compresses the signal with three distinct levels. Karmelsonix system, a commercially obtainable cough counter, used with two microphones namely audio and contact microphone for cough detection [36]. For pediatric patients, couch sideways contactless microphone is implemented for cough recognition [4]. Study of sensor significance [39] exploited the part of ECG, thermal resistor, trunk strap, acceleration sensor, touching base and acoustic microphones in cough finding. Rode NT3 a bed side microphone was placed in two directions for cough detection [41]. Non-contact detection in pediatric ward [42] was deployed with Rode NT3 microphone, preamplifier, A/D converter and mobile pre USB. Sensor-based automatic cough detection system [43] enacted ECG, thermistor, chest belt, accelerometer, oximeter, contact and audio microphones, sensors, analog signal conditioning circuit (front-end), analog-to-digital conversion, communication and storing functional blocks. Mobicough [45] consisted of wireless low-cost microphone connected through Bluetooth to mobile phone. Smart watch

[46] for cough detection with low power accelerometer sensor and audio recorder with support of Android app. Asthmatic voluntary sound [48] deployed with computing system supported with MATLAB 2017b and adobe audition CS6. AI4COVID-19 [51] used AI engine for performing cough symptom of COVID-19. FluSense [52] for influenza like illness sensing deployed squat rate microphone, thermal imaging information, Raspberry Pi and Intel Movidius neural engine. The details of instruments utilized for various cough detection work are summarized in Table 4, and important instruments list is highlighted in Fig. 7.

6 Parameters Achieved in Cough Detection Deployment

In cough detection deployment, the main parameters measured as in Fig. 8 are confidence interval, correlation coefficient, positive predictive value or positive foretelling rate, positive rate or optimistic ratio, negative rate, sensitivity or susceptibility, specificity or selectivity, recall, precision, accuracy and F1 score. Confidence interval denotes the sort of value with in which the correct rate lies.

Generally, it is used for comparison between verbal descriptive scores and visual analogue scales [55]. Correlation coefficient gives the strength of relationship with two methods of cough detection mainly video and audio. Positive predictive value indicates the possibility of the focuses with an affirmative screening examination ensuring a sickness. The interlinking connection between positive, negative rate, sensitivity, specificity and predictive value is portrayed in Fig. 9. Supplementary a comprehensive representation about mathematical assessment of parameters is presented in Table 5.

Sensitivity and specificity refer, respectively, to the actual positive cases and actual negative cases predicted appropriately. Positive predictive value and negative predictive value refer the correctness of predicted value is true positive or negative correspondingly.

7 Dataset Details for Cough Detection

For cough detection, numerous data are recorded, created, and existing data bases are used. Data are collected directly from patients [20], and at times, in certain situations, the recordings from subjects were carried out [21]. Mixed sounds from both healthy and ill patients [23], male and female [29] were collected. Sounds from cough due to various illness such as pneumonia, asthma, chronic disorder, tuberculosis and as well as COVID-19 were used [41], [51].

Cough sounds from adults, pediatric [42] and infants [23] are gathered. Already existing YouTube recordings [9], RALE repository [49], environmental sound classification dataset [45], health mode cough dataset [47], sounds from Freesounds.org

Table 4 Instruments list deployed for cough detection

Author	Year	Instruments installed
Munyard et al.	1994	Accelerometer, positive and negative electrode, microphone, conventional tape recorders and multiparametric cough monitoring system
Chang et al.	1997	Holter monitor, cough processor and tape recorder.
Hamutcu et al.	2002	LR100 cough recording device and conventional tape recorder.
Corrigan et al.	2003	LR100 cough monitor, infrared sound and video recorder
Paul et al.	2004	Accelerometer portable device with no programmed examination software
Coyle et al.	2005	A peripatetic cardiorespiratory observing structure, adapted unimaneuvering, touching base microphone, videoing in pseudoorganized circumstance.
Barry et al.	2006	Hull automatic cough counter using computing system with MATLAB 6.1
Matos et al.	2006	HMM deployed with digital sound recorder and microphone.
Smith et al.	2006	Digital acoustic footage
Martinek J et al.	2008	Portable digital voice recorder, a miniature microphone and plastic foam
Birring S et al.	2008	Leicester cough observer expending allowed arena choker microphone and digital sound tape recorder.
Larson et al.	2011	T-Mobile G1 mobile phone platform
McGuinness K. et al.	2012	VITALOJAK with lapel microphone, trained manual cough counter with compression software
Drugman T et al.	2012	Karmelsonix system, audio and contact microphone
Swarnkar et al.	2013	Couch side contactless microphone
Drugman T et al.	2013	ECG, thermal resistor, trunk strap, acceleration sensor, touching base and acoustic microphones
Kosasih et al.	2014	Two bed side microphone Rode NT3
Amrulloh et al.	2015	Rode NT3 microphone, preamplifier, A/D converter and mobile pre USB.
Drugman T et al.	2016	ECG, thermistor, chest belt, accelerometer, oximeter, contact and audio microphones, sensors, analog signal conditioning circuit (front-end), analog-to-digital conversion, communication and storing functional blocks.
Pham C. et al.	2016	Mobi Cough using wireless low cost microphone, mobile phone and Bluetooth.
Nguyen et al.	2018	Smart watch with accelerometer and audio recorder

(continued)

Table 4 (continued)

Author	Year	Instruments installed
Kvapilova et al.	2019	Health mode cough application in smart phone
Hwan Ing Hee et al.	2019	Computing system with MATLAB 2017b and adobe audition CS6
Imran et al.	2020	AI4COVID-19 in AI engine.
Hossain et al.	2020	FluSense with squat rate microphone, thermal imaging information, Raspberry Pi and neural engine Intel Movidius

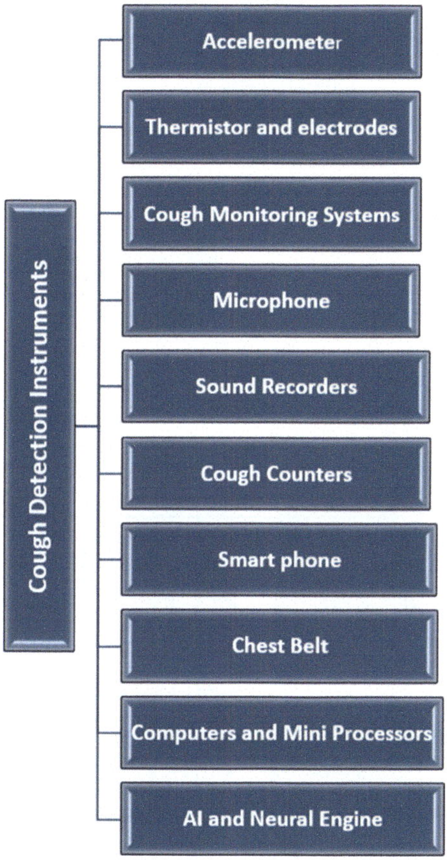

Fig. 7 Imperative implements used for cough recognition

[45], non-speech audio snippets [52] were utilized. In addition, more group of recordings such as Huawei W1 smart watch recordings [45], sounds from weaners [50] were congregated. Cough sound depending on aerial factors was gathered [50]. Sounds from hospital waiting room in recent for influenza like flu symptom checking were also done [52]. A detailed description of data collection is tabulated in Table 6, and the significant data collection depiction is presented in Fig. 10.

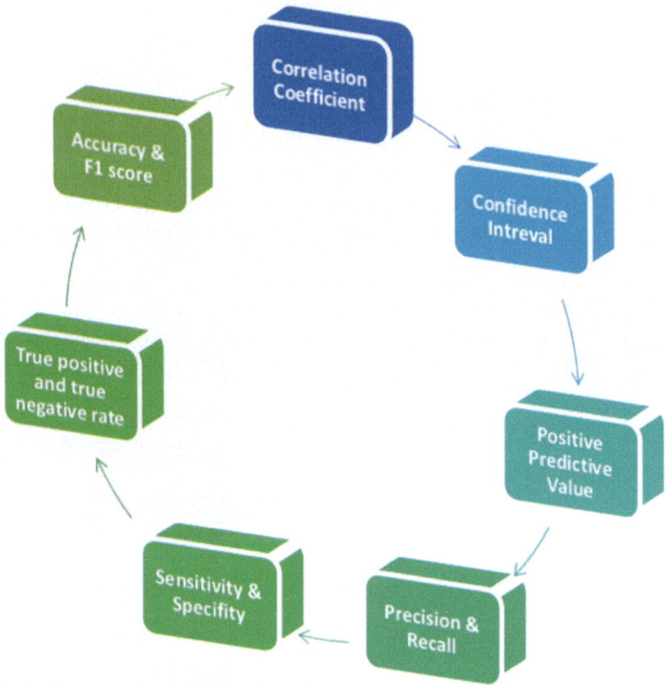

Fig. 8 Parameters list measured in cough detection

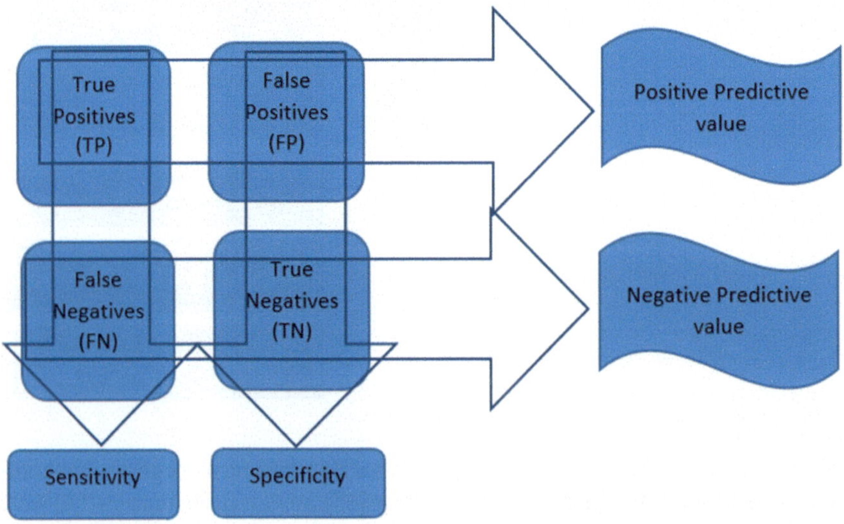

Fig. 9 Interlinking connection of parameters

Table 5 Parameter values and details for cough detection

Author	Year	Parameters description
Munyard et al.	1994	Confidence Interval—95%,
		Correlation coefficient—0.99
Corrigan et al.	2003	Susceptibility 81%
		Positive foretelling rate—0.8
Paul et al.	2004	Confidence Interval—95%
Coyle et al.	2005	Sensitivity—78.1%,
		Specificity—99.6%
Barry et al.	2006	Sensitivity of 80%
		Specificity of 96%
Matos et al.	2006	Sensitivity 82%
Smith et al.	2006	Confidence interval—95%
Martinek J et al.	2008	Sensitivity of 100%
		Specificity of 95%
Birring S et al.	2008	Sensitivity of 91%
		Specificity of 99%
Tracey et al.	2011	Sensitivity 81%
Larson et al.	2011	Susceptibility 92%,
		Mean true optimistic ratio of 92%
		False optimistic ratio of 0.5%.
Chatrzarrin et al.	2011	Accuracy 100%
McGuinness K. et al.	2012	Sensitivity higher than 99%
Drugman T et al.	2012	Sensitivity 95%
		Specificity 95%
Swarnkar et al.	2013	Sensitivity 94.5%
		Specificity 93.4%
Liu et al.	2013	Sensitivity 91%
		Specificity 95%
Swarnkar et al.	2013	Wet tussis susceptibility 84%
		Dry tussis susceptibility 76%
Parker et al.	2013	False positive fault 7%
		False negative fault 8%
Drugman T et al.	2013	Sensitivity 94.5%
		Specificity 94.5%
Lucio et al.	2014	Sensitivity 87.5%
		Specificity 84%
		Recall 86.6%

(continued)

Table 5 (continued)

Author	Year	Parameters description
		Precision 84.3%
Kosasih et al.	2014	Sensitivity (without wavelets) 94%
		Specificity (without wavelets) 63% Sensitivity (with wavelets)
		94%
		Specificity (with wavelets) 88%
Amrulloh et al.	2015	Sensitivity 93%
		Specificity) 97.5%
Drugman T et al.	2016	Sensitivity 94.7%
Pham C. et al.	2016	Recall 91%
		Precision 91%
		Subject independent training 81%
Nguyen et al.	2018	Accuracy 98.75% uncertainty 93.75%
Teyhouee et al.	2019	Region governed by acceptor operating characteristic curvature 92%
Kvapilova et al.	2019	Cough recognition sensitivity determined by human listeners was 90 and 75 at 99.5% specificity preset and 99.9% specificity preset, respectively
Hwan Ing Hee	2019	Sensitivity 82.81%
		Specificity 84.76%
Soujanya Chatterjee et al.	2019	Susceptibility 96.08%
		Selectivity 97.96%
		Exactness 96.99%
Wang et al.	2019	Average recognition rate 95%
Imran et al.	2020	Accuracy 90%
Hossain et al.	2020	Recall 92.26
		Precision 92.26
		F1 Score 92.25

8 Conclusion

In this chapter, an extensive exploration of cough detection methods implemented for various prevailing diseases such as tuberculosis, asthma, wheezing, chronic disorder to newly developed disease coronavirus infection disease in 2019 (COVID-19) is analyzed in a detailed manner. A classic introduction about the famous sick sound is given along with its taxonomy to gather a deep understanding about cough.

Cough-associated medical, non-medical and environment condition are presented. Important features of cough sound such as Mel-frequency cepstral significant, explosive cough sounds, cough seconds, cough breaths, cough epochs, cough intensity,

Table 6 Data collection description list for cough detection

Author	Year	Detailed description of data collection and datasets
Munyard et al.	1994	Collected from 20 subjects
Chang et al.	1997	21 occasions in 18 children aged between six and 15 years
Hamutcu et al.	2002	Recordings collected from 14 children
Corrigan et al.	2003	38 recordings from 30 infants; in which 13 with coughing illness and 17 healthy ones
Paul et al.	2004	Question survey from parents of 100 children with upper respiratory disorder
Coyle et al.	2005	Eight subjects with history of chronic pulmonary disorder which includes six women
Barry et al.	2006	33 fuming observant with twenty male and thirteen female in peer group of 20–54
Matos et al.	2006	Dataset consists of 2155 tussis from nine observants
Smith et al.	2006	Digital recordings from 21 patients
Martinek J et al.	2008	20 health subjects with 15 female aged between
		18 and 56 years and 5 male with age ranging from 26 to 66 years
Birring S et al.	2008	Footages from 15 patients with chronic cough extent beyond 21 days
Tracey et al.	2011	Ten subjects are used
Larson et al.	2011	2500 cough sounds from 17 subjects and recordings from 12 persons
Chatrzarrin et al.	2011	Set of eight highly dry and wet cough was used,
McGuinness K. et al.	2012	Ten patients echoes were documented which comprise six enduring cough, two asthma, one chronic cough and I healthy. In ten patients, four were female.
Drugman T et al.	2012	Two clusters of people were noted. Cluster A consists of 22 subjects. Cluster B comprised of ten supplementary focuses
Swarnkar et al.	2013	13395 separation entailing of cough and supplementary echoes. Further 342 coughs from three subjects
Liu et al.	2013	Designed cough dataset followed by 10 fold cross validation
Swarnkar et al.	2013	536 recorded pediatric cough from 78 patients against validation of 310 recordings from 60 patients and 117 cough events from 18 patients.
Parker et al.	2013	YouTube representing children coughs is utilized
Drugman T et al.	2013	32 healthy subjects are noted
Lucio et al.	2014	411 tussis echoes from 50 characters
Kosasih et al.	2014	815 cough sounds from 91 patients with illnesses as pneumonia, asthma and bronchitis
Amrulloh et al.	2015	1400 cough sounds from 14 pediatric subjects

(continued)

Table 6 (continued)

Author	Year	Detailed description of data collection and datasets
Drugman T et al.	2016	Two clusters of people were noted. Cluster A consists of 22 subjects. Cluster B included ten supplementary focuses.
Pham C. et al.	2016	1000 cough events and numerous noises
Nguyen et al.	2018	Environmental sound classification dataset with 2000 training samples. 40 recording samples in Huawei W1 smart watch in different ambient noise environments. We sampled another 40 sneezing recordings from Freesound.org.
Kvapilova et al.	2019	Health Mode Cough a public dataset with 22 subjects
Hwan Ing Hee	2019	1192 asthma cough sounds from 89 children and healthy 1140 cough sounds from 89 children
Soujanya Chatterjee et al.	2019	RALE repository consisting of 26 lung recordings of newborn to 78 years
Wang et al.	2019	Cough sounds from 84 weaners with aerial factors such as air temperature, relative humidity, ammonia concentration and dust concentration were measured
Imran et al.	2020	Environmental sound classification 50 dataset along with 993 cough sounds and non-cough sounds.
Hossain et al.	2020	21,230,450 non-speech audio snippets from hospital waiting rooms

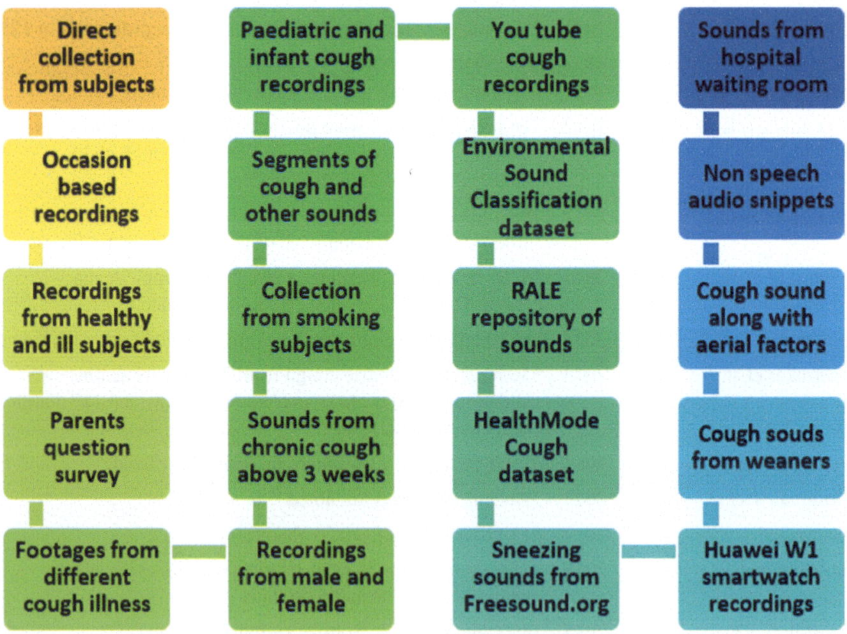

Fig. 10 Significant data collection depiction for cough detection

cough pattern, zero intersection ratio, spectral centroid, spectral bandwidth and spectral roll-off are discussed.

An extensive study of classification and segmentation algorithms such as random forest, KNN, principal component analysis, ANN, SVM, HMM, decision tree, discriminator, accelerometer portable device, universal background model, cough monitor, automatic tagging, cough counter, LRM and GMM deployed is highlighted.

A scrutiny of instruments such as accelerometer, thermistor, cough monitoring systems, microphone, sound recorders, cough counters, smart phones, chest belt, computers, mini processors and AI neural engine utilized in cough detection from conventional stage to the latest edge computing stage is investigated.

The important parameters like correlation coefficient, confidence interval, positive predictive value, precision, recall, sensitivity, specificity, true positive rate, true negative rate, accuracy and F1 score that plays a major role in cough detection are analyzed. Further, dataset involved and created in cough detection such as direct collection from subjects, occasion-based recordings, mixed healthy and ill recordings, cough footages, cough segments, smoking subject collections, environmental sound classification dataset, RALE repository, health mode cough sets, sneezing sounds, non-speech audio snippets, aerial factor cough, weaner cough sounds and Huawei cough sounds is also studied.

References

1. Jans, P., Guarino, M., Costa, A., Aerts, J.M., Berckmans, D.: Evaluation of an algorithm for cough detection in pig houses. IFAC Proc. Volumes **38**(1), 92–96 (2005)
2. Mannino, D.M., Ford, E.S., Redd, S.C.: Obstructive and restrictive lung disease and markers of inflammation: data from the third national health and nutrition examination. Am. J. Med. **114**(9), 758–62 (2003). https://doi.org/10.1016/s0002-9343(03)00185-2
3. Smith, J.A., Ashurst, H.L., Jack, S., Woodcock, A.A., Earis, J.E.: The description of cough sounds by healthcare professionals. Cough. **2**(1), (2006). https://doi.org/10.1186/1745-9974-2-1
4. Swarnkar, V., Abeyratne, U.R., Chang, A.B., Amrulloh, Y.A., Setyati, A., Triasih, R.: Automatic identification of wet and dry cough in pediatric patients with respiratory diseases. Ann. Biomed. Eng. **41**(5), 1016–1028 (2013)
5. Rudraraju, G., Palreddy, S., Mamidgi, B., Sripada, N.R., Sai, Y.P., Vodnala, N.K., Haranath, S.P.: Cough sound analysis and objective correlation with spirometry and clinical diagnosis. Inf. Med. Unlocked. 100319 (2020)
6. De Blasio, F., Virchow, J.C., Polverino, M., et al.: Cough management: a practical approach. Cough **7**, 7 (2011). https://doi.org/10.1186/1745-9974-7-7
7. Shi, Y., Liu, H., Wang, Y., Cai, M., Xu, W.: Theory and application of audio-based assessment of cough. J. Sensors. (2018)
8. Tiwari, V.: MFCS and its applications in speaker recognition. Int. J. Emerg. Technol. **1**, 19–22 (2010). https://www.mendeley.com/research-papers/MFCS-applications-speaker-recognition/
9. Parker, D., Picone, J., Harati, A., Lu, S., Jenkyns, M. H., Polgreen, P.M.: Detecting paroxysmal coughing from pertussis cases using voice recognition technology. PloS One. **8**, 12 (2013)
10. Yin, Y., Mo, H.: The identification method of cough signals using Mel-Frequency cepstrum coefficient. Inf. Technol. pp. 86–91 (2012)

11. Chung, Y., Oh, S., Lee, J., Park, D., Chang, H.-H., Kim, S.: Automatic detection and recognition of pig wasting diseases using sound data in audio surveillance systems. Sensors (Basel) **13**, 12929–12942 (2013). https://doi.org/10.3390/s131012929
12. Du, B., Gao, J., Cao, C.: Objective Recognition of Cough as a Non-invasive biomarker for exposure to cooking oil fumes. Proc. Eng. **205**, 3497–3502 (2017)
13. Shi, Y., Zhang, B., Cai, M., Zhang, X.D.: Numerical simulation of volume-controlled mechanical ventilated respiratory system with 2 different lungs. Int. J. Numer. Methods Biomed. Eng. **33**(9), e2852 (2017)
14. Pavesi, L., Subburaj, S., Porter-Shaw, K.: Application and validation of a computerized cough acquisition system for objective monitoring of acute cough: a meta-analysis. Chest. **120**(4), 1121–1128 (2001)
15. Lee, K.K., Matos, S., Ward, K., Raywood, E., Evans, D.H., Moxham, J., Birring, S.S.: P158 cough sound intensity: the development of a novel measure of cough severity. Thorax **67**(Suppl 2), A130–A131 (2012)
16. Gibson, G.J., Whitelaw, W., Siafakas, N., Supinski, G.S., Fitting, J.W., Bellemare, F. et al.: American Thoracic Society. ATS/ERS statement on respiratory muscle testing. Am. J. Respir. Crit. Care. Med. **166**, 518–624 (2002)
17. Shi, Y., Zhang, B., Cai, M., Xu, W.: Coupling effect of double lungs on a VCV ventilator with automatic secretion clearance function. IEEE/ACM Trans. Comput. Biol. Bioinform. (2017)
18. Abaza, A.A., Day, J.B., Reynolds, J.S., Mahmoud, A.M., Goldsmith, W.T., McKinney, W.G., Frazer, D.G. et al.: Classification of voluntary cough sound and airflow patterns for detecting abnormal pulmonary function. Cough. **5**(1), 8 (2009)
19. Pramono, R.X.A., Imtiaz, S.A., RodriguezVillegas, E.: A cough-based algorithm for automatic diagnosis of pertussis. PLoS ONE **11**(9), e0162128 (2016). https://doi.org/10.1371/journal.pone.0162128
20. Munyard, P., Busst, C., Logan-Sinclair, R., Bush, A.: A new device for ambulatory cough recording. Pediatr. Pulmonol. **18**(3), 178–186 (1994)
21. Chang, A.B., Newman, R.G., Phelan, P.D., Robertson, C.F.: A new use for an old Holter monitor: an ambulatory cough meter. Eur. Respir. J. **10**(7), 1637–1639 (1997)
22. Hamutcu, R., Francis, J., Karakoc, F., Bush, A.: Objective monitoring of cough in children with cystic fibrosis. Pediatr. Pulmonol. **34**(5), 331–335 (2002)
23. Corrigan, D.L., Paton, J.Y.: Pilot study of objective cough monitoring in infants. Pediatr. Pulmonol. **35**(5), 350–357 (2003)
24. Paul, I.M., Yoder, K.E., Crowell, K.R., Shaffer, M.L., McMillan, H.S., Carlson, L.C., Berlin, C.M. et al.: Effect of dextromethorphan, diphenhydramine, and placebo on nocturnal cough and sleep quality for coughing children and their parents. Pediatrics. **114**(1), e85–e90 (2004)
25. Coyle, M.A., Keenan, D.B., Henderson, L.S., Watkins, M.L., Haumann, B.K., Mayleben, D.W., Wilson, M.G.: Evaluation of an ambulatory system for the quantification of cough frequency in patients with chronic obstructive pulmonary disease. Cough. **1**(1), 3 (2005)
26. Barry, S.J., Dane, A.D., Morice, A.H., Walmsley, A.D.: The automatic recognition and counting of cough. Cough. **2**(1), 8 (2006)
27. Matos, S., Birring, S.S., Pavord, I.D., Evans, H.: Detection of cough signals in continuous audio recordings using hidden Markov models. IEEE Trans. Biomed. Eng. **53**(6), 1078–1083 (2006)
28. Smith, J., Owen, E., Earis, J., Woodcock, A.: Effect of codeine on objective measurement of cough in chronic obstructive pulmonary disease. J. Allergy. Clin. Immunol. **117**(4), 831–835 (2006)
29. Martinek, J., Tatar, M., Javorka, M.: Distinction between voluntary cough sound and speech in volunteers by spectral and complexity analysis. J. Physiol. Pharmacol. **59**(6), 433–440 (2008)
30. Birring, S.S., Fleming, T., Matos, S., Raj, A.A., Evans, D.H., Pavord, I.D.: The Leicester Cough Monitor: preliminary validation of an automated cough detection system in chronic cough. Eur. Respir. J. **31**(5), 1013–1018 (2008)
31. Smith, J.: Monitoring chronic cough: current and future techniques. Expert Rev. Respir. Med. **4**(5), 673–683 (2010)

32. Tracey, B.H., Comina, G., Larson, S., Bravard, M., López, J.W., Gilman, R.H.: Cough detection algorithm for monitoring patient recovery from pulmonary tuberculosis. In: 2011 Annual international conference of the IEEE engineering in medicine and biology society (pp. 6017–6020). IEEE (2011)
33. Larson, E.C., Lee, T., Liu, S., Rosenfeld, M., Patel, S.N.: Accurate and privacy preserving cough sensing using a low-cost microphone. In: Proceedings of the 13th International Conference on Ubiquitous Computing, pp. 375–384, (2011)
34. Chatrzarrin, H., Arcelus, A., Goubran, R., Knoefel, F.: Feature extraction for the differentiation of dry and wet cough sounds. In: 2011 IEEE International Symposium on Medical Measurements and Applications (pp. 162–166). IEEE, May 2011
35. McGuinness, K., Holt, K., Dockry, R., Smith, J.: P159 Validation of the VitaloJAK™ 24 hour ambulatory cough monitor. Thorax **67**(Suppl 2), A131–A131 (2012)
36. Drugman, T., Urbain, J., Bauwens, N., Chessini, R., Aubriot, A. S., Lebecque, P., Dutoit, T.: Audio and contact microphones for cough detection. In: Thirteenth Annual Conference of the International Speech Communication Association (2012)
37. Swarnkar, V., Abeyratne, U. R., Amrulloh, Y., Hukins, C., Triasih, R., Setyati, A. (2013, July). Neural network based algorithm for automatic identification of cough sounds. In: 2013 35th Annual International Conference of the IEEE Engineering in Medicine and Biology Society (EMBC) (pp. 1764–1767). IEEE
38. Liu, J.M., You, M., Li, G.Z., Wang, Z., Xu, X., Qiu, Z., Chen, S et al.: Cough signal recognition with gammatone cepstral coefficients. In: 2013 IEEE China Summit and International Conference on Signal and Information Processing (pp. 160–164). IEEE, July 2013
39. Drugman, T., Urbain, J., Bauwens, N., Chessini, R., Valderrama, C., Lebecque, P., Dutoit, T.: Objective study of sensor relevance for automatic cough detection. IEEE J. Biomed. Health. Inform. **17**(3), 699–707 (2013)
40. Lücio, C., Teixeira, C., Henriques, J., de Carvalho, P., Paiva, R. P.: Voluntary cough detection by internal sound analysis. In: 2014 7th International Conference on Biomedical Engineering and Informatics (pp. 405–409). IEEE
41. Kosasih, K., Abeyratne, U.R., Swarnkar, V., Triasih, R.: Wavelet augmented cough analysis for rapid childhood pneumonia diagnosis. IEEE Trans. Biomed. Eng. **62**(4), 1185–1194 (2014)
42. Amrulloh, Y.A., Abeyratne, U.R., Swarnkar, V., Triasih, R., Setyati, A.: Automatic cough segmentation from non-contact sound recordings in pediatric wards. Biomed. Sig. Process. Control. **21**, 126–136 (2015)
43. Mahmoudi, S.A., Possa, P.D.C., Ravet, T., Drugman, T., Chessini, R., Dutoit, T., Valderrama, C.: Sensor-based system for automatic cough detection and classification. In: ICT Innovations Conference (2016)
44. Pham, C.: MobiCough: real-time cough detection and monitoring using low-cost mobile devices. In: Asian Conference on Intelligent Information and Database Systems, pp. 300–309. Springer, Berlin, Heidelberg (2016)
45. Nguyen, K.A., Luo, Z.: Cover your cough: detection of respiratory events with confidence using a smartwatch. In: Conformal and Probabilistic Prediction and Applications (pp. 114–131) (2018)
46. Teyhouee, A., Osgood, N.D.: Cough detection using hidden markov models. In: International Conference on Social Computing, Behavioral-Cultural Modeling and Prediction and Behavior Representation in Modeling and Simulation, pp. 266–276. Springer, Cham, 2019
47. Kvapilova, L., Boza, V., Dubec, P., Majernik, M., Bogar, J., Jamison, J., Karlin, D.R. et al: Continuous sound collection using smartphones and machine learning to measure cough. Dig. Biomarkers. **3**(3), 166–175 (2019)
48. Hee, H.I., Balamurali, B.T., Karunakaran, A., Herremans, D., Teoh, O.H., Lee, K.P., Chen, J. M. et al.: Development of machine learning for asthmatic and healthy voluntary cough sounds: a proof of concept study. Appl. Sci. **9**(14), 2833 (2019)
49. Chatterjee, S., Rahman, M.M., Nemanti, E., Kuang, J.: WheezeD: Respiration phase based wheeze detection using acoustic data from pulmonary patients under attack. In: 13th EAI International Conference on Pervasive Computing Technologies for Healthcare-Demos and Posters. European Alliance for Innovation (EAI) (2019)

50. Wang, X., Zhao, X., He, Y., Wang, K.: Cough sound analysis to assess air quality in commercial weaner barns. Comput. Electron. Agric. **160**, 8–13 (2019)
51. Imran, A., Posokhova, I., Qureshi, H.N., Masood, U., Riaz, S., Ali, K., Nabeel, M.: AI4COVID-19: AI enabled preliminary diagnosis for COVID-19 from cough samples via an App. arXiv preprint arXiv:2004.01275 (2020)
52. Al Hossain, F., Lover, A.A., Corey, G.A., Reich, N.G., Rahman, T.: FluSense: a contactless syndromic surveillance platform for influenza-like illness in hospital waiting areas. Proc. ACM Interact. Mobile. Wearable. Ubiquit. Technol. **4**(1), 1–28 (2020)
53. Raju, P.S., Mahalingam, M., Rajendran, R.A.: Review of intellectual video surveillance through internet of things. In: The Cognitive Approach in Cloud Computing and Internet of Things Technologies for Surveillance Tracking Systems, pp. 141–155. Academic Press (2020)
54. Sambandam Raju, P., Mahalingam, M., Arumugam Rajendran, R.: Design, implementation and power analysis of pervasive adaptive resourceful smart lighting and alerting devices in developing countries supporting incandescent and led light bulbs. Sensors. **19**(9), 2032 (2019)
55. Leconte, S., Ferrant, D., Dory, V., Degryse, J.: Validated methods of cough assessment: a systematic review of the literature. Respiration. **81**(2), 161–174 (2011)

S. R. Preethi is currently working as Assistant Professor in Department of Electronics and Communication Engineering at SRM Valliammai Engineering College. Her research interests are mainly focused on video processing, surveillance, Internet of things, artificial intelligence. She is a Lifetime Fellow of ISTE and CSI.

Dr. A. R. Revathi is currently working as Associate Professor in Department of Information Technology at SRM Valliammai Engineering College. Her research interests are mainly focused on motion detection, human detection and recognition, mining, vision and IoT. She is a lifetime fellow of ISTE and CSI.

Dr. M. Murugan is serving as the Professor of ECE Department and the Vice Principal of SRM Valliammai Engineering College. He is having over 30 years of teaching experience, and his fields of interests are antennas, microwave, satellite communication, optical communication and electromagnetic interference. He is a member of IETE, Life Fellow of ISTE, IEI, ISOI, SEMCEI, SSI and Fellow of CSI and ISCA.

Clinical Deep Dive and Role of Ai/Ml Techniques in Tackling COVID-19

Sangeetha Sundaramoorthy, Vidya Kameshwari, and Selva Kumar Selvaraj

Abstract Novel coronavirus (nCoV) spill over event, with its epicenter in Wuhan, People's Republic of China, has emerged as a public health emergency of international concern. This began as an outbreak in December 2019. Since its transmission is airborne, it has become a very big challenge for controlling the spread. The pandemic has catalyzed the development of novel coronavirus vaccines across the biotech industry, both by pharmaceutical companies and research organizations such as the National Institutes of Health (NIH), USA. It is now one of the top-priority pathogens to be dealt with, because of high transmissibility, severe illness and associated mortality. This chapter highlights the morphological characteristics, the clinical diagnosis and mode of transmission, replication, symptoms, preventions and treatments. This chapter also includes COVID-19 spread analysis using SIR model across few countries and its ability to predict "when would flattening of curve occurs for a country?" also how machine learning (ML)and artificial intelligence (AI) plays a role in estimating the spread. At this moment, appropriate treatment for the virus has not been identified. Combination of antiviral, anti-malarial drugs has been used all over the globe. As of now, social distancing and quarantine are best options to control the pandemic. This chapter is written with aim of providing specific information on COVID-19 which would serve as reference for further studies.

Keywords SARS-CoV-2 · PCR · Artificial Intelligence · Machine learning · Social distance · Myth buster

1 General Introduction on COVID-19

A very recent virus which has come into play named coronavirus also known as SARS-COV-2 which mostly infects birds and mammals. Coronavirus causes a disease known as COVID-19.This virus is already known before many years but has

---

S. Sundaramoorthy (✉) · V. Kameshwari · S. K. Selvaraj
St.Peter's Institute of Higher Education and Research, Avadi, Chennai, Tamil Nadu, India
e-mail: sangeetha.sundaramoorthi@yahoo.com

© The Editor(s) (if applicable) and The Author(s), under exclusive license to Springer Nature Singapore Pte Ltd. 2020

C. Chakraborty et al. (eds.), *Internet of Medical Things for Smart Healthcare*, Studies in Big Data 80, https://doi.org/10.1007/978-981-15-8097-0_9

recently become more mobile or progressive. Let us keep an eye on the morphological structure of COVID-19 disease causing virus.

1.1 Morphological Structure

Coronavirus is a single stranded virus with spherical particle (Diameter-120 nm). It comprises of envelope which consists of lipid bilayer is attached with membrane, envelope and spike structural proteins. It prevents when it was not inside the host cell. Some of the subgroups of virus have hemagglutin esterase which has shorter spike like protein called β coronavirus. The envelope consists of multiple copies of nucleocapsid protein [1].

1.2 Genomic Characteristics

See Fig. 1.

The genome size of RNA virus is one of the largest and it ranges approximately from 27 to 34 m kilobases. It has 5' methylated cap and 3' polyadenylated tail. The genomic organization comprises of 5' leader sequence replicase/transcriptase, spike protein, envelope protein, membrane protein, nucleocapsid 3' UTR poly A tail.

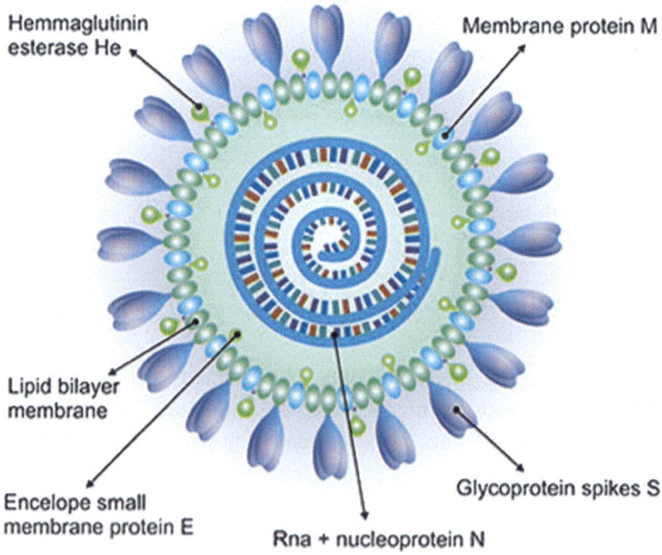

Fig. 1 Coronavirus morphology

1.3 Coronavirus Spike Protein

Coronavirus spike protein is a class one chimeric protein, which interferes with the attachment to the host receptor. Its species differs significantly in N-glycosylated S protein, scaling roughly from 1100 to 1600 in length, with an approximated molecular mass up to 220 kDa. The length of the trimer spike proteins ranges from 18 to 23 nm, whereas its common target is to neutralize vaccines and antibodies. It is divided into two subunits such as globular S1 subunit and S2 subunit. Subunit S1 is responsible for recognizing receptor and S2 for fusion on the membrane. The components of S1 consist of huge receptor-binding domain and it is organized with four domains A,B,C and D in which first two domains such as A and B serve as RBD of S protein and subunit 2 composed of spike molecules which contains the segments that enable fusion of virus cell. This consists of HR1 and HR2 along with that transmembrane domain that are tightly preserved between species around different gene. This recently emerged coronavirus shows difference when compared with older coronavirus identified before. And the difference is the insertions of the N terminal domain, which may confer binding activity of sialic acid, and the key residues variation in the receptor-binding motif in organizing with coronavirus.

1.4 Spike—Receptor Interactions

Studies proved that spike glycoprotein showed that both N and C terminal region of subunit 1 penetrates into host receptors, and thus, it acts as receptor-binding domain. The C terminal region of α and β coronaviruses bounds to proteinaceous receptors [2] (Table 1).

Table 1 Types of coronavirus

Genera	HCoV types	Host receptors
α COVID-19	HCoV-229E APN	(aminopeptidase N, CD13)
α COVID-19	HCoV-NL63 ACE2	Angiotensin-converting enzyme
β COVID-19	HCoV-HKU1 HCoV-HKU1	O-ac Sia
β COVID-19	HCoV-OC43	O-ac Sia
β COVID-19	MERS-CoV	DPP4 (dipeptidyl peptidase
β COVID-19	SARS-CoV ACE2	Angiotensin-converting enzyme

2 Mode of Transmission

Respiratory disease can be circulating through sneeze droplets of various dimensions like greater than 5–10 μm; they are called as respiratory droplet likewise when they are less than 5 μm in diameter it is droplet nuclei. According to the present sign, this virus mainly spreads through respiratory droplets when symptomatic people sneeze or cough [3]. Transmission of droplets takes place if an individual is in close contact with the persons who have problem in respiration and is risky for the person who is in close contact of having his/her face nearby without wearing mask. Not only through this, it may also occur through touching the objects used by the infectious person, and hence, it occurs by both direct and indirect contact. Transmission that occurs through air is different from droplet transmission as it refers to the infectious nuclei that are released from the patients remains in air for lengthy time and was transferred to the healthy individual who were around 1 m. At sometimes in COVID-19, transmission is even possible through the treatments given to the patients that generate aerosols like cardiopulmonary resuscitation, administration of nebulized treatment, endotracheal intubation, NIV, turning the patient to the prone position and bronchoscopy. Some evidences also say that COVID-19 infection will also transmit through feces. But to date, only one positive study was undergone for a single stool specimen [4–6].

2.1 Clinical Symptoms

Coronavirus belongs to the family of viruses which can give rise to the sickness like cold, (SARS) and (MERS). In the year 2019, novel coronavirus was recognized as the causative agent of infection outburst that developed in China. Symptoms of COVID-19 develop after two weeks of exposure which causes cough, fever, difficulty in breathing and shortness of breath. Apart from this major symptoms, sore throat, runny nose and tiredness include. Rarely some patients experienced the loss of smelling and tastelessness. The seriousness of the virus exists from mild to life threatening. Symptomless people also have the chance of spreading the disease. Older people who have chronic complaints such as lung disease, heart disease or diabetes or immunosuppressed patients are at high risk. This resembles other respiratory sickness like influenza which leads to pneumonia and organ failure in several organs [7–9] (Fig. 2).

3 Evidence for Natural Evolution

Researchers investigated that the receptor-binding domain of coronavirus spike proteins had progressed to target a molecular feature on the human cells called ACE2. ACE2 is a receptor which regulates blood pressure in humans. Scientists conclude

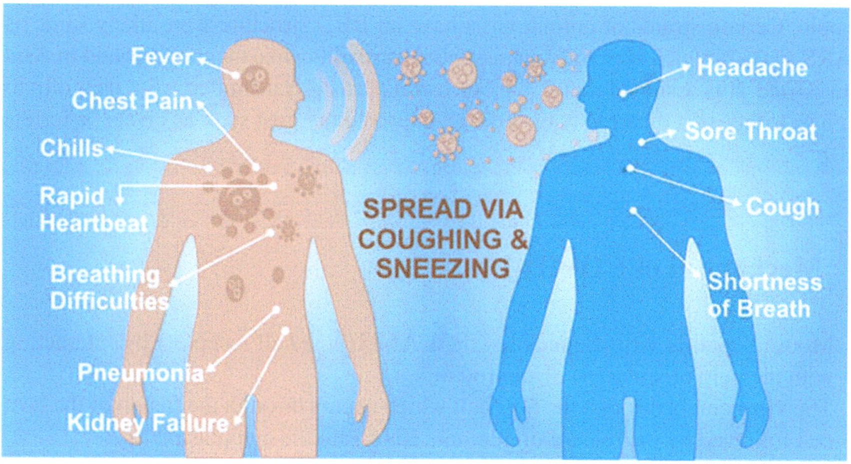

Fig. 2 COVID-19 transmission and symptoms

that SARS-CoV-2 was the naturally produced virus and it is not artificially generated because its spike protein was so active at binding the human cells. And they added, the backbone of SARS-CoV-2 differs substantially compared to other known coronavirus and resembles related viruses that was identified in bats and pangolins. "Observation of mutation in the RBD portion of the spike protein and its distinct backbone of the virus rule out the statement laboratory manipulation as a potential origin for SARS-CoV-2".

3.1 *Possible Origin of Virus*

Scientists have concluded that the most likely origins for SARS-CoV-2 followed one of two possible scenarios. The first scenario is coronavirus developed to its pathogenic stage naturally in animals and then it is transferred to humans. Older history of coronavirus happened by this way, after direct disclosure to civets and camels with humans. Since it is likely to a bat coronavirus, scientists anticipated bats as the most likely reservoir for recently emerged COVID. No cases have documented a transmission directly from bat to human. However, it is assumed that an intermediate host was likely involved between humans and bats.

In this scenario, two unique structural features of SARS-CoV-2's spike protein and the RBD portion that bounds with cells and the cleavage site opens up the virus have developed to their present stage before it enters into humans. As the virus evolved the structure that makes it pathogenic, the current outbreak would perhaps have developed as soon as humans were infected and able to spread between humans.

In the other proposed scenario, a virus that is not pathogenic to animals has jumped into humans and then developed into its current pathogenic state within the people. Certain strains of corona virus have an RBD structure were likely same as SARS-CoV-2, which is isolated in pangolins, armadillo-like mammals found in Asia and Africa. It is assumed that A type of coronavirus is transmitted from pangolin to human, either in a direct way or through intermediate host such as civets or ferrets [10].

4 Mechanism of COVID-19

- Mouse hepatitis virus bounds to CEACAM-1(host cell receptor) by interacting with the help of spike (S) glycoprotein.
- The virus enters through the host cell which occurs through the fusion of the host cell followed by the release of genomic RNA into the cytoplasm.
- Instead of that, MHV will even enter into the host by forming endocytic vesicles, and followed by that fusion occurs with the vesicle membrane.
- Proteolytic processing generates an RNA-dependent RNA polymerase and it happens due to the translation of the positive-strand genomic RNA which gives rise to a large polyprotein.
- A full-length, antisense negative-strand template is generated, by the action of the RNA polymerase.
- Subgenomic negative-strand templates apparently synthesizes subgenomic mRNAs.
- Translation of subgenomic mRNA forms structural viral proteins.
- Multiplication with CEACAM-1 is promoted by S—glycoprotein which forms on the outer region of the host cell.
- Virus develops into the vesicles along with that, virions which is smaller than the virus multiplies in the plasma membrane.
- Replication of the host cell by binding with CEACAM-1, and the virus liberates that causes infection.
- Along with plasma membrane virions are multiplied and the virus is accumulated inside the vesicles.
- Leocapsid protein; ORF, open readingframe [11] (Fig. 3).

5 Diagnostic Test

After the first official WHO's announcement of outbreak of COVID-19, China developed first diagnostic test in less than three weeks, however virus did not had proper identity. After two months, so many diagnostic centers on the market had developed. The Director General of the WHO highlighted a line repeatedly "test, test, test" in the battle against this outburst.

Polymerase chain reaction (PCR) is the most universal test on the detection of genes of the virus. On the aim of lowering the cost and speeding up the diagnosis,

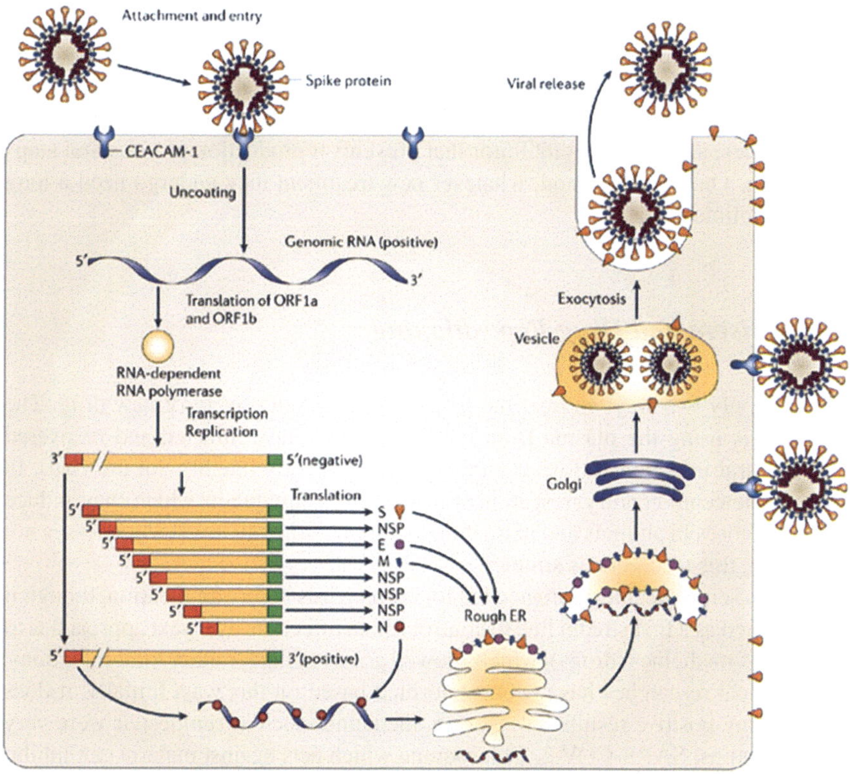

Fig. 3 Coronavirus replication mechanism

some of the other tests are also coming which do not require the samples to be sent to large automated centers, but can be carried out in home and medical care sites. Important trial such as serological test detects antibodies against the virus in the blood. It helps to diagnose the people who are infectious and also even who recover from infection. In addition, it also helps to identify the people already immune to virus and to appreciate the true scale of pandemic. Countries like Singapore and China are already using these serological tests and are expected for the availability of other countries for mass usage [12, 13].

6 New Antivirals

To target certain virus, some of the specific treatments of virus have been recently developed. Monoclonal antibodies similar to our immune system which fights against pathogen were designed in the laboratory.

The spike protein which the virus applies to affect the host cell has been drawn a transparent aim for the sketch of antibodies. The next step is to discover drug that intervenes with the virus which contains vital proteins. Recent research reveals that composition of the protease which SARS-CoV-2 uses the proteins develops new viral particles, along with an inhibitor that prevents reproduction of virus and stops functioning. On the other hand, whatever new treatment they undergo need a long process of clinical trials.

6.1 Antisera and Drug Repositioning

There are only two ways to treat the patients until the discovery of new drug. The first thing is using the plasma from the person who have infected and recovered from the viral infection and whose antibodies are already fought with the virus. In the late nineteenth century, researchers invented a technique in which they induce natural defenses in animals and extract their serum. Although its effectiveness is not guaranteed, this technique is simpler.

Reliable serological tests are needed for coronavirus before application, though it has been used as a first stream line to control Ebola infection. The next approach is to make use of medicines (drugs), which showed good results for other viral infections. Many clinical researches have been performed based on this way. Initially, it does not show any positive results but later on, medicines such as remdesivir were very effective against SARS-COV-2. Chloroquine which acts against malaria can inhibit the infection. WHO promoted both of these compounds (remdesivir, chloroquine) as a large clinical trial project which focuses on four promising therapies. China has already approved the antiviral drug named favilavir (or favipiravir) created by Japanese group Fujifilm for use against other RNA viruses such as influenza in the treatment of COVID-19. Added advantages on using these already approved drugs are that instead of giving approval for new drug, they repositioned the very same drugs for the use of COVID-19.

6.2 The Long-Awaited Vaccine

Epidemiologists stress that the ends SARS-COV-2 lies in obtaining a vaccine, even if the given treatment shows good results effectively against the disease. Even though the efforts are extraordinary, at the time of writing, there are at least 50 candidate vaccines in development against COVID-19. Trails have been started in almost all the industries. Moderna Therapeutics and the US National Institutes of Health created the case for the messenger RNA (mRNA) vaccine. This invention includes instructing the cells to produce proteins from the virus that stimulates immune responses. Initially, around 45 volunteers from Seattle are inoculated. CanSino Biologics located in china developed another vaccine at this stage of clinical trials that works on a harmless virus masked with the proteins of the coronavirus. Pharmaceuticals will begin testing its DNA vaccine in human. However, the safety of the vaccines is being assessed in this first phase. The sad part is even the researchers and WHO accepts that fulfilling all the phases for the approval of a vaccine for COVID-19 will nearly take one or two years [14].

7 "Times of India" Report

COVID-19 has been detected in laboratories through RT-PCR and gene fingerprinting, which is not easy to diagnose. So far only 403 laboratories are functioning to test this novel virus. All these laboratories works by the guiding principle given by noninvasive ventilation (NIV). The tests use more sensitive form of assay called RT-PCR. WHO recommends that the patients who are suspected are hospitalized only after the confirmation of RT-PCR or gene sequencing results [15]. The fast spread of the coronavirus has created the final stage of alert all over the world; thus, WHO has declared this outbreak as pandemic. At the same time, researchers are doing so many trials with the virus to identify new therapies and vaccines for treating the disease. Since the cases are increasing day by day, hospitals have developed their capabilities to care for the patients.

8 Role of Artificial Intelligence (AI) & Machine Learning (ML) Applications in COVID-19 Times

When we hear the term "artificial intelligence," most of us remember, Terminator or Robots which takes over humans, AI is not that, at least for now. AI is a broader science which makes or teaches machines to think and make rational decisions and goal-oriented actions, having said that, still we have a long journey a head to match a 5-year old in mental ability. We are at a nascent but at most important time in AI revolution as new developments and discoveries happen in AI world every hour.

Before we jump into different AI/ML applications which were designed to tackle COVID-19 situation, let us understand what AI really mean, is ML part of AI? And so on.

Artificial Intelligence (AI)

AI is a broad science which deals with simulating or mimicking human like intelligence by machines, i.e., teaching machines to think and act like humans do. We see lot of AI system in our day-to-day lives; sometimes, we use or consume their services without even realizing that they are a type of AI systems. When we talk to "Siri" on apple phones, when we drive a Tesla car, when Amazon or Netflix understands

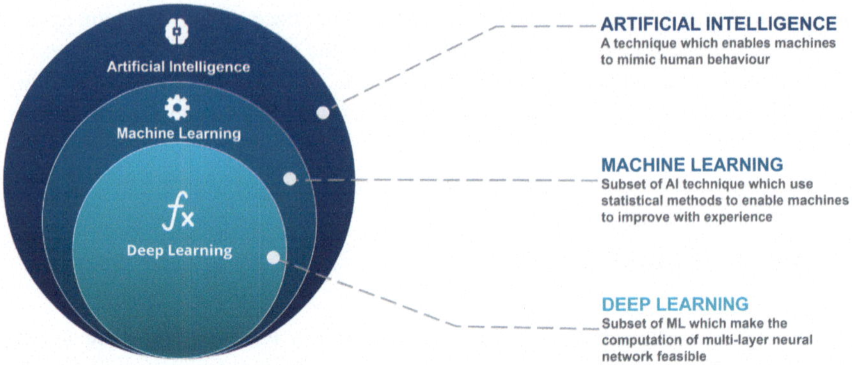

Fig. 4 AI/ML conceptual representation

your better and customizes offers and discounts or gmail helps you with next letter to complete your email and so many to quote, all of these are AI systems (Fig. 4).

Machine Learning (ML)

ML (a subset of AI) is a field of study where computers learn from data and act without explicit programs. ML uses statistical methods to analyze data, find patterns and learn outcomes and decisions with minimal human intervention. ML is the latest buss word and most sought after technology at least nine out of ten companies would be actively investing in ML technologies. Applications like email filtering, fraud analytics, and understanding customer churn, customer segmentation, Image, speech recognition, medical diagnosism etc. are all ML applications. Above diagram shows ML being a subset of AI.

Deep Learning

Deep Learning being a subset of ML uses layered structures of algorithms called an artificial neural network (ANN). The design of an artificial neural network is inspired by the biological neural network of the human brain, leading to a process of learning that is far more capable than that of standard machine learning models. Deep learning is suitable for problems which are more complex and often require huge amount of training data for, e.g., image analysis to differentiate a cat and dog or to detect different objects in an image, language translation, and speech recognition are all better performed using deep learning methodologies.

To give to better understand similarities and differences, below are some of real world examples of ML and deep learning (Table 2).

Table 2 AI, ML Use Cases

Some real world use cases of ml and deep learning	
Machine learning	Deep learning
Prediction of customer satisfaction score of a product	Virtual personal assistance like Siri, Alexa or Google which are trained to understand voice and make decisions
Detection of fraud in banking or insurance transactions	Chatbots which can understand your text and respond based on your questions. Chatbots can be text or voice based.
Estimating sales based on various factors such as region, season, promotions, etc.	Image recognition, facial recognition, face detections, predicting age based on facial features
Prediction of cyberattacks	Object detections from images, object tracking, self-driving cars
Customer segmentation based on various factors such as recency, frequency, monetary (RFM)	Speech recognition, voice to text, text to voice, language translation
Email spam and malware filtering	Video surveillance, video analysis, motion tracking, actions identifications
Product recommendation system	Understanding emotions from tweets, text
Market basket analysis	Text, music generation

8.1 Role of AI/ML During COVID-19 Times

Technology has played a very important role during COVID-19 situations, right from spread analysis, diagnosis, treatment and vaccine developments doctors and technicians rely on various technologies. Since the outbreak, we are witnessing increasing use of technologies like virtual laboratories, telemedicine which helps to maintain social distancing at the same time reach out to masses in quick turnaround time. Many digital platforms from countries around the globe are providing right information and directions for their citizens in real time. Digital platforms have reached out to people from all touch points including televisions, laptops mobile devices, etc. which caters information and statistics on COIVD-19 spread, safe zones, precautions measures, safety procedures, diagnostic centers near you, medical support live lines and contacts, etc. Upsurge of many virtual assistance and chatbots nearly answers almost all COVID-19-related questions helps governments to address huge number of people at the same time.

Now let us see few AL/ML technologies which are used for tackling COVID-19 with little more details. Following use cases helps you to understand the problem and how AI/ML technology address them. However, we will not go very deep to their working principles and techniques here.

(i) **Use Case 1: Social distancing using computer vision**

Back Ground:

It is a known fact that social distancing is the best approach to prevent the spread of COVID-19; after several rounds of lock down, countries are easing up and allowing trades and business operations with the condition of maintaining safe social distancing among customers and staffs. In response to it, there is a huge demand especially from retail and manufacturing sectors for camera surveillance to signal breech of social distancing and to provide heat map of store locations where usually people crowd up.

Problem:

With help of CCTV cameras, enable retail stores to detect social distancing violations and provide floor zones where most of violations happen so that stores can ease up aisles for better customer navigations.

Solution Approach

Using computer vision technology, it is possible to analyze each frame in a video from CCTV camera and teach model to detect objects (Pedestrians or customers in this case) so it a two-step process.

Step 1: Train the model with large number of images with humans in it and provide coordinates (locations in x-axis and Y-axis) of bounding box where humans are present. Since we are training the model, this process is called training process.

Step 2: After training the model, on giving a new image to the model. Model can clearly identify humans and their location in the newly provided (Figs. 5, 6 and 7).

Step 3: Calculate distance between all rectangle box centroids; when the distance is less than stipulated safe distance, then highlight those persons with different color to show as violations of social distancing (Fig. 8).

Step 4: Record violations coordinates for a span of time and plot them as heat map, which eventually says where (which location) violations have widely happened. This will help the authorities to take step to avoid congestions in those locations (Fig. 9).

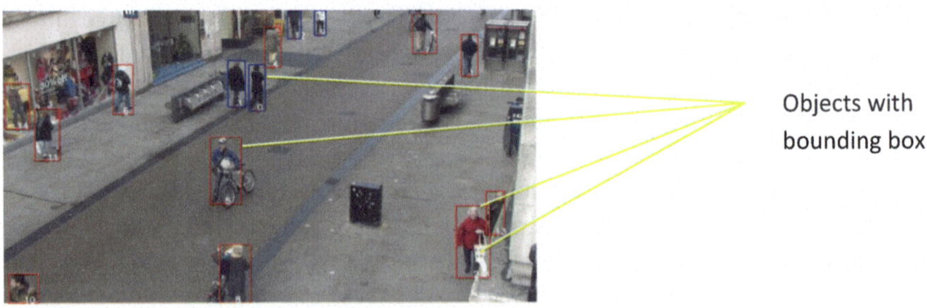

Fig. 5 Sample training image with pedestrians and marked bounding boxes

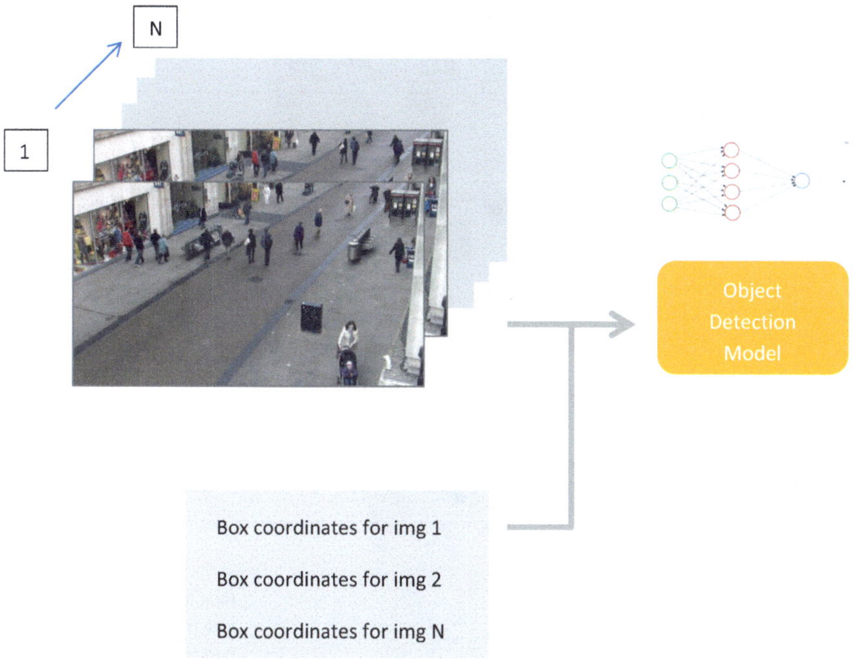

Fig. 6 Training process of object detection deep learning neural network

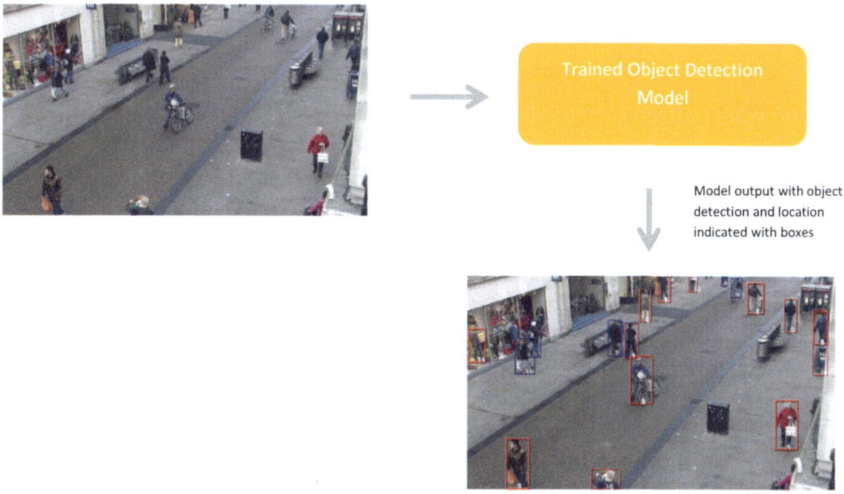

Fig. 7 Inference process of object detection deep learning neural network

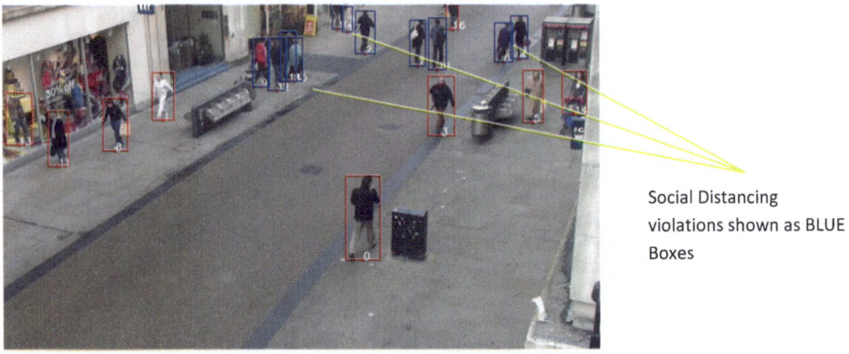
Social Distancing
violations shown as BLUE
Boxes

Fig. 8 Final output shows persons violating social distancing

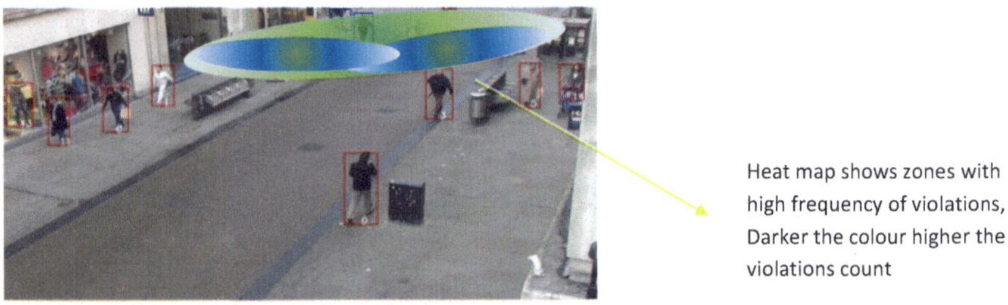
Heat map shows zones with
high frequency of violations,
Darker the colour higher the
violations count

Fig. 9 Heat map showing zones with high frequency of social distancing violations

If you want to deep dive on deep learning model working, below are pointers to guide you for further reading

- Object detection used for this experiment is called "detectron" which is latest high performance object detection from Facebook research and it is available as open source.
- Refer following Facebook research github for full implementation codes and notes.
  https://github.com/facebookresearch/detectron[16]
- Distance measure used is called Euclidean distance; there will be slight variations to real measures. To obtain real measures, camera calibrations and camera angle and transformation would be required for accuracy.
- Refer following Facebook research github for full implementation codes and notes.

(ii) **UseCase 2: COVID-19 Myth Busters Using Text Analytics (Natural Language Processing)**

Back Ground:

During COVID-19 situations, digital platform was widely used to spread vital information; at the same time, same media were used to spread false news, rumors and myths. Rumors and myths became a challenge for governments; hence, many governments posted myth busters on their web portals and communications.

Problem:

Many technology companies and NGOs used AI technology to produce self-serving personal assistance or chatbots to answer them whether a given user statement or questions is a myth or a fact. Point to note is people can frame questions in many (example below) ways but still chatbots need to identify if it is a myth or fact.

Example of user question or Phrase People can frame a same question in many as shown in below sample

- Can lemon fight COVID-19?
- Is lemon good to prevent coronavirus?
- Do lemon and garlic are good to fight COVID?

Solution Approach

Convert sentences (Covid Myths) to high-dimensional vectors using pretrained model (Universal Sentence Encoder) high-dimensional vectors will enable us to compare semantic similarity between two sentences are phrases.

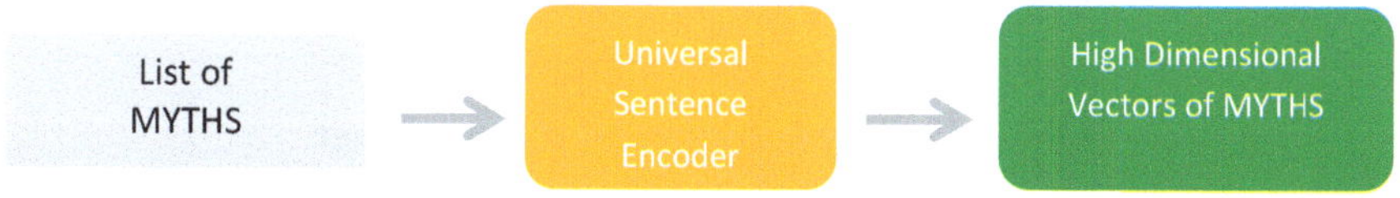

When people post a new question, question will be converted to high-dimensional vector and will be matched with already created MYTH vectors; if there is a close match, then given statement is likely to be a myth else it is not (at least not matching with entire myth list we have trained). When chatbots are linked to this service, it can take questions and respond back with its prediction, i.e., whether it a myth or not.

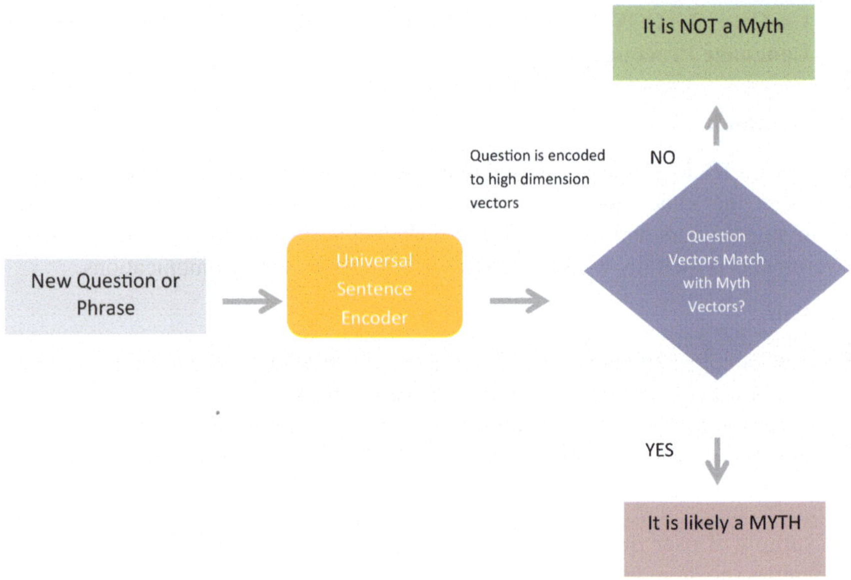

For deep dive sentence encoding, refer to below pointers for further study

- Sentence encoder used in this experiment is TensorFlow Hub's "Universal Sentence Encoder." It is available as ***Open Source***.
- It is trained on a variety of data sources and a variety of tasks with the aim of dynamically accommodating a wide variety of natural language understanding tasks.
- Refer following link for code and notes.
  https://tfhub.dev/google/universal-sentence-encoder/1 [17]

(iii) **UseCase3: COVID-19 diagnosis using chest x-ray image**

Back Ground:

Kaggle is an online community of data scientist and machine learning practitioners; Kaggle is known for pushing existing boundaries and paves way for new discoveries in area of data science by its completions. Kaggle competitions are mostly based on real word problem and it seeks solution from world wide data science practitioners, enthusiasts and students.

Kaggle launched a completion to build a model for computers to identify COVID-19, pneumonia from chest x-ray images.

Problem:

Computer needs to classify chest x-ray images as "normal" or COVID-19 or pneumonia.

Solution Approach

In computer vision problem specifically known as "image classification," where computer model is trained do differentiate specific class (say cat or dog, in this case COVID-19 or pneumonia or normal) from the image. Solution involves following steps.

Step1: Train the model with large number of chest x-ray images which are of COVID-19, pneumonia and normal cases and their respective case names (class0-COVID-19, Class1-Pnuemonioa, Class2-Normal). Model learns the image features and their corresponding classes. After significant iterations of training, model learns to classify any new chest x-ray image as any of the closely matching three classes.

Step2: After training the model, on giving a new chest x-ray image to the model. Model can clearly classify the given image as any one of the following classes.

- Class0- COVID-19
- Class1-Pnuemonia
- Class2-Normal

Following figures show the training and inference steps in making an image classifier model (Figs. 10 and 11).

For more deeper reading on chest x-ray classification Kaggle completionFollow the link https://www.kaggle.com/bachrr/covid-chest-xray [18]

(iv) **Use Case 4: COVID-19 chatbot**

Back Ground:

COVID-19 situation clogged all manually operated help lines seeking COVID-19 information; many governments relied on AI technology to build virtual assistance and chatbots to cater information to large mass in real time. This solution was several times cheaper and efficient and no manual effort required. Chatbots can operate during lock downs and available 24/7 for people's service.

Problem:

Governments and NGOs wanted to develop a chatbot accessible from their PCs and handheld devices to answer questions on various themes which includes the following.

- COVID-19 self-diagnosis by a survey.
- COVID-19 precaution and safety tips.

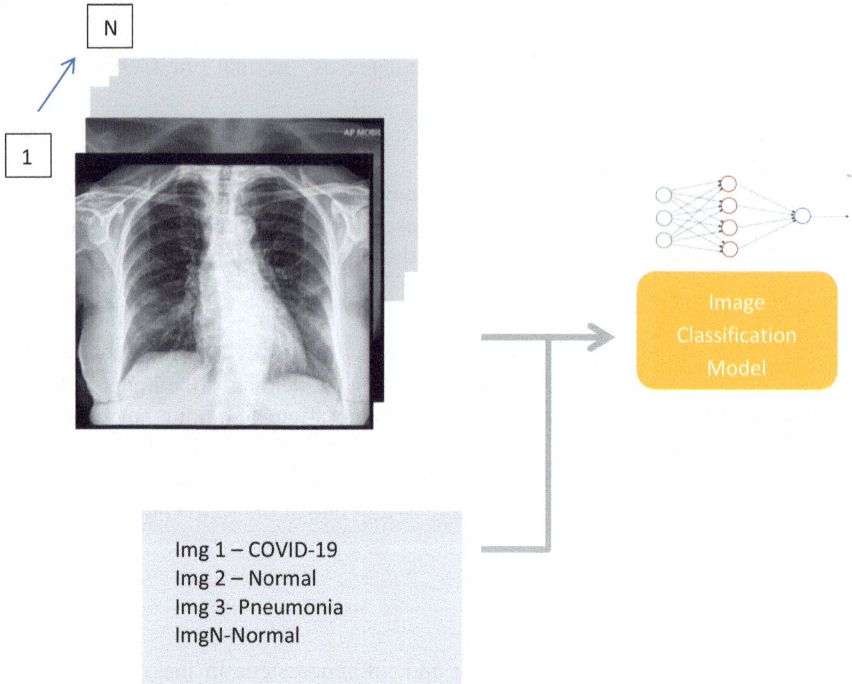

Fig. 10 Training process of image classification deep learning neural network

- COVID-19 spread statistics.
- Lockdown situations, red zones, etc.
- COVID-19 testing centers near me.
- Medical and help centers near me.

Solution Approach

Text-based or voice-based chatbots are suited for answering various questions from huge number of people at the same time and be available 24/7. Chatbots are computer programs which are specially trained to respond to questions from a specific area. One of the leading AI chatbots such as IBM's Watson for instance is trained on large volumes of data to make it a general purpose chatbot which is ready to answer almost all questions from any given area. However, in order to make chatbots more relevant, chatbots must be trained in a specific tasks data to make it equipped to answer most of the questions from an given area.

In this section, we can see some of the solutions built from different governments for addressing one or many of above mentioned themes.

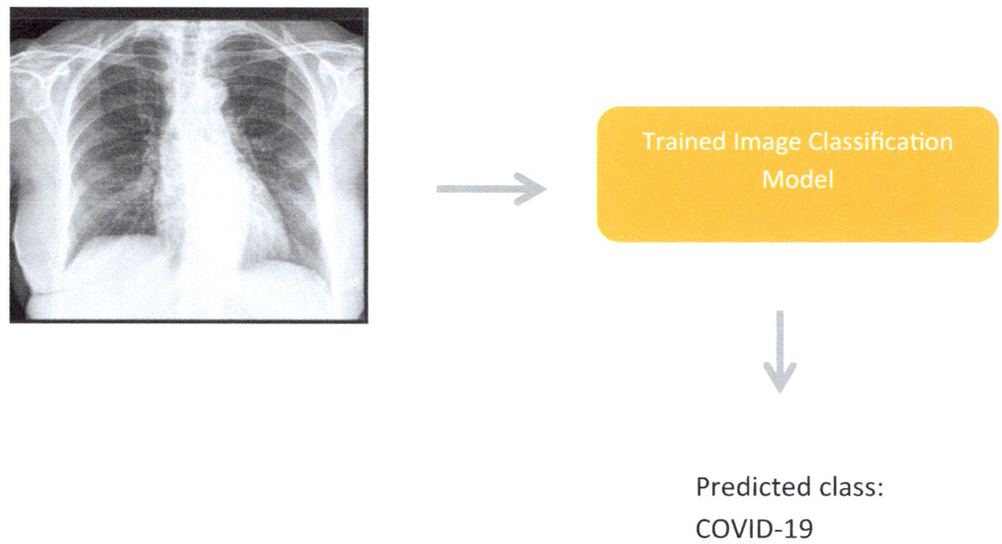

Fig. 11 Inference process of image classification deep learning neural network

"Arogya Setu" Mobile App from Indian Government for COVID-19 Self-diagnosis

Helps people to take self-assessment by answer a series of questions which are adapted based on people's responses. All accepting the inputs for the questions; app provides a risk score and relevant support information for the users.

This app is equipped uses Bluetooth to alert if any COVID-19 positive people in closer proximity (Fig. 12).

"Self-check Bot from Centers for Disease Control and Prevention

Similar self-check for COVID-19 from https://covid19healthbot.cdc.gov/ [19] (Fig. 13)

World Health Organization (WHO) COVID-19 self-help BOT in Facebook

World Health Organization has launched COVID-19 Self-help BOT in its Facebook page https://www.facebook.com/WHO/ [20] (Fig. 14)

(v) **Use Case 5: COVID-19 spread analysis using SIR model**

Back Ground:

During this tough lock down times, million dollar questions from every one of us is "When will all this end?", i.e., exactly when my country or state's infection curve will flatten? To answer this questions, mathematician and machine learning enthusiastic all over the globe adopted different approaches to accurately model the infection, recovery and death trends of a nation or state.

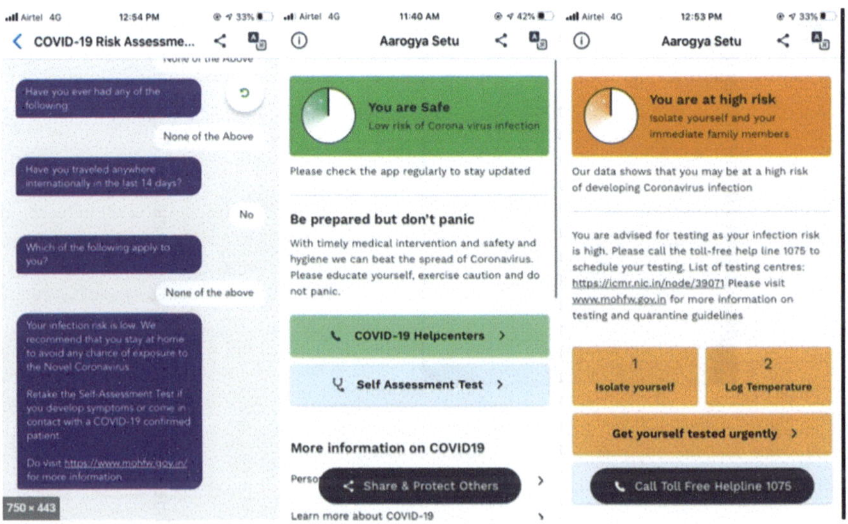

Fig. 12 Arogya Setu mobile app sample screen shots

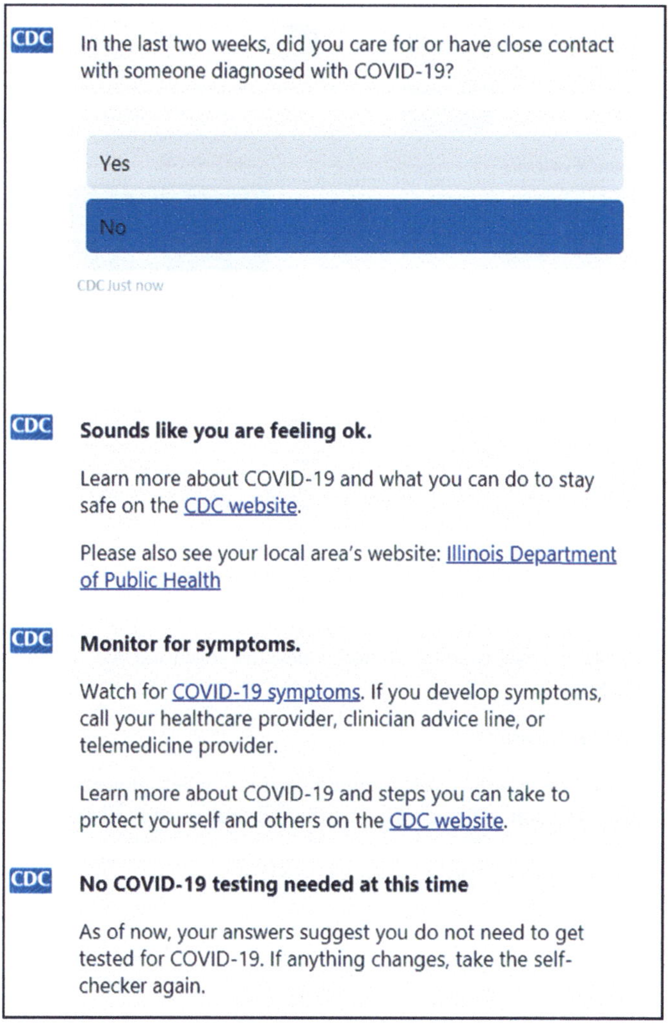

Fig. 13 CDC's COVID-19 self-check BOT sample screen shots

Problem:

Develop a model to accurately predict number of infections, recovery and death of a country/state given a date/time or to predict when infection curve will begin to flatten out.

Solution Approach

There are several ways to approach this problem using ML forecasting methods such as time series analysis, "Susceptible Infected Recovery" (SIR) mathematical models and modified SIR models with ML optimization techniques. In this experiment, we

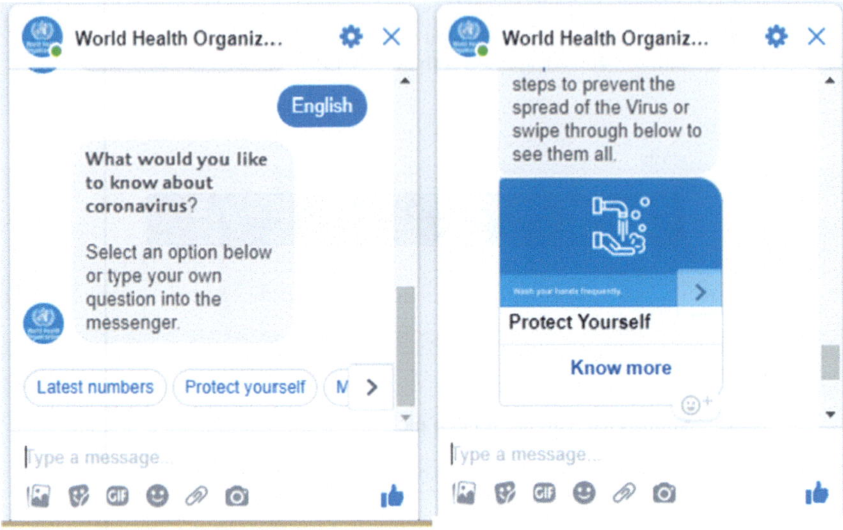

Fig. 14 WHO's COVID-19 self-help BOT sample screen shots

shall read about basic SIR mathematical model and modified SIR model with ML optimization techniques.

SIR Mathematical Model:

SIR model is based on ordinary differential equations where population is split into three compartments such as susceptible, infected and recovered (including death) where people will move from compartment to compartment (Fig. 15).

Let us first define the variables involved in this model

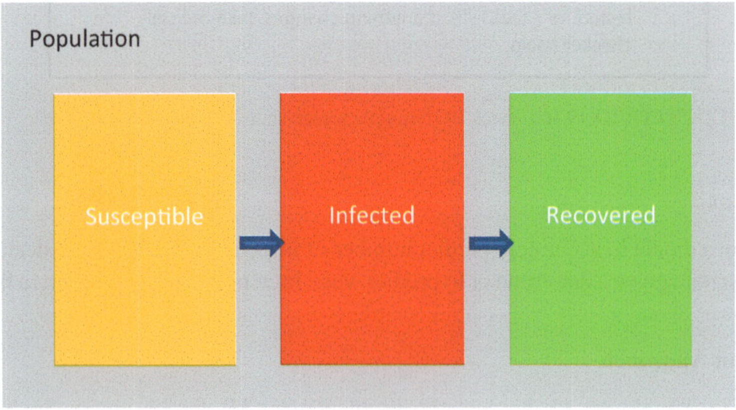

Fig. 15 SIR model compartments

Time (t)—Independent variable, measured in days
S = S(t)—Number of susceptible people
I = I(t)—Number of susceptible people
R = R(t)—Number of recovered people

Some of assumptions and points to note

- We assume every infected person has fixed "b" of contacts with other people
- On an average, each infected individual generates b s(t) new infected individuals per day
- fixed fraction k of the infected group will recover during any given da

Susceptible differential equation is arrived with assumption and constantly "b" number of contacts is made with susceptible.

$$\frac{\mathrm{d}s}{\mathrm{d}t} = -bs(t)I(t)$$

Recovery differential equation is arrived with assumption that infected people gets recovered at "K" constant rate.

$$\frac{\mathrm{d}r}{\mathrm{d}t} = ki(t)$$

Infected differential equation is arrived as follows

$$\frac{\mathrm{d}s}{\mathrm{d}t} + \frac{\mathrm{d}i}{\mathrm{d}t} + \frac{\mathrm{d}r}{\mathrm{d}t} = 0$$

$$\frac{\mathrm{d}i}{\mathrm{d}t} = bs(t)i(t) - ki(t)$$

Let us try to illustrate above model with an example, assume a state as susceptible number is 7,900,000 and infected is 10 and recovered is 0, assume $k = 1/3$ and $b = 1/2$. Let take this initial conditions and try to plot the values.

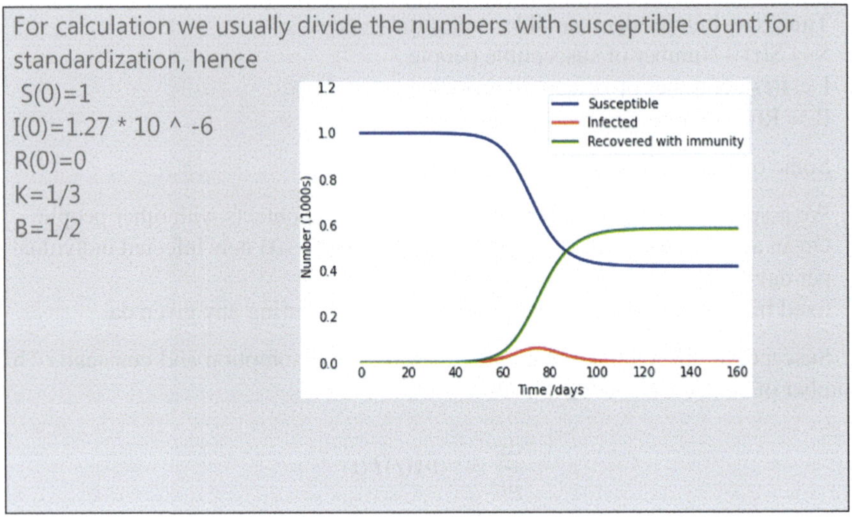

We can observe that infection curve (RED curve) peaks nearly at 75–78 days after which curves tappers off; complete recovery is achieved from nearly 100th day.

SIR Mathematical Model with ML optimization

We can observe that in above model has a static infection (b) and recovery rate (k) but in real world especially COVID-19 spread could not be modeled with constant infection and recovery rate. Hence, ML optimization techniques were used to obtain closely matching infection and recovery rate based on the actual spread data available since December 2019. COVID-19 spread is so dynamic, changes from time to time and too many unknown variables involved to accurately modeling the infection spread.

9 Prevention

As we know there is no vaccine for this virus till date, prevention is the only option the worlds have. WHO and CDC have proposed the following prevention methods.

- Avoid public gathering, religious meetings, parties, etc.
- Maintain safe distance of 6 feet to 2 meters with person having symptoms.
- Vulnerable people need to be isolated, if there is a virus spread in the vicinity.
- Frequent hand wash with soap for 20 s and alcohol-based sanitizers are recommended as a preventive measure [21].
- Use triple-layered (N95) mask while going out.
- Cover nose and mouth while sneezing or coughing.
- Frequent touching of areas around nose, mouth and eyes with non-sanitized hand need to be avoided.

- Do not use shared items from person having symptoms
- Frequently clean floors, surfaces which comes into contact with more people
- People with sickness need to stay indoors and quarantine themselves for 14 days.
- Avoid public transport if you are sick. [22–25].

10 Treatment of Coronavirus-Covid-19

So far, no specific treatments were given for covid-19 since the research is still going on. Initially patients were treated with HIV antidote in Jaipur. Later on lopinavir and ritonavir were practiced with patients in the proportion of 4:1. Researchers suggested giving chloroquine (a drug used for malaria) and oseltamivir (treats swine flu). Ayurveda experts suggest people to take natural herbs to improve the immune system. Recently those who are moderately ill were given antiviral drug lopinavir along with antibiotic azithromycin and anti-malarial drug chloroquine. For severely affected patients, a drug named actemra is given, which is used to treat rheumatoid arthritis but shows good results in patients who suffer from pneumonia with COVID-19.

References

1. Covid 19 basics - symptoms,spread, and others essential Information on corona virus and new Covid 19, Harvard health publishing, 2020– Available from https://www.health.harvard.edu/diseases-and-conditions/covid-19-basics
2. R.J.G. Hulswit, C.A.M. de Haan, and B.-J. Bosch Coronavirus Spike Protein and Tropism Changes, Advances in virus research,2016: 96: 29–57
3. van Doremalen, N., et al.: Aerosol and surface stability of HCoV-19 (SARS-CoV-2) compared to SARS-CoV-1. New England J. Med. (2020). https://doi.org/10.1056/NEJMc2004973
4. Corona virus disease 2019 – How it spreads, CDC, 2020, Available from: https://www.cdc.gov/coronavirus/2019-ncov/prevent-getting-sick/how-covid-spreads.html 7
5. Liu, J., Liao, X., Qian, S., et al.: Community transmission of severe acute respiratory syndrome coronavirus 2, Shenzhen, China, 2020. Emerg. Infect. Dis. (2020). https://doi.org/10.3201/eid2606.200239
6. WHO – Modes of transmision of virus causing Covid 19: implications for IPC precautions recommendation – scientific brief, 29/3/2020
7. Huang, C., Wang, Y., Li, X., et al.: Clinical features of patients infected with 2019 novel coronavirus in Wuhan. China. Lancet **395**, 497–506 (2020)
8. Corona virus disease 2019 – How it spreads, CDC, 2020, Available from: https://www.cdc.gov/coronavirus/2019-ncov/prevent-getting-sick/how-covid-spreads.html
9. Corona virus disease 2019 – what to do if you are sick, CDC, 2020, Available from:https://www.cdc.gov/coronavirus/2019-ncov/if-you-are-sick/steps-when-sick.html
10. Kristian G. Andersen, Andrew Rambaut, W. Ian Lipkin, Edward C. Holmes, Robert F. Garry. The proximal origin of SARS-CoV-2. Nature Medicine, 2020; DOI: https://doi.org/10.1038/s41591-020-0820-9
11. Stanley, G. Sawicki, Dorothe L. Sawicki, Stuart G. Siddell—A contemporary view of corona virus replication, journal of virology 2016, https://doi.org/10.1128/JVI.01358-06

12. WHO-Laboratory testing for coronavirus disease (COVID-19) in suspected human cases interim guidance
13. WHO-global surviellance for covid 19 caused by human infection with covid 19 virusb – interm guidence
14. Corona virus disease 2019 – protect yourself, CDC, 2020, Available from:https://www.cdc.gov/coronavirus/2019-ncov/prevent-getting-sick/prevention.html
15. World Health Organization. Report of the WHO-China Joint Mission on Coronavirus Disease 2019 (COVID-19) 16–24 February 2020 [Internet]. Geneva: World Health Organization; 2020 Available from: https://www.who.int/docs/default- source/coronaviruse/who-china-joint-mission-on-covid-19-final-report.pdf
16. Object detection used for this experiment is called "Detectron" which is latest high performance object detection from Facebook Research and it is available as open source https://github.com/facebookresearch/detectron
17. Tensor Flow Hub's "Universal Sentence Encoder." https://tfhub.dev/google/universal-sentence-encoder/1
18. Deep reading on chest x-ray classification Kaggle completion. https://www.kaggle.com/bachrr/covid-chest-xray
19. Self-check Bot from Centers for Disease Control and Prevention. https://covid19healthbot.cdc.gov/
20. World Health Organization COVID-19 self-help bot in its Facebook https://www.facebook.com/WHO/
21. List N: Disinfectants for Use Against SARS-CoV-2 (COVID-19) - https://www.epa.gov/pesticide-registration/list-n-disinfectants-use-against-sars-cov-2-covid-19
22. Preventing the spread of the corona virus - Harvard health publishing, 2020, Available from: https://www.health.harvard.edu/diseases-and-conditions/preventing-the-spread-of-the-coronavirus
23. Corona virus disease 2019 – protect your self, CDC, 2020, Available from:https://www.cdc.gov/coronavirus/2019-ncov/prevent-getting-sick/prevention.html 8
24. Corona virus disease 2019 – what to do if you are sick, CDC, 2020, Available from:https://www.cdc.gov/coronavirus/2019-ncov/if-you-are-sick/steps-when-sick.html 9
25. WHO-Infection prevention and control during health care when novel coronavirus (nCoV) infection is suspected

A Review on Use of Data Science for Visualization and Prediction of the COVID-19 Pandemic and Early Diagnosis of COVID-19 Using Machine Learning Models

Shiv Kumar Choubey and Harshit Naman

Abstract On December 30, 2019, the WHO China office was informed of a pneumonia-like disease with unknown etiology, from the Wuhan city of China. This disease was found to be caused by a new type of coronavirus. The virus was named severe acute respiratory syndrome coronavirus 2 (SARS-Cov-2) and the disease caused by it was named as COVID-19. On March 11, the WHO declared COVID-19 a pandemic. The testing for COVID-19 disease can be broadly classified into two main techniques, firstly, by testing the patient's blood for immunoassays and second by PCR. The above two techniques are quite costly. Due to this, large-scale testing in developing countries like India is not practically possible. The novel coronavirus is highly infectious, and it spreads from one person to another even before the symptoms have appeared. So, the early detection of the virus will be a great way to stop this global pandemic from causing any more devastation and controlling its spread. In this paper, we review the role of technologies like artificial intelligence and deep learning in early detection, diagnosis, analysis (cure), and socio-economic impact of COVID-19. The purpose of this review paper is to provide a concise but judicious source of information to look over all the possible solutions. *Technologies used:* Artificial neural networks—Artificial neural networks are based on human brain and nervous system. An artificial neural network consists of several neurons and an activation function. ANNs have been used in diagnosis and early detection of several diseases like dengue and pneumonia. The same can be done in the case of COVID-19 by training the algorithm with suitable datasets. Deep Learning—Deep learning is a subclass of machine learning consisting of algorithms that are based on artificial neural networks. Deep learning is a very efficient way to handle large amount of data. Python libraries like Tensorflow are used in Linux-based systems for executing deep learning algorithms. *Visualization of the Pandemic* Several dashboards emerged gradually providing a global overview of the pandemic. Some of these are Upcode

S. K. Choubey (✉) · H. Naman
Department of Electronics and Communication Engineering, Birla Institute of Technology Mesra, Patna Campus 800014, India
e-mail: skchoubey@bitmesra.ac.in

H. Naman
e-mail: be15253.18@bitmesra.ac.in

© The Editor(s) (if applicable) and The Author(s), under exclusive license to Springer Nature Singapore Pte Ltd. 2020

C. Chakraborty et al. (eds.), *Internet of Medical Things for Smart Healthcare*, Studies in Big Data 80, https://doi.org/10.1007/978-981-15-8097-0_10

and NextStrain. Technologies like Python, Excel, R, and Tableau are used here for extracting data and visualizing them in the form of graphs and tables for the general public to understand. *Early Detection and Diagnosis* Artificial neural networks and deep learning can be used for early detection and diagnosis of the disease. The X-rays and CT images of the patients can be used as datasets. As of now the number of patients of COVID-19 in the world has increased to more than half a million, thus the dataset for training the neural networks and algorithms is quite large. This situation can be capitalized to make highly accurate neural networks using deep learning algorithms. The data can be extracted from press releases on the Internet and government databases by Web scraping. Libraries like Tensorflow can be used in training the models. *Tracking and Prediction* Artificial intelligence can be used to track and predict the spread of the coronavirus pandemic. We will try to throw some light on the past works in the area of epidemic prediction using AI. In 2015, neural networks were made for prediction of the Zika virus pandemic. These neural networks need to be trained again in accordance with the datasets of COVID-19. For example, Carnegie Mellon University algorithms used for predicting seasonal flu are being retrained with the datasets of COVID-19.

Keywords Coronavirus · COVID-19 · Data visualization · Artificial neural network · Deep learning · Pneumonia · Chest X-ray · CT images · AutoML · Artificial intelligence

1 Introduction

On December 30, 2019, the WHO China office was informed of pneumonia-like disease with unknown etiology, from the Wuhan city in Hubei province of China. On January 7, 2020, the Chinese authorities isolated the virus and notified the world about a new type of coronavirus. This virus has been named severe acute respiratory syndrome coronavirus 2 (SARS-Cov-2), and its origins were identified to be a wet market in Wuhan city. The disease spread to the nearby countries of Japan and the Republic of Korea. On March 11, the WHO declared COVID-19 a pandemic as it spread across the world at an unimaginable rate, paralyzing the healthcare systems around the world. The epicenter of the pandemic shifted from Wuhan China to Italy and then to the USA [1].

We can classify testing for COVID-19 into two main techniques, firstly, by testing the patient's blood for immunoassays or coronavirus-related antibodies and proteins, and the second method is by identifying the genetic code of the virus. In the second process, the genetic material of the suspicious content is replicated by reverse transcription-polymerase chain reaction or RT-PCR. The above two techniques are quite cumbersome as well as costly [2]. Due to this, extensive scale testing in developing countries like India is not practically possible. As of now, ₹4500 is the estimated cost for COVID-19 tests in India. India has a population of more than 1.3 billion people, which makes testing even more costly [3].

So the question that arises is how helpful is extensive scale testing in eradicating this infection. The answer lies in the nature and behavior of this disease. The novel coronavirus is highly infectious; it spreads from one person to another even before the symptoms have appeared; this makes it more dangerous. So, the early detection of the virus will be a great way to stop this global pandemic from causing any more devastation and controlling its spread. South Korea implemented significant scale testing and decreased the number of cases per day to a very nominal value [4].

In this paper, we study and review the role of technologies like artificial intelligence and deep learning and their role in early detection and diagnosis of COVID-19.

2 Key Concepts

2.1 Data Science

Data science is one of the most sought after fields in the current software industry. There are many misconceptions about data science and its relationship with artificial intelligence models. Data science involves an assortment of several steps involved in the data science pipeline. These steps depend on the task assigned. So, how can we define data science? We can define data science as the science of collecting, storing, processing, describing, and modeling data. We can now discuss each of them and their implementation in the present scenario with proper examples.

Collecting data

Data collection and its role—Data collection is the process of collecting data(numerical, text, video, and audio) based on the question that is to be answered and the environment on which work is being done.

Environment type	1. Data is already collected	2. Data exists but is not owned and organized	3. Data needs to be collected
Technologies and skills involved	SQL queries, Java, Python	Web crawler, SQL	Programming, statistics

This step probably forms the background for all other upcoming actions. The collection of data from authentic and precise sources is necessary for designing effective models.

For example, in several models and designs for the detection of COVID-19, algorithms are made to differentiate CT scans and X-ray images of lungs of a COVID-19 patient with a healthy sample. In some cases, these are used for distinguishing between regular Pneumonia and COVID-19. These algorithms are nothing but neural networks that need to be trained on proper datasets. As of now, there are more than three million cases of COVID-19 in the world, providing scientists with a large dataset to train the algorithms. The precision of detection depends on several factors. One of them is the number of parameters being considered during the evaluation. How are these parameters chosen? The parameters are determined such that all the internal and external symptoms can be covered, such as body temperature, the effects on blood sugar level, the oxygen level in the blood, and CT images of lungs. These can be considered as potential parameters. Most of the governments keep the data regarding these parameters in a structured manner and are available for research purposes. Most of these come under our category 1 and 2 in the above table. The available data can be accessed from the database by basic SQL queries and then manipulated according to use by languages like Java and Python. If our data falls under the second environment, we have to put some more effort and collect data from Web sites by Web scraping using Python. The third case is the most cumbersome, as in this case, data needs to be collected; in many instances, this data is collected by surveys and other traditional methods that prolong the process.

Storing data

In various projects related to the pandemic and its behavior, we mostly come across relational and operational databases.

Patient ID	Name	Ailment	Contact details
00001	ABC	COVID	87955XXX14
00002	XYZ	COVID	1515XXXX25

The above table is an example of an operational or transactional database (the details are just for visualization purposes). In operational databases, data is arranged in the form of tables. Tableau and Excel are standard software used for the manipulation of operational databases. Generally, data such as patient records, medical examination reports, and drug dosage records are stored in operational databases. Operational databases are used to save data in real time.

Relational databases have predefined relationships between the data items stored. SQL is used for general queries and for gathering reports from data. Relational databases are helpful in many inferential statistics problems.

Data from multiple databases.

We are taking the example of a bank. A bank offers several services such as bank accounts, credit cards, and investments. If we want to study the preferences of customers in different services, we need to consider the data related to various services together.

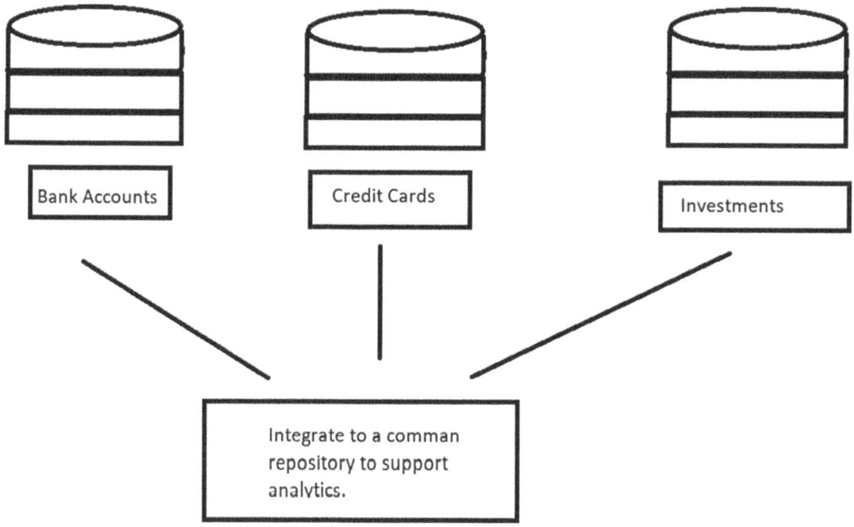

Data warehouses consist of **structured** data from several databases integrated into a shared repository. Data lakes are similar structures except for the fact that data collected in them is raw and unstructured.

Processing data

Data wrangling or data munging

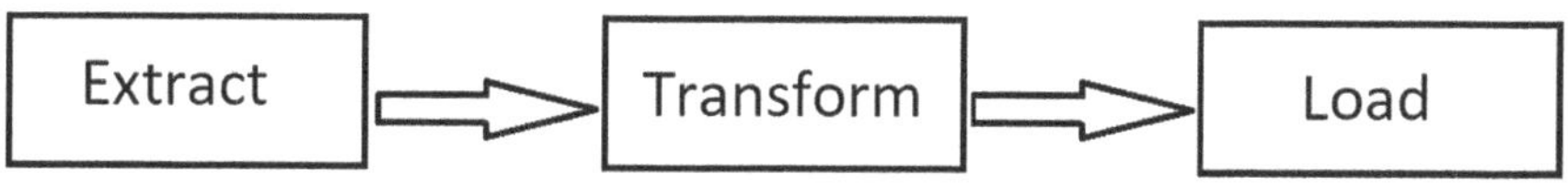

Above are the steps involved in data wrangling. In the first step, data is extracted from the database of the concerned organization. This data is mostly in tabular format. The information is then converted to some data interchange format, such as JavaScript Object Notation format (JSON). The data interchange format is then used to load data into the concerned algorithm.

Data cleaning

Data cleaning can be summarized in four primary steps:

- Filling missing values
- Standardizing keyword tags
- Correcting spelling and other manual errors
- Identify and remove outliners.

Data scaling, normalizing, and standardizing

Data scaling is done according to the project. Units for the quantities given in the procured dataset might not be suitable for the project calculations. We may scale the data to suitable units. Normalizing is essential in the analysis of data. There might be cases where reporting mean and variance of the data using graphs might be difficult without normalizing it.

There are more than three million cases of COVID-19 in the world as of May 12, 2020. The dataset of such enormous size needs a lot of computing power. In these cases, performance becomes a critical issue. Distributed computing is quite useful in such cases. Softwares, such as Hadoop (Map-Reduce), expand can be used for Big Data analysis.

Describing Data

Describing data can be mainly divided into two parts:

- Visualizing data
- Summarizing data.

Tables and excel sheets are not suitable for visualizing data. Visualizing can be done using graphs and bar charts. For example, in later sections, we will be discussing several works related to the presentation of new data regarding the number of patients admitted, discharged, and deceased in real time. Excel sheets and tables are not feasible for representing data in such cases as it would be a cumbersome process to look for information in such format. Charts and graphs would be better as they provide a one look summary of the data to the common users.

When government agencies and research institutes are studying the situation of the pandemic, some common questions that pop up regularly are, "What is the typical number of cases registered daily?" "What is the typical variation in the number of cases registered daily?" This is where the summarizing of data steps in. Data can be summarized using specific quantities that define different queries regarding the data such as mean, median, mode, standard deviation, and variance. In the first question mentioned above mean of the cases registered can be the appropriate answer. Some of the important tools used here are descriptive statistics, iterative processes, and explanatory data analysis.

Modeling data

Statistical modeling-statistical modeling is used to identify underlying relationships between variables.

Let us suppose there is a new drug in the market; there are many questions associated with the medication that can be answered by statistics, like "Is the new drug effective in reducing blood sugar levels?" There are several techniques to answer these questions; one of them is by plotting these quantities against each other and finding the relationship between them. Suppose we get a normal distribution for the above quantities. Normal distribution can be defined using mean and variance only. In the case of COVID-19, a significant relationship is the one between age and number of days of treatment. Statistical modeling can be summarized in four points:

- Modeling underlying data distribution.
- Modeling underlying relations in data.

- Formulate and test hypotheses. (e.g., Is the drug effective?).
- Giving statistical guarantees.

Algorithmic modeling

It is an alternative to statistical modeling. Statistical modeling is used for sensitive fields like agriculture, where we have to give statistical guarantees. The drawback of statistical modeling is that we are left with only simple models, and we cannot take any complex relationships in the picture. Let y be the number of days required for the treatment of a patient; it is highly unlikely that the number of days of treatment will be related to only one parameter or that it will have a linear relationship with any of the parameters. Algorithmic modeling will help establish complex relationships between y and quantities such as blood pressure, body temperature, blood sugar level, age, gender, and other relevant parameters.

2.2 Machine Learning

The algorithms used in algorithmic modeling are machine learning algorithms. In machine learning, we choose very complex functions to show the relationship between the quantities. In the machine learning paradigm, real-world inputs and outputs are used to predict outputs for data that are new to the machine. Sometimes, the outputs may not be specified. There are several learning processes.

Supervised learning

The dataset consists of both inputs as well as outputs. We train the algorithm using raw input and target output. The trained algorithm is used to find the output for input data that is new to the algorithm.

Unsupervised learning

Unsupervised learning involves the training of dataset using raw input data without labeled outputs. Unsupervised learning looks for undetected patterns and correlations in the data without the help of any labeled outputs.

Reinforcement learning

Reinforcement learning is used to train algorithms using reward and punishment techniques. Raw input data is fed into the algorithm, and the system is rewarded for every correct output and punished for every wrong output. The trained algorithm is then used to detect output for new input.

Some important terms are used extensively in the machine learning paradigm:

Features—The measurable properties of a data object are called features. These are used as the input variable(s) for making necessary predictions. Features are essential for making efficient predictions about the data.

Example: Patient's age, blood sugar level, body temperature, etc.

Target/Label—The value that is to be predicted using machine learning is known as the target. It is the desired outcome of the machine learning exercise.

Example: Number of days required for recovery, chances of being diagnosed with COVID-19.

Model—The hypothesis that defines the relationship between the features and target is known as model.

Training-exposure of the model to features and expected targets. The process by which the machine establishes a relationship between the labels and the features.

Prediction-applying the model to unseen data and predicting the target (labels based on data).

Gathering and Cleaning Data
Choose and train Model
Evaluate the Model
Predicting the Target

Machine Learning Pipeline

Deep learning

Deep learning is part of machine learning. It consists of algorithms mainly based on artificial neural networks with representation learning. Deep learning is an essential asset for us when we have to deal with a large amount of high dimensional data. In this case, we use a specific class of complex ML models and algorithms, collectively known as deep learning.

2.3 *Artificial Intelligence*

We can study artificial intelligence and its role in any task under the following sub-sections:

Problem solving

In general problem-solving tasks, starting point and destination are provided, and we need to find a path linking the two. For example, tree algorithm can be used to solve a maze problem.

Knowledge representation

Knowledge representation is done using propositional and first-order logic (if-else statements).

Reasoning, decision making, and expert systems

Expert systems are used in various medical applications.

Expert systems have been employed in the identification of diseases for some time now. We can consider the example of dengue. A set of rules is specified based on symptoms of the disease. We define functions like hasRash(Patient), hasVomiting(Patient), hasHighFever(Patient), and target function hasDengue(Patient). All of these functions are generally of Boolean type. Now, how does it work? hasRash(Patient) AND hasVomiting(Patient) AND hasHighFever(Patient) → hasDengue(Patient). These functions have more logical functions working abstractly. For example, there might be an underlying function is TempGreater102(Patient) such that is TempGreater102(Patient) → hasHighFever(Patient). This function is also of the Boolean return type.

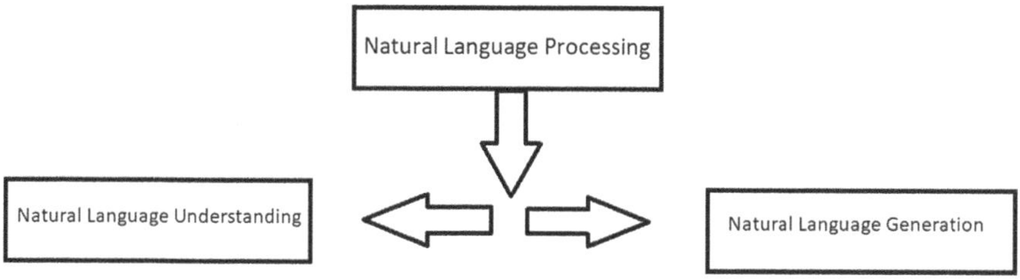

How can we pull this off? There are three significant steps in making expert systems.

1. Formulation of rules by domain experts.
2. Encoding the rules using knowledge representation.
3. Execution of rules and encoding done by a program.

Communication, perception, and actuation

Communication in AI is done by natural language processing; it consists of two sections. Natural language understanding is when a machine interprets human commands in the form of voice or handwritten text. Natural language generation is the generation of replies or responses by the device for the user. Perception is done by computer vision technology, microphones, and other audio-visual sources. Physical robots mostly do actuation. These robots are primarily data-driven hence involve a lot of concepts of data science. These robots can perform complex actuations by learning from simulations or by mimicking human examples.

2.4 Statistics

Statistics is the science of collecting, describing, and drawing inferences from the data. The population is the total collection of all objects that we are interested in studying. A sample is the subgroup of the population that we study to draw conclusions about the population. Generally, we are interested in some parameters of the sample.

How to select a sample?

"A sample and resulting statistic will be useful only if it is a correct and fair representation of the population." For example, let us assume a new medication for COVID-19 has come into the market, and we want to study its effect on the number of days required for treatment. If we take the sample as a group of university students here, then we will not get proper conclusions. The sample here is a group of university students; they have similar age, eating habits, sleep schedules, etc. Thus, the effect of the drug on them would not reflect the general effectiveness of the drug against COVID as it has to be used by a large number of people with different habits and lifestyle inclinations.

3 Contributions of AI and Data Science Against COVID-19 (Actual and Potential)

3.1 Visualization of the Pandemic

Data dashboards do visualization of the pandemic. Several data dashboards have been developed across the world to provide the world with the latest data about the number of people affected by the pandemic. The data provided by all of these dashboards is almost the same. The difference is the underlying machinery and the type of presentation. Presentation skills matter in case of visualizing a pandemic. These data dashboards are meant to be a resource for the public to analyze what level of precautions are to be taken. They must be highly readable, i.e., minimum effort is needed by the public for interpreting the data. These dashboards are nothing but landing pages with maps and visuals depicting where the virus has spread and the numbers on the latest recoveries and deaths. All databases are not the same; some are easy to navigate, some not all people look to same dashboards, and data is not available for all MIT technology review even posted a rank list of these dashboards. Many people raised their concerns regarding the safety of data of the patients, as the data of most dashboards is open-sourced. MIT technology review even posted a rank list of these dashboards.

Some of the best dashboards are:

Upcode

Upcode was ranked the best dashboard by MIT technology review. Upcode is not the best in terms of designs and looks, but it is very informative and easy to use. It uses the data provided by the Singapore Ministry of Health. It is quite transparent about data. The information from the dataset is compiled in the form of charts and graphs. The trends across gender, age, nationality, and location in the city are illustrated in a very understandable manner. The platform also shows the average days required for recovery.

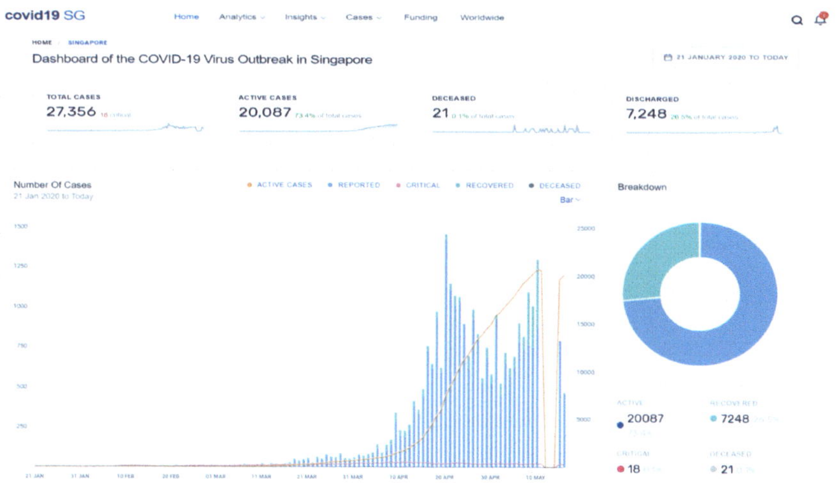

The above picture shows the number of cases with respect to time in the form of a bar graph. The pie chart shows active, critical, and recovered cases. Upcode maintains its data with utmost accuracy after rigorous verification.

There is only one problem with Upcode; it represents only Singapore, due to privacy reasons [5].

NextStrain

Trevor Bedford et al. have made a bioinformatics based dashboard. It is a bit more technical than most of the dashboards. The general public might have a little difficulty in interpreting it. However, researchers, scientists, and other enthusiasts might find it very useful. The team of epidemiologists and engineers at NextStrain collect data from the laboratories around the world, working on the genome of the virus, and integrate them into a central genome tree.

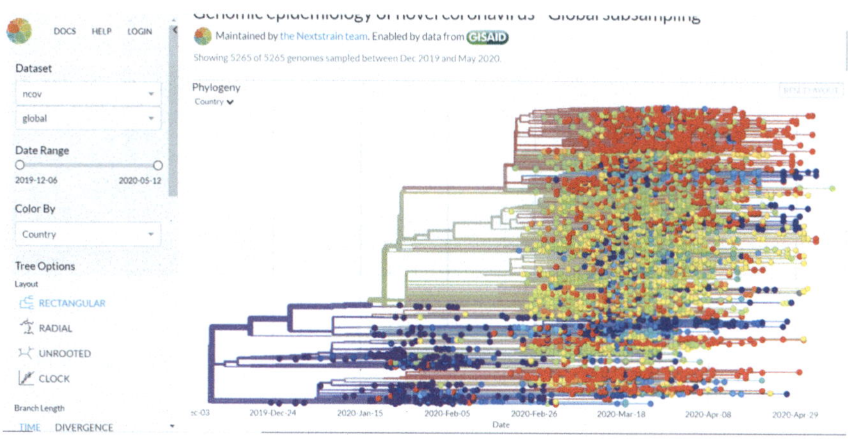

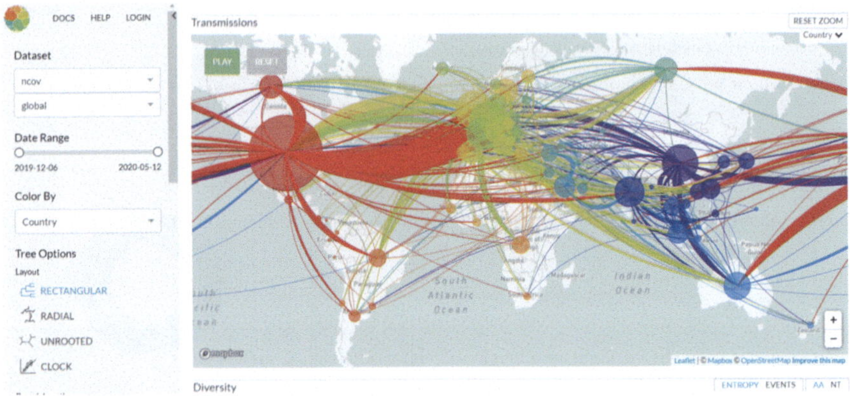

NextStrain provides a very impressive map depicting the status of transmission around the world. This map is one of its kinds. It gives governments and other higher authorities to control international travel from concerned countries, which could be very useful in controlling the infection [6].

JHU CSSE

The dashboard designed by JHU CSSE is inspired by the previous dashboard made for tracking measles in the USA. It is one of the dashboards with the highest utility value for people from different parts of the world. It provides precise information about the cases from almost every remote location on earth. Many other dashboards have taken inspiration from it.

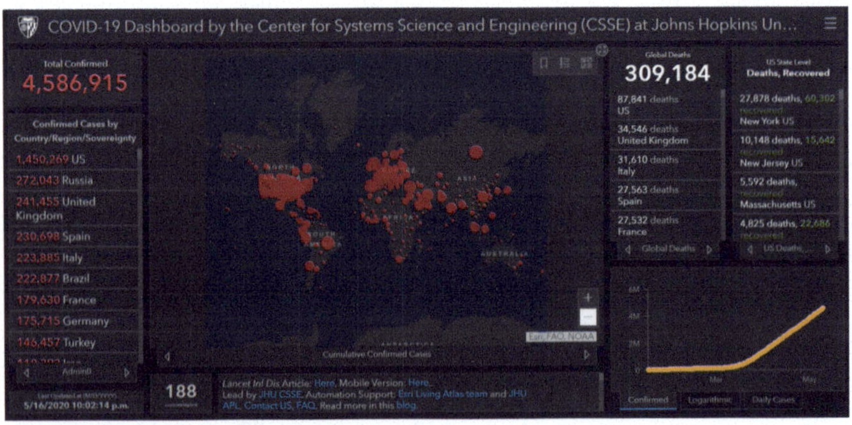

A screenshot of Dashboard designed by JHU CSSE

However, this dashboard has been updated thrice since its inception and can be considered as a work in progress [7].

3.2 India's COVID-19 Tracker

Similar to Upcode, a country centric dashboard was designed for India. India's COVID-19 tracker is different from other dashboards as it is updated at a faster pace than most of the dashboards in the world. This is because unlike other dashboards of its kind COVID-19 tracker is crowd-sourced. It gathers its information from state bulletins, press information bureau, and ANI reports, which are more recent as the Ministry of Health Affairs, India, updates its data at a scheduled time. It also has a section that suggests the nearest stores for buying essentials based on the selected location [8].

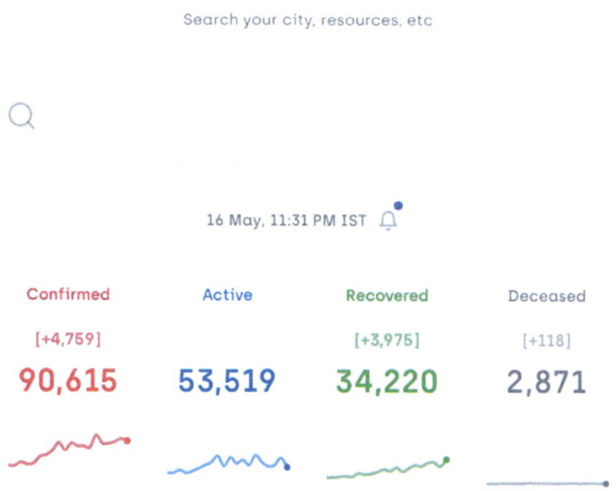
Search your city, resources, etc
16 May, 11:31 PM IST
Confirmed
[+4,759]
90,615
Active
53,519
Recovered
[+3,975]
34,220
Deceased
[+118]
2,871

A screenshot of COVID 19 tracker's landing page

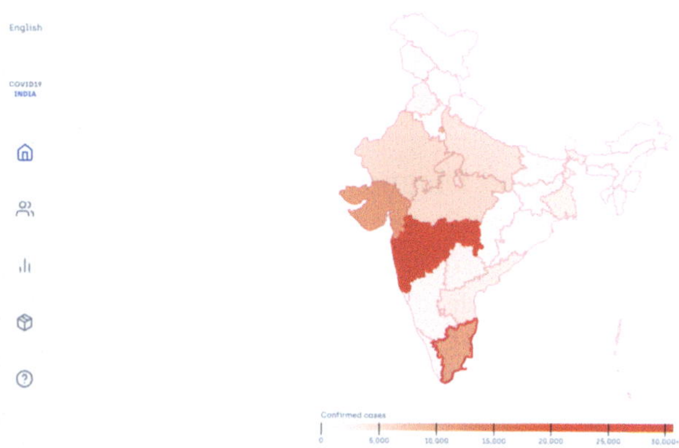

COVID 19 Tracker's Map indicating affected areas in India and severity using different color zones.

3.3 What Do All These Have in Common?

All the dashboards share several standard features such as the bar showing all the statistics about the cases registered, deceased, and recovered, the world map with the distribution of cases around the world, a chart showing the number of cases registered with time, etc. These are some essential pieces of information that are necessary for everyday people. Apart from these, some unique features like information about average recovery time, location of shops for essentials may be added.

3.4 Major Technologies Used

Data dashboards are mainly based on several data science concepts. Most of these concepts are discussed earlier in detail. We can relate most of them to the uses here. The data is collected mainly from sources of health ministries of different countries. Some dashboards, as we studied, were crowd-based (collecting data from press reports and other press resources) and some even scrape data from Web sites. The tools required are different for different sources. We can classify the sources mainly into three categories here:

Environment type	1. Data is already collected Ex-data from databases of health ministries	2. Data exists but is not owned and organized Ex-data from other Web sites and dashboards	3. Data needs to be collected Ex-data from crowd-based sources such as press reports
Technologies and skills involved	SQL Queries, Java, Python	Web crawler, SQL	Programming, Statistics

Tableau, Python, or Excel can easily do the visualization part.

4 Early Detection and Diagnosis

Early detection and diagnosis of COVID-19 can be beneficial in controlling the spread of the disease. The mortality rate of COVID-19 low compared to other diseases like Ebola, HIV, etc. What is it about COVID that makes it more formidable? The problem with COVID-19 is that it has a long incubation period. It is highly contagious during this period, and the patient may not even know that he is suffering from COVID and might spread the infection to hundreds of people daily. Early detection and diagnosis will help significantly in controlling the disease. Early detection is also necessary so that treatment can be started as early as possible. The replication mechanism of the SARS-COV 2 is enabling it to mutate. Mutations make it difficult for the immune system of the body to detect and fight against it. This is making it more difficult for scientists to come up with a vaccine for COVID-19.

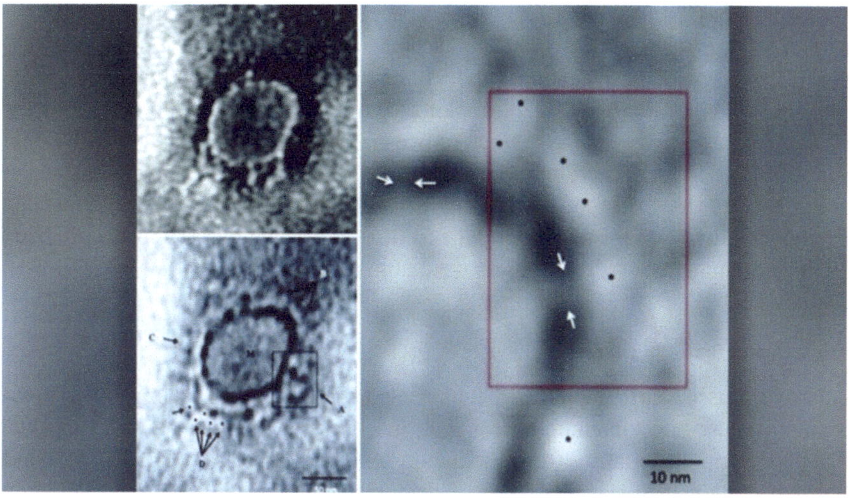

Transmission electron microscopy imaging of Covid-19 | Photo from Indian Journal of Medical Research

The image shows the TEM image of coronavirus. The Indian Journal of Medical Research released it [9].

Artificial intelligence has been used earlier for the diagnosis of diseases like dengue. Image-based medical diagnosis will be beneficial in the identification of the illness, x-rays, and computed tomography can be used as inputs. The dataset for identification has grown significantly, with more than three million cases of COVID-19 around the world.

Reverse transcription-polymerase chain reaction (RT-PCR) is the most common method for diagnosis on COVID-19 being used these days. It is very costly and time taking, and sometimes inaccurate. Several machine learning methods are being used by researchers to find efficient improvements for RT-PCR tests.

Metsky et al. have used machine learning algorithms along with clustered regularly interspaced short palindromic repeats (CRISPR) technology to develop the assay designs and experimental details of 67 different viruses, including SARS-COV2. They are confident that this technology will be helpful in the fast detection of the disease and will lighten the burden from the diagnosis industry. The ML algorithms used are very specific and will eliminate the probability of false-positive cases. The authors state that this process will be useful not only for SARS-COV2 but for an extensive range of genomes [10].

Lack of accuracy in the testing facility is one of the most prominent reasons for the rapid spread of COVID-19. For example, if a person suffering from COVID is found to be negative due to inaccuracy can go on spreading the disease to hundreds of people daily.

RopezLincon et al. have used a different approach to improve the RT-PCR by using a convolutional neural network (CNN). These are used to classify the nucleic acid-based on associativity with SARS-COV2. SARS-COV2 is very similar to viruses such as SARS-COV1, MERS-COV, etc. Hence, identifying gets difficult. Missing information due to noise in the signal contributes to the difficulty. The convolutional neural network used here generates the features of the virus, including the genome sequence. The authors use a 21-base pair convolution over the whole genome (as opposed to previous approaches which only examine sequences of fixed length) and visualize the network's convolution and max-pooling layers to understand which particular sequences help to identify SARS-COV2. The authors also deploy a classification model (ex-logistic regression) to distinguish the cases into hospitalized and asymptomatic cases. The authors were able to identify SARS-COV2 with 99% accuracy [11].

Image-based medical diagnosis

We have discussed earlier that RT-PCR has several demerits such as limited resources for running tests, specimen collection, and inaccuracies. High costs of testing kits prevent developing countries from conducting tests on a large scale. RT-PCR is found to have accuracy as low as 60%–70%. Diagnosis using RT-PCR requires excluding several negative tests, and equipment being in short supply makes it very exorbitant. Novel coronavirus causes a severe infection in the lower respiratory tract in 50%–75% of the cases, which can be detected by CT findings [12].

There are several radiological patterns that COVID-19 leaves; these can be found in several medical imageries. Identifying these patterns is difficult and time-consuming for even expert radiologists. ML algorithms can be used for fast analysis of the medical imagery, thus making it a strong candidate for fast diagnostic processes. Although the extent to which ML and medical imagery can be used for diagnosis is still under discussion [13, 14].

Machine learning brings several possibilities in the picture. Classification algorithms based on an artificial neural network can use deep learning that can be used to make binary (healthy vs. COVID) and multi-class (healthy vs. COVID vs. other types of Pneumonia) classifications. These approaches can use different architectures, such as ResNet [15], UNet ++ [16], and inception [17].

Ophir Gozes et al. have used automated AI-based tools for the analysis of CT images for the identification of COVID-19. The authors claim to state that this technique can be used to distinguish COVID-19 patients with non-patients. The authors used 2D and 3D deep learning models and combined existing AI models with medical imagery such as CT to create a system that can identify COVID with 98.2% sensitivity and 92.2% specificity. They used multiple international datasets, including datasets from affected areas in China. The testing dataset includes 157 patients [18].

X-ray images of the chest can also be used for COVID-19 detection. Machinery for X-ray imaging is more accessible and portable than that of CT imaging. X-ray imaging is also more cost-efficient than CT imaging. It can be used along with similar architecture (ResNet, convolutional neural network, etc.) as the one used in CT imaging techniques.

Turing Ozturk et al. have coupled artificial intelligence with radiological imaging for accurate detection of COVID-19. They presented a model that can automatically detect COVID-19 once raw X-ray is presented. The model is designed to perform binary (COVID vs. healthy) and multi-level classification (COVID vs. healthy vs. Pneumonia) with 98.08% accuracy for binary classes and 87.02% accuracy for multi-class classes [19].

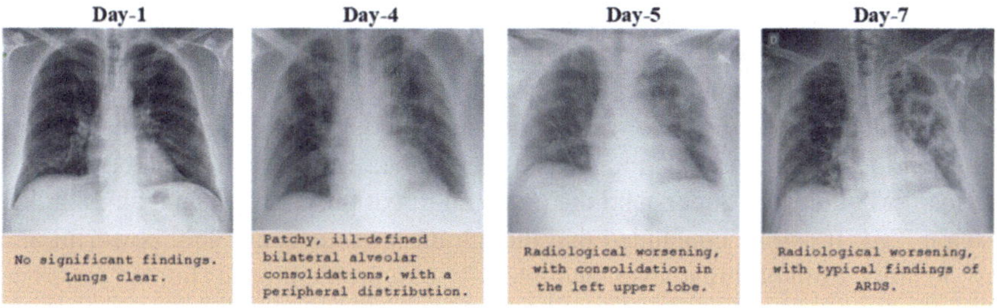

Chest X-ray images of a 50-year-old COVID-19 patient with Pneumonia over a week [20]

Diagnosis of COVID is a very important and sensitive task; minute errors might result in catastrophic results. Image-based medical diagnosis has come up with satisfactory results, but it has a long way to go before we can consider it as a replacement for clinical diagnostic machinery. The image-based medical diagnosis must comply with certain standards that are set by medical associations worldwide. The models should be tested on larger, more diverse datasets. We observe that most of the papers we reviewed were tested on very small datasets and did not comply with most of the regulations set by medical associations. Therefore, these diagnosis techniques should be properly evaluated before implementing them in the medical diagnosis field [21].

5 Early Warnings and Alerts

In the case of early warnings and alerts, the Canadian AI model 'BlueDot' has done a commendable job in predicting the outbreak early. BlueDot is a Canadian health monitoring company. According to certain articles [22] and their statements, BlueDot predicted the outbreak of coronavirus pandemic in China and the world on December 31, 2019 and sent a report to its customers, after nine days on January 9, 2020, WHO declared COVID-19 a pandemic.

BlueDot collects a large amount of data from several sources like official statements of health organizations, press reports, digital media reports, airplane ticket records, and even animal health data. They use big data to handle such a huge amount of data. They use natural language processing and machine learning algorithms to isolate important data [22].

The MIT-based AI HealthMap used AI to map the spread of COVID-19 across the world. It took data from sources similar to BlueDot except for the fact that it took data from social media Web sites as well. The authorities in HealthMap clarified later that all the data that was procured and used was public. One of the most important facts here is that HealthMap predicted the outbreak even before BlueDot on 30th December itself. These AI models like BlueDot and HealthMap are very important tools for giving early warnings, but without human input, they cannot predict the intensity of the threat correctly. Let us take HealthMap; for example, HealthMap rated the COVID-19 threat to be 3 out of 5, and now more than 3 million people are suffering from it [22]. Thirty minutes after HealthMap, a scientist from ProMed (International society for infectious diseases) raised the alarm about COVID and understood its potential to become an epidemic. At the same time, it took the automated systems of HealthMap days to understand the potential threat posed by this pneumonia-like disease [23]. It can be concluded that though these systems are very powerful and fast, identification of threat level, and intensity of a problem needs human expertise for correct prediction.

6 Tracking and Prediction

Artificial intelligence software can be used for tracking pandemics and their spread over different countries with time. In 2015, Zika virus had spread in Brazil, and eventually, in the rest of the Americas, this posed a major challenge to the health agencies there. They were not able to predict the spread of the virus and contain it later in 2019, and Mahmood Akhtar et al. have designed a dynamic neural network model to predict the outbreaks in real time. The model used the data from air travel details, socio-economic, and population data to predict the regions and states to be most affected by the virus. This model was applied to the Zika virus data, and it predicted the high-risk areas with an accuracy of 85% and a prediction range of 12 weeks [24]. Models like these can be used for tracking the COVID-19 pandemic; we need to train these ANN-based models with the new dataset of the current pandemic. Carnegie Mellon University has employed a similar model to predict the outbreak of seasonal flu; their team updates the model with a new dataset every year. This year they are updating the model with the dataset of COVID-19.

However, there are several challenges in implementing AI systems for tracking purposes in this situation. If we study the social media activity after the outbreak of COVID, it can be found that there is a lot of panic in the people regarding the sickness. Many AI systems worked by collecting the data from social media posts, the number of related searches on the Internet, etc. Due to the excess panic among people, searches related to symptoms are occurring unnecessarily even without any serious illnesses. Symptoms of COVID are contributing to this problem as some of the symptoms of COVID overlap with symptoms of several diseases that are not that serious [25].

Lack of historical data is another problem that poses a challenge to implement these technologies. The rate of spread of COVID-19 is way higher than any other pandemic that humanity has observed. The Spanish flu of 1918 had a similar contagious nature, but the records of that pandemic are not readily available, and the virus causing it was also quite different from SARS-COV2.

Tracking and prediction will help the governments in analyzing, planning, and preparing for the pandemic. It will also be helpful in finding out how much the preventive measures such as quarantine, lockdowns, and social distancing are working for flattening the epidemiological curve.

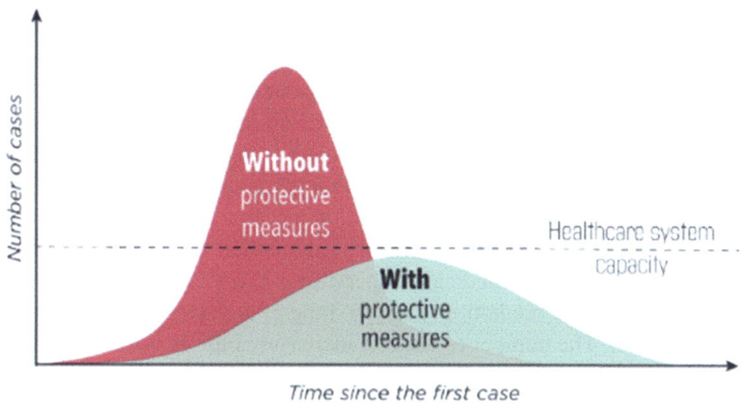

A curve showing the number of cases with time with and without the protective measures [26].

6.1 Clustering

The outbreak of COVID in any region or country depends on several factors like demographics, air travel history, government policies, climate, etc. On the basis of these factors, countries, and regions can be divided into clusters. Data from one of the regions can be used to predict the scenario of the outbreak in other countries.

Carrillo Larco et al. have used unsupervised machine learning algorithms (k-means) to define clusters for countries based on the level of air pollution, socio-economic coverage, and healthcare infrastructure. The model classified 155 countries into clusters. The model worked well in classifying the countries in terms of the number of cases but in terms of the number of deaths or fatality rates [27].

Zixin Hu et al. have studied data from 31 provinces in China fed to a modified autoencoder (MAE) for broadcasting purposes. The authors then extracted the data from the autoencoder's latent data layers and fed it into a k-means clustering algorithm, which grouped them into clusters for further analysis.

7 Patient Outcome Prediction

The number of patients suffering from COVID-19 is increasing day by day; we have seen the top-rated healthcare systems such as that of Italy collapse because of the overwhelming pressure of the ever-increasing number of cases. We observe that most of the cases consist of mild symptoms and may even go undetected, but some of the cases may develop into acute respiratory distress syndrome (ARDS). AI can help in analyzing and narrowing down factors that lead to ARDS and, eventually, death due to respiratory failure. There have been several papers suggesting the use of medical data such as blood tests, age, and other medical data for evaluating the risk of development of ARDS at the later stages. Several clinical indicators have been identified by ML methods.

Li Yan et al. have studied electronic records of more than two thousand patients and screened out records of twenty-nine patients. They tested these records using a prediction model based on the XGBoost machine learning algorithm. Their model is shortlisted lactic dehydrogenase (LDH), lymphocyte, and high-sensitivity C-reactive protein (hs-CRP) out of more than three hundred features. The authors claim that their model predicts mortality of a patient with more than 90% accuracy [28].

Several studies show that medical imagery, like X-ray and CT imaging, can be used for patient outcome prediction. Zhenyu Tang et al. have used CT imaging for severity assessment. The number of cases is increasing rapidly, and manual severity assessment will become extremely difficult and will eat up an important time of treatment. The authors claim that their model to have an accuracy of 0.875 [29].

8 Fake News and Misinformation

According to WHO, an infodemic may be defined as a scenario where there are surplus sources of information with unknown accuracy, which may be problematic for people who are looking for correct information when they need it. Social media can be our most important tool against this pandemic if we use it correctly. The promotion of social distancing and other preventive measures using social media can be very useful. The social media platforms host accounts of almost two billion active users. These numbers give us an estimate of their effect. There are several posts on social media propagating misinformation, selling fake coronavirus cures; there have even been several cyber attacks on databases of hospitals. The United Nations has warned people to verify any information regarding vaccines and cures with authentic sources such as the Web site of WHO [30].

Artificial intelligence can be used for the detection of fake news regarding COVID-19. Adrian Groza used description logics (DLs) to differentiate between the news on the basis of the source of information. The system detects inconsistencies between trusted and non-trusted medical sources [31].

9 Treatment and Cure

AI is being used in the pharmaceutical and drug-making industry for a long time before the outbreak of COVID-19. AI can be used for easing several tasks such as studying the structure of different viruses and proteins, studying the effects of different drugs on viruses, etc. With these extremely helpful features, AI can help in resurfacing past drugs that may be effective in this scenario or even discovering new drugs that may be effective against this disease. Google's AI software DeepMind predicted the structure of proteins associated with SARS-COV2. However, they specify that there is no experimental verification about the accuracy of the predicted structures. The structure of proteins is a very important asset for making a useful drug. The Web site also mentions that the system correctly predicted the structure of the protein spikes on the SARS-COV2, which was verified using the data from the Protein Data Bank, which signifies that the accuracy of the software is better compared to any previous software [32].

Bo Ram Beck et al. have used deep learning for drug resurfacing for discovering effective treatment of COVID-19. The authors used a deep learning-based drug target interaction model called the molecular transformer-drug target interaction model (MT-DTI). The model showed that atazanavir, an antiretroviral that was used for preventing human immunodeficiency virus (HIV), is one of the best candidates against SARS-COV2. Molecule transformer-drug target interaction (MT-DTI) predicted the effectiveness of the drug on the basis of affinity between the drug and the protein spikes of the virus. Scientists at benevolent AI, an AI company from the UK identified Baricitinib, a drug used for rheumatoid arthritis could be used for the treatment of COVID-19 [33].

Konstantin Avchaciov et al. have used deep learning methods to find a number of drugs that could be used against COVID-19, including some of the drugs currently used for lung cancer treatments [34].

The drugs that we have discussed are not very likely to be used in the near future. The main reason behind this being a large number of checks and screenings that drugs have to go through. Every drug has to satisfy certain regulations set by the medical associations of the world before coming into the market for general use. All these screening processes take a lot of time.

10 Resources for Data

Machine learning and deep learning models require a very large amount of data and computing power to create effectively functional algorithms.

Data from the cases

Almost every section that we have discussed in this paper requires data about the number and location of the cases. Several datasets for these purposes are provided by organizations such as WHO and Centers for Disease control for every country. These have been hosted on public repositories by organizations like GITHUB and institutions like Johns Hopkins JSSE. Apart from location and number, there are several complementary datasets that may or may not be available in a structured form, such as the socio-economic impact of the virus and the perception of people about the virus. Efforts are being made to extract and study the de-identified large-scale data to study the local impact and evolution of the disease in Italy [35] and North America [36].

Data from Scientific Research

Machine learning methods can be used to extract and explicate data about coronavirus from written materials. The publications about transmission, incubation, and stability of the viruses, vaccines, and health care are available on several databases like WHO global research database on COVID-19. We also have the COVID-19 Open Research Dataset (CORD-19), which currently has over 52,000 relevant research articles making it the largest open dataset available. NLP techniques can be applied to develop text mining tools and resources that can help extract data for the medical community to find answers to key scientific questions regarding the nature and progress of COVID-19.

Data from social media

Several times the data from social media and news reports can be used to complete the data for scientific purposes. (Datasets like COVID-19 Twitter dataset) These datasets are maintained by tweets about COVID-19; these may be helpful in tracking down the spread of misinformation about the pandemic. The dataset COVID-19 real-world worry dataset is maintained with the emotional responses of people about the pandemic. These datasets are useful in judging the reaction of the people toward the pandemic, for preventing panic and unnecessary social gatherings.

There are repositories like the COVID-19 Coronavirus News Article database and the COVID-19 Television Coverage Dataset that can be used to study the working and evolution of the paper and television media as the pandemic advances.

Clinical data

Datasets for clinical data are not as readily available as other datasets. Some CT scans and X-ray images that we discussed in the medical imagery diagnosis section may be open-sourced and available to the public. Efforts are being made to make relevant data crowd-sourced and open-sourced such as the COVID chest X-ray dataset. However, using and maintaining these datasets are quite difficult. We have discussed several steps involved in the data science pipeline; in this case, the steps like data collection and model training may be performed by a computer scientist, but data cleaning, giving annotations and data labeling require professional medical expertise and may be performed only by doctors and clinicians. To fulfill the need for this much-needed data, the number of initiatives and repositories are increasing the Data4COVID Living Data Repository [37] and the COVID-19 Dataset Clearinghouse [38] some of them.

11 Conclusion

This review shows that ML and AI have the potential to contribute to a wide range of domains against the COVID-19 pandemic. Particularly, we have discussed their role in visualization, diagnosis, tracking and prediction, drug delivery, patient outcome detection, and detection of fake news. However, we note that most of the models do not have operational maturity at this stage. To improve this scenario, we need to take certain steps as a community. Firstly, more open-sourced repositories should be available with relevant datasets; secondly, as we have observed that we need interdisciplinary co-ordination to make proper models. Therefore, medical professionals and data scientists need to coordinate their work. Thirdly, all the sectorial and international differences should be set aside, and different companies, countries, and research institutes should join hands to achieve a common goal. We hope that this review will help the research community in knowing where we are standing know and how much more do we have to work. We also hope that this review will provide an insight into the areas that are achievable using data science methods and show us the domains where these methods might be nothing more than a great risk.

References

1. Situation Report 1 WHO https://www.who.int/docs/default-source/coronaviruse/situation-reports/20200121-sitrep-1-2019-ncov.pdf?sfvrsn=20a99c10_4 Accessed 1st May 2020
2. Ai, T., Yang, Z., Hou, H., Zhan, C., Chen, C., Lv, W., et al.: Correlation of chest CT and RT-PCR testing in coronavirus disease 2019 (COVID-19) in China: a report of 1014 cases. Radiology **2020**, 200642 (2019)
3. Scroll.in Why does Coronavirus Test cost 4500 in India? https://scroll.in/article/961002/why-does-the-coronavirus-test-cost-rs-4500-in-india Accessed 14th May 2020
4. Trust, Testing and Tracing: How South Korea succeeded where the US stumbled in coronavirus response. https://abcnews.go.com/Health/trust-testing-tracing-south-korea-succeeded-us-stumbled/story?id=70433504 Accessed 14th May 2020
5. Dashboard for COVID 19 outbreak in Singapore. https://www.againstcovid19.com/singapore/dashboard Accessed 16th May 2020
6. Genomic epidemiology of novel coronavirus - Global subsampling https://nextstrain.org/ncov/global Accessed 16th May 2020
7. Dashboard by the Center for Systems Science and Engineering (CSSE) at John Hopkins University. https://www.arcgis.com/apps/opsdashboard/index.html#/bda7594740fd40299423467b48e9ecf6 Accessed 16th May 2020
8. Coronavirus outbreak in India https://www.covid19india.org/ Accessed 16th May
9. Prasad, S., Potdar, V., Cherian, S., Abraham, P., Basu, A.: ICMR-NIV NIC Team. Transmission electron spectroscopy of SARS-COV-2 Indian J. Med. Res. **151**(2 & 3), 241–243 (Feb and Mar 2020)
10. Metsky, H.C., Freije, C.A., Kosoko-Thoroddsen, T.S.F., Sabeti, P.C., Myhrvold, C.: CRISPR-based surveillance for COVID-19 using genomically-comprehensive machine learning design. bioRxiv preprint bioRxiv:20200226967026. 2020
11. Lopez-Rincon, A., Tonda, A., Mendoza-Maldonado, L., Claassen, E., Garssen, J., Kraneveld, A.D.:Accurate identification of Sars-Cov-2 from viral genome sequences using deep learning. bioRxiv preprint bioRxiv:20200313990242v1. 2020

12. Kanne, J.P., Little, B.P., Chung, J.H., Elicker, B.M., Ketai, L.H.: Essentials for radiologists on COVID-19: an update—Radiology Scientific Expert Panel. Radiology. p. 200527 (2020)
13. Ng, M.Y., Lee, E.Y., Yang, J., Yang, F., Li, X., Wang, H. et al.: Imaging profile of the COVID-19 infection: radiologic findings and literature review. Radiology: Cardiothoracic Imaging. **2**(1), e200034 (2020)
14. Weinstock, M.B, RJeaEchenique, A.: Chest x-ray findings in 636 ambulatory patients with COVID-19 presenting to an urgent care center: a normal chest x-ray is no guarantee. J. Urgent Care Med. p. 13–18 (2020)
15. He, K., Zhang, X., Ren, S., Sun, J.: Deep residual learning for image recognition. In Proceedings of the IEEE Conference on Computer Vision And Pattern Recognition, p. 770–778 (2016)
16. Szegedy, C., Liu, W., Jia, Y., Sermanet, P., Reed, S., Anguelov, D. et al.: Going deeper with convolutions. In Proceedings of the IEEE conference on computer vision and pattern recognition. pp. 1–9 (2015)
17. Zhou, Z., Siddiquee, M.M.R., Tajbakhsh, N., Liang, J.: Unet ++: A nested u-net architecture for medical image segmentation. In Deep Learning in Medical Image Analysis and Multimodal Learning for Clinical Decision Support, p. 3–11. Springer, 2018
18. Gozes, O., Frid-Adar, M., Greenspan, H., Browning, P.D., Zhang, H., Ji, W. et al.: Rapid AI development cycle for the coronavirus (COVID-19) pandemic: initial results for automated detection & patient monitoring using deep learning CT Image analysis. arXiv preprint arXiv: 200305037. 2020
19. Ozturk, Tulin, Talo, Muhammed, Yildirim, Eylul Azra, Baloglu, Ulas Baran, Ozal Yildirim, U., Acharya, Rajendra: Automated detection of COVID-19 cases using deep neural networks with X-ray images. Comput. Biol. Med. **121**, 103792 (2020). https://doi.org/10.1016/j.compbiomed.2020.103792. ISSN 0010–4825
20. Edgar Lorente, COVID-19 pneumonia—evolution over a week. https://radiopaedia.org/cases/COVID-19-pneumonia-evolution-over-a-week-1?lang¼us. Accessed 16th May
21. Nagendran, M., Chen, Y., Lovejoy, C.A., Gordon, A.C., Komorowski, M., Harvey, H. et al.: Artificial intelligence versus clinicians: systematic review of design, reporting standards, and claims of deep learning studies. bmj. 368 (2020)
22. ARS Electronica https://ars.electronica.art/index.html Accessed 16th May 2020
23. Can AI flag disease outbreaks faster than humans? Not quite AP News https://apnews.com/100fbb228c958f98d4c755b133112582 Accessed 16th May 2020
24. Akhtar, M., Kraemer, M.U.G., Gardner, L.M.: A dynamic neural network model for predicting risk of Zika in real time. BMC Med. **17**, 171 (2019)
25. Artificial Intelligence against COVID-19: an Early Reviewhttps://towardsdatascience.com/artificial-intelligence-against-covid-19-an-early-review-92a8360edaba Accessed 16th May 2020
26. Relief Central Epidemic(Epi) Curves for Coronavirus COVID 19 https://relief.unboundmedicine.com/relief/view/Coronavirus-Guidelines/2355041/all/Epidemic__Epi__Curves_for_Coronavirus_COVID_19 Accessed 16th May 2020
27. carrillo-larco r, castillo-cara m. using country-level variables to classify countries according to the number of confirmed covid-19 cases: an unsupervised machine learning approach [version 1; peer review: awaiting peer review]. welcome open research. 2020;5(56). https://doi.org/10.12688/wellcomeopenres.15819.1
28. Zixin Hu, Qiyang Ge, Shudi Li, Li Jin, MomiaoXiong, Artificial Intelligence Forecasting of Covid-19 in China. arXiv, 2020
29. Prediction of criticality in patients with severe Covid-19 infection using three clinical features: a machine learning-based prognostic model with clinical data in Wuhan Li Yan, Hai,Tao Zhang, Yang Xiao, Maolin Wang, Chuan Sun, Jing Liang, Shusheng Li, Mingyang Zhang, Yuqi Guo, Ying Xiao, Xiuchuan Tang, Haosen Cao, Xi Tan, Niannian Huang, Bo Jiao, Ailin Luo, Zhiguo Cao, Hui Xu, Ye Yuanmed Rxiv 2020.02.27.20028027; doi:https://doi.org/10.1101/2020.02.27.20028027
30. Tang, Z., Zhao, W., Xie, X., Zhong, Z., Shi, F., Liu, J. et al.: Severity assessment of coronavirus disease 2019 (COVID-19) using quantitative features from chest CT images. arXiv preprint arXiv:200311988. 2020

31. WHO website Emergencies Coronavirus disease https://www.who.int/emergencies/diseases/novel-coronavirus-2019?gclid=CjwKCAjw_LL2BRAkEiwAv2Y3SbUEvAwKpNUpsJPSreZUGtQGlCBedIXdmXmOirYAiNuXCjbSR5VAtxoCqjoQAvD_BwE Accessed 17th May 2020
32. Adrian Groza, Detecting the fake news regarding Coronavirus by reasoning on COVID 19 ontology arXiv:2004.12330 2020
33. DeepMind https://deepmind.com/research Accessed 17th May 2020
34. Beck, B.R., Shin, B., Choi, Y., Park, S., Kang, K.: Predicting commercially available antiviral drugs that may act on the novel coronavirus (2019-nCoV), Wuhan, China through a drug-target interaction deep learning model. bioRxiv preprint bioRxiv:20200131929547. 2020
35. Potential new treatment for COVID 19 uncovered by BenevolentAI enters trials https://techcrunch.com/2020/04/14/potential-new-treatment-for-covid-19-uncovered-by-benevolentai-enters-trials/ Accessed 17th May 2020
36. COVID 19 Mobility Monitoring Project https://covid19mm.github.io/in-progress/2020/03/13/first-report-assessment.html Accessed 17th May 2020
37. Safegraph US consumer activity during COVID 19 Pandemic https://www.safegraph.com/dashboard/covid19-commerce-patterns?is=5e7a3815f20d617a17a33173 Accessed 17th May 2020
38. DataforCOVID Repository https://docs.google.com/document/d/1JWeD1AaIGKMPry_EN8GjIqwX4J4KLQIAqP09exZ-ENI/edit Accessed 17th May 2020

Fuzzy Cellular Automata Model for Discrete Dynamical System Representing Spread of MERS and COVID-19 Virus

Sumita Basu and Sreeya Ghosh

Abstract Dynamical system is the mathematical model for computing changes over time of any physical, biological, economic or social phenomena. Usually discrete dynamical system is described mathematically by difference equations and the solution of such difference equation gives the exact value of the changing variable over time. Another widely used computation model that predicts the trend of the dynamical system is Cellular Automata. Crisp Cellular Automata model which makes use of exactly measurable variables and parameters have been studied widely. However, our practical experience tells us that getting exact measurement of any physical, biological, economic or social phenomena is difficult, if not impossible. The inexactness arising due to imprecision or vagueness is called fuzzy uncertainty and was introduced by Zadeh [22]. The discrete dynamical system where the measurements of variables and/or parameters are imprecisely defined are modelled by *Fuzzy Difference Equations* or *Fuzzy Cellular Automata*. We have found fuzzy triangular number solutions of fuzzy one dimensional first order finite difference equation and corresponding fuzzy cellular automata model. This technique have been used to find a fuzzy cellular automata model for the dynamical system representing MERS and COVID-19 virus spread. The model so obtained reveals the trend of growth and gradation of the infection.

S. Basu (✉)
Bethune College, 181 Bidhan Sarani, Kolkata 700006, India
e-mail: sumi_basu05@yahoo.co.in

Guest Faculty, Department of Mathematics, The Heritage College, Kolkata 700107, India

S. Ghosh
Department of Applied Mathematics, University of Calcutta, Kolkata 700009, India
e-mail: sreeya135@gmail.com

© The Editor(s) (if applicable) and The Author(s), under exclusive license to Springer Nature Singapore Pte Ltd. 2020

C. Chakraborty et al. (eds.), *Internet of Medical Things for Smart Healthcare*, Studies in Big Data 80, https://doi.org/10.1007/978-981-15-8097-0_11

1 Introduction

Spread of any virus, results in the change of the number of persons infected by the corresponding virus. The total population being large it becomes almost impossible to distinguish the critically infected and mildly infected persons precisely. Hence fuzzy numbers are used to quantify the critical/mildly infected population. We know a dynamical system representing growth may be modelled by a first order linear difference equation when the variables are crisp. We have formulated fuzzy first order difference equation and found the solutions to include fuzzy variables.

Cellular Automata (CA) model of a dynamical system reveals the trend of change of the variable studied in the corresponding dynamical system. So we have designed the fuzzy CA model for growth of infected population. Application of fuzzy CA modelling to MERS and COVID-19 virus spread which is an imprecise dynamical system is also included in this chapter.

Cellular Automata model was introduced by von Neumann and Ulam [16, 18] for designing self replicating systems which later saw applications in Physics, Biology and Computer Science.

Neumann conceived a CA as a two-dimensional mesh of finite state machines called cells which are locally interconnected with each other. Each of the cells change their states synchronously depending on the states of some neighbouring cells (for details see [17, 18] and references therein). The local changes of each of the cells together induce a change of the entire mesh. Later one dimensional CA, i.e a CA where the elementary cells are distributed on a straight line was studied. Stephen Wolfram's work in the 1980s contributed to a systematic study of one-dimensional CA, providing the first qualitative classification of their behaviour [19, 20].

The applications of discrete fuzzy dynamical systems have been studied by many authors, including Barros et al. in the setting of theoretical aspects and ecological applications [1], in asymptotic stability of attractors [2]. Fuzzy Cellular Automata (FCA) models have been studied by Cattaneo et al. [10], Basu et al. [3], Betel et al. [5].

Buckley et al. (see [6–9]) solved second order linear constant coefficient difference equation of the form

$$y(k+2) + ay(k+1) + by(k) = g(k) \tag{1}$$

for $k = 0, 1, 2, \ldots$ where a, b are constants with $b > 0$ and $g(k)$ continuous for $k \geq 0$ having initial conditions $y(0) = \tilde{\gamma}_0$ and $y(1) = \tilde{\gamma}_1$ where $\tilde{\gamma}_0$ and $\tilde{\gamma}_1$ are triangular fuzzy numbers. The chapter reports existence of three different types of solution namely classical solution ($\tilde{y}_t^C$), extension principle solution ($\tilde{y}_t^E$) and intervel arithmetic solution ($\tilde{y}_t^I$).

Section 2 is devoted to fundamental results used in this chapter. In Sect. 3 we report our work on solutions of one-dimensional fuzzy first order finite difference equation (FFDE). Crisp CA model and Fuzzy CA (FCA) model for FDE and FFDE were studied by us and are included in Sect. 4. We have designed FCA models which are temporally hybrid representing the spread of MERS and COVID-19 virus in Sect. 5.

2 Basic Concepts

2.1 Cellular Automaton

Cellular Automaton(CA) is a computation model of a dynamical system where the smallest computation unit is a *finite state semi automaton*. Thus a CA is a finite dimensional network of finite state semi automaton known as 'cells'.

The mathematical definition of a finite state semi automaton is given as:

Definition 2.1 A **Finite State Semi Automaton** (*abbrev.* **FSSA**) is a three tuple $A = \{Q, X, \mu\}$, where,

- Q is a finite set of memory elements sometimes referred as internal states
- X is the input alphabet
- $\mu : Q \times X \to Q$, is the rule by which an internal state on encountering an input alphabet changes to another internal state. μ is also called transition function.

Thus a CA is a computation model where finite/countably infinite number of cells are arranged in an ordered n-dimensional grid. Each cell receives input from the neighbouring cells and changes according to the transition function. The transitions at each of the cells together induce a change of the grid pattern [15].

Here we have considered only synchronous homogeneous one-dimensional CA. A typical one-dimensional CA is given below.

…	…	A_{i-1}	A_i	A_{i+1}	…	…

Fig. A

A typical grid of a one-dimensional CA

A CA does not have any external input and hence is self-evolving. However the different possible combinations of the state of a cell at any ith grid point along with the states of its adjacent cells can be considered as inputs for the cell at the ith grid point.

Each cell works synchronously leading to evolution of the entire grid through a number of discrete time steps. If the set of memory elements of each FSSA is $\{0, 1\}$ then a typical pattern evolved over time t (represented along horizontal axis) may be as shown in Table 1.

A formal definition of a CA [14] is given below:

Definition 2.2 Let Q be a finite set of memory elements also called the **state set**. The memory elements of the cells belonging to the set Q are placed on an ordered line.

Table 1 C_t is the configuration of the CA(represented along vertical axis) at time t

Grid Position (i)	Time			
	$t = 0$	$t = 1$	$t = 2$	...
⋮	⋮	⋮	⋮	⋮
A_{i+2}	0	0	1	...
A_{i+1}	0	1	0	...
A_i	1	0	1	...
A_{i-1}	0	1	0	...
⋮	⋮	⋮	⋮	⋮
Configuration →	C_0	C_1	C_2	...

A **global configuration** is a mapping from the group of integers $\mathbb{Z}$ to the set Q given by $C : \mathbb{Z} \to Q$.

The set $Q^{\mathbb{Z}}$ is the set of all global configurations where $Q^{\mathbb{Z}} = \{C | C : \mathbb{Z} \to Q\}$. A mapping $\tau : Q^{\mathbb{Z}} \to Q^{\mathbb{Z}}$ is called a **global transition function**.

A **CA** (denoted by $\mathcal{C}_{\tau}^{Q}$) is a triplet $(Q, Q^{\mathbb{Z}}, \tau)$ where Q is the finite state set, $Q^{\mathbb{Z}}$ is the set of all configurations, τ is the global transition function.

Remark 1 For a particular state set Q and a particular global transition function τ a triple $(Q, Q^{\mathbb{Z}}, \tau)$ denoted by $\mathcal{C}_{\tau}^{Q}$ defines the set of all possible cellular automata on (Q, τ). However, the evolution of a CA at times is dependent on the initial configuration (starting configuration) of the CA. A particular CA $\mathcal{C}_{\tau}^{Q}(C_0) \in \mathcal{C}_{\tau}^{Q}$ is defined as the quadruple $(Q, Q^{\mathbb{Z}}, \tau, C_0)$ such that $C_0 \in Q^{\mathbb{Z}}$ is the initial configuration of the particular CA $\mathcal{C}_{\tau}^{Q}(C_0)$.

At any time t, configuration $C_t \in Q^{\mathbb{Z}}$ and $\tau(C_t) = C_{t+1}$.

With reference to Table 1, $C_0 = \ldots 001000\ldots$; $\tau(C_0) = \tau(\ldots 0100 \ldots) = \ldots 1010 \ldots = C_1$; $\tau(C_1) = \ldots 0101 \ldots = C_2$ etc.

CA defined above have the same global transition function $\tau : Q^{\mathbb{Z}} \to Q^{\mathbb{Z}}$ for all time t. However there are a special class of CA called *temporally hybrid CA* where the global transition function varies over time. The formal definition is given with reference to Definition 2.2.

Definition 2.3 A **Temporally Hybrid CA** (denoted by $\mathcal{C}_{\tau_t}^{Q}$) is a triplet $(Q, Q^{\mathbb{Z}}, \{\tau_t\})$ where Q is the finite state set, $Q^{\mathbb{Z}}$ is the set of all configurations, τ_t is a global transition function.

Evolution of a CA is mathematically expressed by the global transition function. However, this global transition is induced by transitions of the cells at each grid point of the CA. The transition of the state of the cell at the ith grid point of a CA at a particular time, depends on the state of the ith cell and its adjacent cells. These adjacent cells constitute the neighbourhood of the ith cell. The transition of the cell at each grid point is called local transition.

Definition 2.4 For $i \in \mathbb{Z}, r \in \mathbb{N}$, let $S_i = \{i-r, \ldots, i-1, i, i+1, \ldots, i+r\} \subseteq \mathbb{Z}$. S_i is the neighbourhood of the ith cell. r is the radius of the neighbourhood of a cell.

It follows that $\mathbb{Z} = \bigcup_i S_i$
A restriction from $\mathbb{Z}$ to S_i induces the following:

1. Restriction of C to c_i is given by $c_i : S_i \to Q$; and c_i may be called **local configuration** of the ith cell.
2. Restriction of $Q^{\mathbb{Z}}$ to Q^{S_i} is given by $Q^{S_i} = \{c_i | c_i : S_i \to Q\}$; and Q^{S_i} may be called the **set of all local configurations** of the ith cell.

The mapping $\mu_i : Q^{S_i} \to Q$ is known as a **local transition function** for the ith automaton having radius r. Thus, $\forall i \in \mathbb{Z}$, $\mu_i(c_i) \in Q$. So, if the local configuration of the ith cell at time t is denoted by c_i^t, then $\mu_i(c_i^t) = c_i^{t+1}(i)$.

Remark 2 If $\tau(C) = C^*$ then $C^*(i) = \tau(C)(i) = \mu_i(c_i)$. So we have,

1. $C_{t+1}(i) = \tau(C_t)(i) = \mu_i(c_i^t) = c_i^{t+1}(i)$
2. $\tau(C) = \ldots \mu_{i-1}(c_{i-1}).\mu_i(c_i).\mu_{i+1}(c_{i+1}) \ldots$
3. If all $\mu_i's$ are identical then the CA is **homogeneous**.
4. For a temporally hybrid CA the $\mu_i's$ are time dependent.

Definition 2.5 If for a particular CA, $|Q| = 2$ so that we can write $Q = \{0, 1\}$, then the CA is said to be a **binary CA** or a **Boolean CA**.

2.2 *Fuzzy Set, Fuzzy Number, α-cut*

Definition 2.6 A **universal set** S is defined as a collection of elements or objects in the universe of discourse. The universal set may be finite, countable or uncountable.

A fuzzy set is a subset of the universal set whose boundary cannot be precisely defined.

Definition 2.7 If S is the universal set then a **fuzzy set** $\widetilde{A}$ in S is a set of ordered pairs: $\widetilde{A} = \{(x, \mu_{\widetilde{A}}(x)) | x \in \widetilde{A} \subseteq S\}$.$\mu_{\widetilde{A}}(x)$ is called the **membership function** or grade of membership of x in $\widetilde{A}$ and is given by $\mu_{\widetilde{A}} : \widetilde{A} \to [0, 1], x \in \widetilde{A}$.

Definition 2.8 A fuzzy number is a convex and normalized fuzzy subset of set of real numbers $\mathbb{R}$.

Definition 2.9 **Triangular fuzzy number** is a fuzzy number represented with three points as follows

$$\widetilde{A} = (a_1/a_2/a_3)$$

$$\mu_{\widetilde{A}}(x) = \begin{cases} 0 & \text{if } x < a_1, \\ \frac{x-a_1}{a_2-a_1} & \text{if } a_1 \le x \le a_2 \\ \frac{a_3-x}{a_3-a_2} & \text{if } a_2 \le x \le a_3 \\ 0 & x > a_3 \end{cases} \tag{2}$$

Definition 2.10 Given a fuzzy set $\widetilde{A}$ in S and any real number $\alpha \in [0, 1]$, then the *α-cut*, denoted by $\widetilde{A}[\alpha]$ is the crisp set $\widetilde{A}[\alpha] = \left\{x \in \widetilde{A} \mid \mu_{\widetilde{A}}(x) > \alpha\right\}$.

Thus on setting the left and right reference functions of $\widetilde{A}$ as $\alpha = \frac{x-a_1}{a_2-a_1}$ and $\alpha = \frac{a_3-x}{a_3-a_2}$, it follows that

$$\widetilde{A}[\alpha] = [a_1 + (a_2 - a_1)\alpha, a_3 - (a_3 - a_2)\alpha]$$

Multiplication of two fuzzy numbers is defined as follows:

Definition 2.11 For two fuzzy numbers $\tilde{A}$ and $\tilde{B}$, if for some $\alpha \in (0, 1]$, we have, $\tilde{A}[\alpha] = [a_1(\alpha), a_2(\alpha)]$ and $\tilde{B}[\alpha] = [b_1(\alpha), b_2(\alpha)]$ then their product is (see [9]),

$$\tilde{A}[\alpha].\tilde{B}[\alpha] = [c_1(\alpha), c_2(\alpha)]$$

where, $c_1(\alpha) = \min\{a_1(\alpha)b_1(\alpha), a_1(\alpha)b_2(\alpha), a_2(\alpha)b_1(\alpha), a_2(\alpha)b_2(\alpha)\}$ and $c_2(\alpha) = \max\{a_1(\alpha)b_1(\alpha), a_1(\alpha)b_2(\alpha), a_2(\alpha)b_1(\alpha), a_2(\alpha)b_2(\alpha)\}$.

2.3 *Fuzzy Cellular Automaton*

A fuzzy CA is a generalization of Boolean CA defined as follows:

Definition 2.12 A one-dimensional **fuzzy CA (FCA)** is a one-dimensional CA where the local transition function is a fuzzy transition function. So the formal definition is as follows:

An **FCA** (denoted by $C^{\mathcal{F}}$) is a four-tuple $(\tilde{Q}, \tilde{Q^{\mathbb{Z}}}, \tilde{f}, \tilde{C_0})$, where,

- $\tilde{Q} \subset [0, 1]$ is the state set
- $\tilde{Q^{\mathbb{Z}}}$ is the set of all configurations
- $\tilde{f}$ is the local transition function which is fuzzy in nature such that if r be the radius of the neighbourhood then $\tilde{f} : \widetilde{Q^{2r+1}} \to \tilde{Q}$
- $\tilde{C_0}$ is the initial configuration which is a fuzzy number.

Table 2 Fuzzy transition rule for Wolfram code 200

$c_{i-1}c_ic_{i+1}$	μ	$\tilde{f}$
000	0	$1 - \min(\neg c_{i-1}, \neg c_i, \neg c_{i+1})$
001	0	$1 - \min(\neg c_{i-1}, \neg c_i, c_{i+1})$
010	0	$1 - \min(\neg c_{i-1}, c_i, \neg c_{i+1})$
011	1	$\min(\neg c_{i-1}, c_i, c_{i+1})$
100	0	$1 - \min(c_{i-1}, \neg c_i, \neg c_{i+1})$
101	0	$1 - \min(c_{i-1}, \neg c_i, c_{i+1})$
110	1	$\min(c_{i-1}, c_i, \neg c_{i+1})$
111	1	$\min(c_{i-1}, c_i, c_{i+1})$

The local transition function $\tilde{f}$ is a fuzzification of Boolean function.

Disjunctive Normal Form-fuzzification of the transition fuction of a classical Boolean CA gives a **Fuzzy transition function**. The Boolean operators AND, OR, NOT in the DNF expression of the Boolean rule can be fuzzified using different fuzzy operators. Here we have replaced $(a \wedge b)$ by $\min(a, b)$, $(a \vee b)$ by $\max(a, b)$ and $\neg a$ by $(1 - a)$ (see [11]).

For Example: Let us consider the Boolean local transition function for some ith cell to be **Rule 200** of Wolfram (see [21]) as shown in (Table 2).

The DNF for RULE 200 is

$$(c_{i-1} \wedge c_i \wedge c_{i+1})_{(111)} \vee (c_{i-1} \wedge c_i \wedge \neg c_{i+1})_{(110)} \vee (\neg c_{i-1} \wedge c_i \wedge c_{i+1})_{(011)}$$

Thus fuzzifucation of the DNF gives the fuzzy transition rule $\tilde{f}$ for Wolfram code 200 as

$$\max\{\min(c_{i-1}, c_i, c_{i+1})_{(111)}, \min(c_{i-1}, c_i, 1 - c_{i+1})_{(110)}, \min(1 - c_{i-1}, c_i, c_{i+1})_{(011)}\}$$

3 Fuzzy First-Order Difference Equation & Its Solution

Buckley found solutions of fuzzy second order difference equation. In this section we restrict our discussion to fuzzy first order linear difference equation and could give fuzzy triangular number solution using extension principle method, interval arithmetic method and classical solution as introduced by Buckley.

Let us consider a first order linear difference equation for $t = 0, 1, 2, \ldots$ of the form

$$y_{t+1} = \lambda y_t \tag{3}$$

where λ is a constant.

If we fuzzify the crisp equation (3) and solve, we are attempting to get the classical solution $\tilde{y}_t^C$. When we first solve Eq. (3) and then fuzzify the crisp solution we obtain $\tilde{y}_t^E$ (solution using extension principle) and $\tilde{y}_t^I$ (α cuts and interval arithmetic). Buckley established the fact that $\tilde{y}_t^C$, $\tilde{y}_t^E$ $\tilde{y}_t^I$ and may differ if more than one fuzzy numbers are used. However, they produce same result if a fuzzy number appears only once in the fuzzy expression. For a difference equation, too often the classical solution fails to exist.

3.1 Solution of FFDE When λ Is Constant and $\tilde{y}_0$ Is a Triangular Fuzzy Number

Fuzzification of FDE (3) gives the following FFDE

$$\tilde{y}_{t+1} = \lambda \tilde{y}_t \tag{4}$$

The solution of FFDE (4) will be as follows:

$$\tilde{y}_t = \lambda^t \tilde{y}_0 \tag{5}$$

A triangular fuzzy solution of the FDE (3) at time t is a **classical solution** denoted by $\tilde{y}_t^C$ if it satisfies FFDE (4) and is a triangular fuzzy number. For some $\alpha \in (0, 1]$, α-*cut* operation on $\tilde{y}_t^C$ gives

$$\tilde{y}_t^C[\alpha] = [y_{t1}(\alpha), y_{t2}(\alpha)] \tag{6}$$

where, $y_{t1}(\alpha) = \lambda^t y_{01}(\alpha)$ and $y_{t2}(\alpha) = \lambda^t y_{02}(\alpha)$.

Now, $\tilde{y}_t^C$ is a triangular fuzzy number if,

$$\frac{\partial y_{t1}(\alpha)}{\partial \alpha} > 0, \quad \frac{\partial y_{t2}(\alpha)}{\partial \alpha} < 0, \text{ and } y_{t1}(1) = y_{t2}(1) \;\; \forall t \geq 1$$

Theorem 3.1 *An FFDE given by* $\tilde{y}_{t+1} = \lambda \tilde{y}_t$ *will have a classical solution* $\tilde{y}_t^C$ *provided* $\lambda > 0$.

Proof Let $\tilde{y}_0 = (a_1/a_2/a_3)$. Then $a_1 \leq a_2 \leq a_3$.

If $\tilde{y}_t^C$ is a classical solution of the given FFDE, then we get

$$\tilde{y}_t^C = \lambda^t \tilde{y}_0. \tag{7}$$

Therefore, for some $\alpha \in (0, 1]$, α-*cut* on the classical solution will be

$$\tilde{y}_t^C[\alpha] = \lambda^t \tilde{y}_0[\alpha], \quad \text{for } t = 0, 1, 2, \ldots, \tag{8}$$

$$So,\ \ y_{t1}(\alpha) = \{a_1 + (a_2 - a_1)\alpha\}\lambda^t\ ;\ y_{t2}(\alpha) = \{a_3 - (a_3 - a_2)\alpha\}\lambda^t$$

$$\text{i.e.,}\ \ \frac{\partial y_{t1}(\alpha)}{\partial \alpha} = (a_2 - a_1)\lambda^t > 0\ ;\ \frac{\partial y_{t2}(\alpha)}{\partial \alpha} = -(a_3 - a_2)\lambda^t < 0$$

$$\text{and,}\ \ y_{t1}(1) = \{a_1 + (a_2 - a_1).1\}\lambda^t = a_2\lambda^t = \{a_3 - (a_3 - a_2).1\}\lambda^t = y_{t2}(1)$$

Hence all the conditions for the existence of a classical solution is satisfied provided $\lambda > 0$. □

A solution to FDE (3) is

$$y_t = \lambda^t y_0 \tag{9}$$

Fuzzification of (9) is

$$\tilde{y}_t = \lambda^t \tilde{y}_0 \tag{10}$$

Solution (10) is an **extension principle solution** denoted by $\tilde{y}_t^E$ if it is a triangular number which is possible provided,

$$\frac{\partial \tilde{y}_t}{\partial \tilde{y}_0} > 0\ \forall t \geq 1\ or\ \frac{\partial \tilde{y}_t}{\partial \tilde{y}_0} < 0\ \forall t \geq 1$$

Let $\tilde{y}_0 = (a_1/a_2/a_3)$. Then for some $\alpha \in (0, 1]$, α-*cut* operation gives a crisp closed bounded interval such that $\tilde{y}_0[\alpha] = [y_{01}(\alpha), y_{02}(\alpha)]$ where,

- $y_{01}(\alpha) = a_1 + (a_2 - a_1)\alpha$ is a monotonic increasing function of α
- $y_{02}(\alpha) = a_3 - (a_3 - a_2)\alpha$ is a monotonic decreasing function of α
- $y_{01}(1) = y_{02}(1)$.

Further, for some $\alpha \in (0, 1]$, α-*cut* operation on $\tilde{y}_t$ gives

$$\tilde{y}_t[\alpha] = \lambda^t \tilde{y}_0[\alpha] \tag{11}$$

So, α-*cut* operation on $\tilde{y}_t^E$ gives

$$\tilde{y}_t^E[\alpha] = [y_{t1}^E(\alpha), y_{t2}^E(\alpha)]$$

where,

- $y_{t1}^E(\alpha) = min\{\lambda^t y_0 \mid y_0 \in \tilde{y}_0[\alpha]\} = \lambda^t(a_1 + (a_2 - a_1)\alpha)$
- $y_{t2}^E(\alpha) = max\{\lambda^t y_0 \mid y_0 \in \tilde{y}_0[\alpha]\} = \lambda^t(a_3 - (a_3 - a_2)\alpha)$.

Remark 3 For an FFDE given by $\tilde{y}_t = \lambda^t \tilde{y}_0$ we get $\tilde{y}_t^C[\alpha] = \tilde{y}_t^E[\alpha]$

Theorem 3.2 *An FFDE given by $\tilde{y}_t = \lambda^t \tilde{y}_0$ will have an extension principle solution $\tilde{y}_t^E$ provided $\lambda > 0$.*

Proof If $\tilde{y}_t^E$ is an extension principle solution of the given FFDE, then it holds that either

$$\frac{\partial \tilde{y}_t}{\partial \tilde{y}_0} = \lambda^t > 0\, \forall t \geq 1 \; or, \; \frac{\partial \tilde{y}_t}{\partial \tilde{y}_0} = \lambda^t < 0\, \forall t \geq 1$$

Hence the condition for the existence of an extension principle solution is satisfied provided $\lambda > 0$. □

A solution to an FFDE at time t is an **interval arithmetic solution** denoted by $\tilde{y}_t^I[\alpha] = [y_{t1}^I(\alpha), y_{t2}^I(\alpha)]$ if for some $\alpha \in (0, 1)$, $\tilde{y}_t^I[\alpha]$ is an interval which is possible provided

$$\forall t \geq 0, \; y_{t1}^I(\alpha) \neq y_{t2}^I(\alpha)$$

where,

- $y_{t1}^I(\alpha) = \lambda^t y_{01}(\alpha) \; = \; \lambda^t(a_1 + (a_2 - a_1)\alpha)$
- $y_{t2}^I(\alpha) = \lambda^t y_{02}(\alpha) \; = \; \lambda^t(a_3 - (a_3 - a_2)\alpha)$

For $\alpha = 1$, $\tilde{y}_t^I$ reduces to the point solution y_t.

Theorem 3.3 *An FFDE given by $\tilde{y}_t = \lambda^t \tilde{y}_0$ will have an interval arithmetic solution $\tilde{y}_t^I$ provided $\lambda \neq 0$ and for $\alpha \in (0, 1)$, $y_{01}(\alpha) < y_{02}(\alpha)$.*

Proof If $\tilde{y}_t^I$ is an interval arithmetic solution of the given FFDE, if

$$\lambda^t y_{01}(\alpha) \neq \lambda^t y_{02}(\alpha)$$

$$\Leftrightarrow \lambda \neq 0 \; and \; y_{01}(\alpha) \neq y_{02}(\alpha)$$

Since $\alpha \in (0, 1)$ and $a_1 < a_2 < a_3$, from the definition of $\tilde{y}_0[\alpha]$ it follows that

$$y_{01}(\alpha) < y_{02}(\alpha)$$

Hence the theorem. □

Remark 4 Since the solution of FFDE $\tilde{y}_t = \lambda^t \tilde{y}_0$ has only one fuzzy number $\tilde{y}_0$, an **interval arithmetic solution** of this FFDE at any time t denoted by $\tilde{y}_t^I$ will produce the same result as that of $\tilde{y}_t^E$ (see [8, 9]).

Remark 5 Clearly, if $\tilde{y}_t$ be a solution of FFDE $\tilde{y}_t = \lambda^t \tilde{y}_0$ at time t, then for some $\alpha \in (0, 1]$,

$$\tilde{y}_t[\alpha] = \tilde{y}_t^c[\alpha] = \tilde{y}_t^E([\alpha] = \tilde{y}_t^I[\alpha]$$

3.2 Solution of FFDE When y_0 Is Constant and the Parameter λ Is a Fuzzy Triangular Number

In this section we will fuzzify the FDE $y_{t+1} = \lambda y_t, t = 0, 1, 2\ldots$ by considering the parameter λ to be fuzzy, and denote it by $\tilde{\lambda}$ where $\tilde{\lambda}$ is a triangular fuzzy number. If y_0 be the crisp initial value then we obtain FFDE which maybe written as

$$\tilde{y}_1 = \tilde{\lambda} y_0 \tag{12}$$

$$\tilde{y}_{t+1} = \tilde{\lambda}\tilde{y}_t \quad for\ t = 1, 2\ldots \tag{13}$$

Thus recursively we get,

$$\tilde{y}_t = \tilde{\lambda}^t y_0 \tag{14}$$

where $\tilde{\lambda^t}$ is a triangular shaped fuzzy number since product of two triangular fuzzy numbers is a triangular shaped fuzzy number (see [9]).

Let $\tilde{\lambda} = (b_1/b_2/b_3)$ such that $b_1 < b_2 < b_3$. Then for some $\alpha \in (0, 1]$, α-*cut* operation gives a crisp closed bounded interval such that $\tilde{\lambda}[\alpha] = [\lambda_1(\alpha), \lambda_2(\alpha)]$ where,

- $\lambda_1(\alpha) = b_1 + (b_2 - b_1)\alpha$ is a monotonic increasing function of α
- $\lambda_2(\alpha) = b_3 - (b_3 - b_2)\alpha$ is a monotonic decreasing function of α
- $\lambda_1(1) = \lambda_2(1)$.

Clearly, if $\alpha \neq 1$, $\lambda_1(\alpha) < \lambda_2(\alpha)$.
Now, $\lambda_1(\alpha) \geq 0 \Leftrightarrow$ either $b_1 \geq 0$ or $|b_1| < (b_2 - b_1)\alpha$.
Again, $\lambda_2(\alpha) \leq 0 \Leftrightarrow$ either $b_3 \leq 0$ or $|b_3| < (b_3 - b_2)\alpha$.

We have found three types of solutions, namely, (i) the classical solution (ii) the extension principle solution and (iii) the interval arithmetic solution.

A solution to an FFDE at time t is a **classical solution** denoted by $\tilde{y}_t^c$ if it is a triangular shaped fuzzy number. Further, for some $\alpha \in (0, 1]$, α-*cut* operation on $\tilde{y}_t^c$ gives

$$\tilde{y}_t^c[\alpha] = [y_{t1}(\alpha), y_{t2}(\alpha)] \tag{15}$$

where, $y_{t1}(\alpha) = (\lambda_1(\alpha))^t y_0$ and $y_{t2}(\alpha) = (\lambda_2(\alpha))^t y_0$.

Theorem 3.4 *An FFDE given by $\tilde{y}_t = \tilde{\lambda^t} y_0$ will have a classical solution $\tilde{y}_t^c$ provided either $y_0 > 0$ and $\lambda_1(\alpha) > 0$ or $y_0 < 0$ and $\lambda_2(\alpha) < 0$ where $\tilde{\lambda}[\alpha] = [\lambda_1(\alpha), \lambda_2(\alpha)]$.*

Proof Let $\tilde{\lambda} = (b_1/b_2/b_3)$. Then $b_1 < b_2 < b_3$.

If $\tilde{y}_t^c$ is a classical solution of the given FFDE, then we get

$$\tilde{y}_t^c = \tilde{\lambda^t} y_0. \tag{16}$$

Therefore, for some $\alpha \in (0, 1]$, α-*cut* on the classical solution will be

$$\tilde{y}_t^c[\alpha] = (\tilde{\lambda}[\alpha])^t y_0, \quad for\ t = 1, 2, \ldots, \tag{17}$$

$$So, \quad y_{t1}(\alpha) = \{b_1 + (b_2 - b_1)\alpha\}^t y_0 \ ; \ y_{t2}(\alpha) = \{b_3 - (b_3 - b_2)\alpha\}^t y_0$$

$$Thus, \quad \frac{\partial y_{t1}(\alpha)}{\partial \alpha} = t\{b_1 + (b_2 - b_1)\alpha\}^{t-1}(b_2 - b_1)y_0 \ ,$$

$$\frac{\partial y_{t2}(\alpha)}{\partial \alpha} = -t\{b_3 - (b_3 - b_2)\alpha\}^{t-1}(b_3 - b_2)y_0$$

$$and, \quad y_{t1}(1) = \{b_1 + (b_2 - b_1).1\}^t y_0 = b_2^t y_0 = \{b_3 - (b_3 - b_2).1\}^t y_0 = y_{t2}(1)$$

Now, $\frac{\partial y_{t1}(\alpha)}{\partial \alpha} > 0$ and $\frac{\partial y_{t2}(\alpha)}{\partial \alpha} < 0$ if

- Case I : $y_0 > 0$ and $\{b_1 + (b_2 - b_1)\alpha\} > 0$
  Moreover, $\{b_1 + (b_2 - b_1)\alpha\} > 0 \Rightarrow \{b_3 - (b_3 - b_2)\alpha\} > 0$ since $b_3 > b_2 > b_1$.
- Case II : $y_0 < 0$ and $\{b_3 - (b_3 - b_2)\alpha\} < 0$
  Moreover, $\{b_3 - (b_3 - b_2)\alpha\} < 0 \Rightarrow \{b_1 + (b_2 - b_1)\alpha\} < 0$ since $b_1 < b_2 < b_3$.

Hence all the conditions for existence of a classical solution are satisfied provided either $y_0 > 0$ and $\lambda_1(\alpha) > 0$ or $y_0 < 0$ and $\lambda_2(\alpha) < 0$. □

A solution to an FFDE at time t is an **extension principle solution** denoted by $\tilde{y}_t^E$ provided

$$\tilde{y}_t{}^E = \tilde{\lambda}^t y_0 \tag{18}$$

$$\frac{\partial \tilde{y}_t{}^E}{\partial \tilde{\lambda}} > 0, \ \forall t \geq 1 \ or \ \frac{\partial \tilde{y}_t{}^E}{\partial \tilde{\lambda}} < 0, \ \forall t \geq 1$$

Further, for some $\alpha \in (0, 1]$, α-*cut* operation on $\tilde{y}_t^E$ gives

$$\tilde{y}_t^E[\alpha] = [y_{t1}^E(\alpha), y_{t2}^E(\alpha)]$$

where,

- $y_{t1}^E(\alpha) = min\{\lambda^t y_0 \mid \lambda \in \tilde{\lambda}[\alpha]\} \ = \ (b_1 + (b_2 - b_1)\alpha)^t y_0$
- $y_{t2}^E(\alpha) = max\{\lambda^t y_0 \mid \lambda \in \tilde{\lambda}[\alpha]\} \ = \ (b_3 - (b_3 - b_2)\alpha)^t y_0$.

Theorem 3.5 *An FFDE given by $\tilde{y}_t = \tilde{\lambda}^t y_0$ will have an extension principle solution $\tilde{y}_t^E$ provided $\lambda_1(\alpha) > 0$ and $y_0 \neq 0$ where $\tilde{\lambda}[\alpha] = [\lambda_1(\alpha), \lambda_2(\alpha)]$.*

Proof If $\tilde{y}_t^E$ is an extension principle solution of the given FFDE, then it holds that either

$$\frac{\partial \tilde{y}_t{}^E}{\partial \tilde{\lambda}} > 0, \ \forall t \geq 1 \quad Or, \quad \frac{\partial \tilde{y}_t{}^E}{\partial \tilde{\lambda}} < 0, \ \forall t \geq 1$$

Now, $\frac{\partial \tilde{y}_t^E}{\partial \tilde{\lambda}} = t\tilde{\lambda}^{t-1} y_0$. Thus, $\forall t \geq 1$,

$$\frac{\partial \tilde{y}_t^E}{\partial \tilde{\lambda}} > 0 \ if \ \tilde{\lambda} > 0, y_0 > 0, \quad Or, \quad \frac{\partial \tilde{y}_t^E}{\partial \tilde{\lambda}} < 0 \ if \ \tilde{\lambda} > 0, y_0 < 0.$$

Consequently, $\tilde{\lambda} > 0 \Rightarrow \lambda_1(\alpha) > 0$.

Hence the condition for the existence of an extension principle solution is satisfied provided $\lambda_1(\alpha) > 0$ and $y_0 \neq 0$. □

An **interval arithmetic solution** of an FFDE at any time t is denoted by $\tilde{y}_t^I$. Further, for some $\alpha \in (0, 1]$, *α-cut* operation on $\tilde{y}_t^I$ gives

$$\tilde{y}_t^I[\alpha] = [\lambda_1(\alpha), \lambda_2(\alpha)]^t y_0 = [y_{t1}^I(\alpha), y_{t2}^I(\alpha)] \tag{19}$$

Theorem 3.6 *An FFDE given by $\tilde{y}_t = \tilde{\lambda}^t y_0$ will have an interval arithmetic solution $\tilde{y}_t^I$ for $t \geq 1$ provided $y_0 \neq 0$ and $\lambda_1(\alpha) < \lambda_2(\alpha)$ where $\tilde{\lambda}[\alpha] = [\lambda_1(\alpha), \lambda_2(\alpha)]$.*

Proof If $y_0 = 0$ or $\lambda_1(\alpha) = \lambda_2(\alpha)$ then the solution of the given FFDE will reduce to crisp constant and $\tilde{y}_t^I$ will not exist.

However, if $y_0 \neq 0$ and $\lambda_1(\alpha) < \lambda_2(\alpha)$ then $\tilde{y}_1^I = [\lambda_1(\alpha)y_0, \lambda_2(\alpha)y_0]$ and $\forall t \geq 2$, $\tilde{y}_t^I = [y_{t1}^I(\alpha), y_{t2}^I(\alpha)]$ obtained will be as follows:

Case I: $y_0 > 0$

- $\lambda_1(\alpha) \geq 0$
  $\tilde{y}_2^I = [\lambda_1(\alpha), \lambda_2(\alpha)][\lambda_1(\alpha)y_0, \lambda_2(\alpha)y_0] = [\lambda_1^2(\alpha)y_0, \lambda_2^2(\alpha)y_0]$
  $\tilde{y}_3^I = [\lambda_1(\alpha), \lambda_2(\alpha)][\lambda_1^2(\alpha)y_0, \lambda_2^2(\alpha)y_0] = [\lambda_1^3(\alpha)y_0, \lambda_2^3(\alpha)y_0]$
  Therefore by induction we get,
  $\tilde{y}_t^I = [\lambda_1(\alpha), \lambda_2(\alpha)]\tilde{y}_{t-1}^I = [\lambda_1^t(\alpha)y_0, \lambda_2^t(\alpha)y_0]$
- $\lambda_2(\alpha) \leq 0$
  $\tilde{y}_2^I = [\lambda_1(\alpha), \lambda_2(\alpha)][\lambda_1(\alpha)y_0, \lambda_2(\alpha)y_0] = [\lambda_2^2(\alpha)y_0, \lambda_1^2(\alpha)y_0]$
  $\tilde{y}_3^I = [\lambda_1(\alpha), \lambda_2(\alpha)][\lambda_2^2(\alpha)y_0, \lambda_1^2(\alpha)y_0] = [\lambda_1^3(\alpha)y_0, \lambda_2^3(\alpha)y_0]$
  $\tilde{y}_4^I = [\lambda_1(\alpha), \lambda_2(\alpha)][\lambda_1^3(\alpha)y_0, \lambda_2^3(\alpha)y_0] = [\lambda_2^4(\alpha)y_0, \lambda_1^4(\alpha)y_0]$
  Therefore by induction we get,
  $\tilde{y}_t^I = [\lambda_1(\alpha), \lambda_2(\alpha)]\tilde{y}_{t-1}^I = [\lambda_2^t(\alpha)y_0, \lambda_1^t(\alpha)y_0]$ or $[\lambda_1^t(\alpha)y_0, \lambda_2^t(\alpha)y_0]$ according as t is even or t is odd.
- $\lambda_1(\alpha) < 0, \lambda_2(\alpha) > 0$ and $\lambda_1^2(\alpha) < \lambda_2^2(\alpha)$
  $\tilde{y}_2^I = [\lambda_1(\alpha), \lambda_2(\alpha)][\lambda_1(\alpha)y_0, \lambda_2(\alpha)y_0] = [\lambda_1(\alpha)\lambda_2(\alpha)y_0, \lambda_2^2(\alpha)y_0]$
  $\tilde{y}_3^I = [\lambda_1(\alpha), \lambda_2(\alpha)][\lambda_1(\alpha)\lambda_2(\alpha)y_0, \lambda_2^2(\alpha)y_0] = [\lambda_1(\alpha)\lambda_2^2(\alpha)y_0, \lambda_2^3(\alpha)y_0]$
  $\tilde{y}_4^I = [\lambda_1(\alpha), \lambda_2(\alpha)][\lambda_1(\alpha)\lambda_2^2(\alpha)y_0, \lambda_2^3(\alpha)y_0] = [\lambda_1(\alpha)\lambda_2^3(\alpha)y_0, \lambda_2^4(\alpha)y_0]$
  Therefore by induction we get,
  $\tilde{y}_t^I = [\lambda_1(\alpha), \lambda_2(\alpha)]\tilde{y}_{t-1}^I = [\lambda_1(\alpha)\lambda_2^{t-1}(\alpha)y_0, \lambda_2^t(\alpha)y_0]$
- $\lambda_1(\alpha) < 0, \lambda_2(\alpha) > 0$ and $\lambda_1^2(\alpha) > \lambda_2^2(\alpha)$
  $\tilde{y}_2^I = [\lambda_1(\alpha), \lambda_2(\alpha)][\lambda_1(\alpha)y_0, \lambda_2(\alpha)y_0] = [\lambda_1(\alpha)\lambda_2(\alpha)y_0, \lambda_1^2(\alpha)y_0]$
  $\tilde{y}_3^I = [\lambda_1(\alpha), \lambda_2(\alpha)][\lambda_1(\alpha)\lambda_2(\alpha)y_0, \lambda_1^2(\alpha)y_0] = [\lambda_1^3(\alpha)y_0, \lambda_1^2(\alpha)\lambda_2(\alpha)y_0]$

$\tilde{y}_4^I = [\lambda_1(\alpha), \lambda_2(\alpha)][\lambda_1^3(\alpha)y_0, \lambda_1^2(\alpha)\lambda_2(\alpha)y_0] = [\lambda_1^3(\alpha)\lambda_2(\alpha)y_0, \lambda_1^4(\alpha)y_0]$
Therefore by induction we get,
$\tilde{y}_t^I = [\lambda_1(\alpha), \lambda_2(\alpha)]\tilde{y}_{t-1}^I = [\lambda_1^{t-1}(\alpha)\lambda_2(\alpha)y_0, \lambda_1^t(\alpha)y_0]$ or $[\lambda_1^t(\alpha)y_0, \lambda_1^{t-1}(\alpha)\lambda_2^t(\alpha)y_0]$ according as t is even or t is odd.

Case II: $y_0 < 0$

- $\lambda_1(\alpha) \geq 0$
  $\tilde{y}_2^I = [\lambda_1(\alpha), \lambda_2(\alpha)][\lambda_1(\alpha)y_0, \lambda_2(\alpha)y_0] = [\lambda_2^2(\alpha)y_0, \lambda_1^2(\alpha)y_0]$
  $\tilde{y}_3^I = [\lambda_1(\alpha), \lambda_2(\alpha)][\lambda_2^2(\alpha)y_0, \lambda_1^2(\alpha)y_0] = [\lambda_2^3(\alpha)y_0, \lambda_1^3(\alpha)y_0]$
  Therefore by induction we get,
  $\tilde{y}_t^I = [\lambda_1(\alpha), \lambda_2(\alpha)]\tilde{y}_{t-1}^I = [\lambda_2^t(\alpha)y_0, \lambda_1^t(\alpha)y_0]$
- $\lambda_2(\alpha) \leq 0$
  $\tilde{y}_2^I = [\lambda_1(\alpha), \lambda_2(\alpha)][\lambda_1(\alpha)y_0, \lambda_2(\alpha)y_0] = [\lambda_1^2(\alpha)y_0, \lambda_2^2(\alpha)y_0]$
  $\tilde{y}_3^I = [\lambda_1(\alpha), \lambda_2(\alpha)][\lambda_1^2(\alpha)y_0, \lambda_2^2(\alpha)y_0] = [\lambda_2^3(\alpha)y_0, \lambda_1^3(\alpha)y_0]$
  $\tilde{y}_4^I = [\lambda_1(\alpha), \lambda_2(\alpha)][\lambda_2^3(\alpha)y_0, \lambda_1^3(\alpha)y_0] = [\lambda_1^4(\alpha)y_0, \lambda_2^4(\alpha)y_0]$
  Therefore by induction we get,
  $\tilde{y}_t^I = [\lambda_1(\alpha), \lambda_2(\alpha)]\tilde{y}_{t-1}^I = [\lambda_1^t(\alpha)y_0, \lambda_2^t(\alpha)y_0]$ or $[\lambda_2^t(\alpha)y_0, \lambda_1^t(\alpha)y_0]$ according as t is even or t is odd.
- $\lambda_1(\alpha) < 0, \lambda_2(\alpha) > 0$ and $\lambda_1^2(\alpha) < \lambda_2^2(\alpha)$
  $\tilde{y}_2^I = [\lambda_1(\alpha), \lambda_2(\alpha)][\lambda_1(\alpha)y_0, \lambda_2(\alpha)y_0] = [\lambda_2^2(\alpha)y_0, \lambda_1(\alpha)\lambda_2(\alpha)y_0]$
  $\tilde{y}_3^I = [\lambda_1(\alpha), \lambda_2(\alpha)][\lambda_2^2(\alpha)y_0, \lambda_1(\alpha)\lambda_2(\alpha)y_0] = [\lambda_2^3(\alpha)y_0, \lambda_1(\alpha)\lambda_2^2(\alpha)y_0]$
  $\tilde{y}_4^I = [\lambda_1(\alpha), \lambda_2(\alpha)][\lambda_2^3(\alpha)y_0, \lambda_1(\alpha)\lambda_2^2(\alpha)y_0] = [\lambda_2^4(\alpha)y_0, \lambda_1(\alpha)\lambda_2^3(\alpha)y_0]$
  Therefore by induction we get,
  $\tilde{y}_t^I = [\lambda_1(\alpha), \lambda_2(\alpha)]\tilde{y}_{t-1}^I = [\lambda_2^t(\alpha)y_0, \lambda_1(\alpha)\lambda_2^{t-1}(\alpha)y_0]$
- $\lambda_1(\alpha) < 0, \lambda_2(\alpha) > 0$ and $\lambda_1^2(\alpha) > \lambda_2^2(\alpha)$
  $\tilde{y}_2^I = [\lambda_1(\alpha), \lambda_2(\alpha)][\lambda_1(\alpha)y_0, \lambda_2(\alpha)y_0] = [\lambda_1^2(\alpha)y_0, \lambda_1(\alpha)\lambda_2(\alpha)y_0]$
  $\tilde{y}_3^I = [\lambda_1(\alpha), \lambda_2(\alpha)][\lambda_1^2(\alpha)y_0, \lambda_1(\alpha)\lambda_2(\alpha)y_0] = [\lambda_1^2(\alpha)\lambda_2(\alpha)y_0, \lambda_1^3(\alpha)y_0]$
  $\tilde{y}_4^I = [\lambda_1(\alpha), \lambda_2(\alpha)][\lambda_1^2(\alpha)\lambda_2(\alpha)y_0, \lambda_1^3(\alpha)y_0] = [\lambda_1^4(\alpha)y_0, \lambda_1^3(\alpha)\lambda_2(\alpha)y_0]$
  Therefore by induction we get,
  $\tilde{y}_t^I = [\lambda_1(\alpha), \lambda_2(\alpha)]\tilde{y}_{t-1}^I = [\lambda_1^t(\alpha)y_0, \lambda_1^{t-1}(\alpha)\lambda_2^t(\alpha)y_0]$ or $[\lambda_1^{t-1}(\alpha)\lambda_2(\alpha)y_0, \lambda_1^t(\alpha)y_0]$ according as t is even or t is odd.

Hence the theorem. □

3.3 Solution of an FFDE When λ Is Time Dependent and $\tilde{y}_0$ Is a Triangular Fuzzy Number

In this section we restrict our discussion to fuzzy first order nonlinear difference equation and its fuzzy solution.

Let us consider a first order nonlinear difference equation for $t = 0, 1, 2, \ldots$ of the form

$$y_{t+1} = \lambda(t)y_t \tag{20}$$

A solution of (20) is calculated by mathematical induction and is as follows:

$$\tilde{y_n} = \prod_{t=0}^{t=n-1} \lambda(t)\tilde{y_0} \tag{21}$$

3.4 *Solution of an FFDE When λ Is Time Dependent and Is a Triangular Fuzzy Number Whereas y_0 Is Crisp*

Let $\lambda(\tilde{t}) = (b_1(t)/b_2(t)/b_3(t))$, where $b_1(t) < b_2(t) < b_3(t)$.

From (20) y_t will be fuzzy for $t \geq 1$ and will be denoted by $\tilde{y_t}$. It is observed that $\tilde{y_1} = (b_1(0)y_0/b_2(0)y_0/b_3(0)y_0)$ is a fuzzy triangular number. So,

$$\tilde{y_1}[\alpha] = [b_1(0)y_0 + (b_2(0) - b_1(0))y_0\alpha, b_3(0)y_0(b_3(0) - b_2(0))y_0\alpha] \tag{22}$$

For $t \geq 2$ we can get an interval estimation solution (represented by α-*cut*) step by step as follows:

$$\tilde{y}^I_{t+1}[\alpha] = [y^I_{(t+1)1}(\alpha), y^I_{(t+1)2}(\alpha)] = [\lambda^t_1(\alpha), \lambda^t_2(\alpha)]\tilde{y}^I_t[\alpha] \tag{23}$$

So by using product of intervals [9] we get, $\tilde{y}^I_2[\alpha] = [b_1(1) + (b_2(1) - b_1(1))\alpha, b_3(1)(b_3(1) - b_2(1))\alpha][b_1(0)y_0 + (b_2(0) - b_1(0))y_0\alpha, b_3(0)y_0(b_3(0) - b_2(0))y_0\alpha]$.

4 CA Models for First Order FDE and FFDE

Here CA modelling have been formulated for dynamical systems represented by one-dimensional first order linear difference equations having time independent coefficients. We will use interval arithmetic solution of the FFDE to design the respective FCA.

4.1 *First Order FDE and CA Models*

Let a one dimensional linear discrete dynamical system be represented by the FDE (3). Here y_t is the state of the system at time t, and λ is the rate of evolution of the system from one time step to another .
If initially $y(t = 0) = y_0$, then we get

$$y_t = \lambda^t y_0, \quad for\ t = 1, 2, \ldots \tag{24}$$

If the initial phase point is real then all possible phase points are real.

Let the phase points be arranged in the increasing order of their values and be denoted in terms of variable 'x' as follows: For any real valued y_t, $\exists i \in \mathbb{Z}$, such that $y_t = x_i$,

$$y_{t+1} = \begin{cases} x_{i+1} & if \;\; y_t < y_{t+1} \\ x_{i-1} & if \;\; y_{t+1} < y_t \end{cases}$$

Let the phase space of the system be given by
$X = \{x_i \mid i \in \mathbb{Z}\}$. The values of the phase points are such that for $i \in \mathbb{Z}$

$$\ldots < x_{i-2} < x_{i-1} < x_i < x_{i+1} < x_{i+2} < \ldots$$

Crisp CA models for FDE (3) have been designed (see [12, 13]) as follows: The ith cell of the CA representing the phase point x_i, is denoted by A_i and the state of the cell A_i at a particular time t is denoted by $A_i(t)$.

$A_i(t)$ is said to be in the ON stage or '1' state represented by a 'black' cell provided at time t the system is at x_i, otherwise it is in the OFF stage or '0' state represented by a 'white' cell in the following figures.

Here $y_0 > 0$ has been considered.

For different values of λ in the given FDE, different homogeneous CA models can be constructed as follows:

- Case 1: $\lambda = 1$
  The dynamical system becomes $y_{t+1} = y_t$. Here, $y_t = y_0, \forall t = 1, 2, \ldots$.
  The only phase point corresponding to y_0 is x_0 and it is represented by cell A_0. Hence we get a null boundaried (denoted by B), 1-celled CA following
  RULE 4$((1 - (c_{i+1} \vee c_{i+1})) \wedge c_i)$ of Wolfram code (Fig. 1a).
- Case 2: $\lambda > 1$
  Here we get a monotonically divergent system as

  $$y_0 < y_1 < y_2 < \cdots < +\infty$$

  Thus the phase points are $x_0, x_1, x_2, \ldots$ and correspondingly we get a countably infinite celled homogeneous CA following
  RULE 16$(c_{i-1} \wedge (1 - c_i) \wedge (1 - c_{i+1}))$ of Wolfram code (Fig. 1b).
- Case 3: $0 < \lambda < 1$
  Here we get a monotonically convergent system as

  $$y_0 > y_1 > y_2 > \cdots > 0$$

  Thus the phase points are $x_0, x_{-1}, x_{-2} \ldots$ and correspondingly we get a countably infinite celled homogeneous CA following
  RULE 2$((1 - c_{i-1}) \wedge (1 - c_i) \wedge c_{i+1})$ of Wolfram code (Fig. 1c).

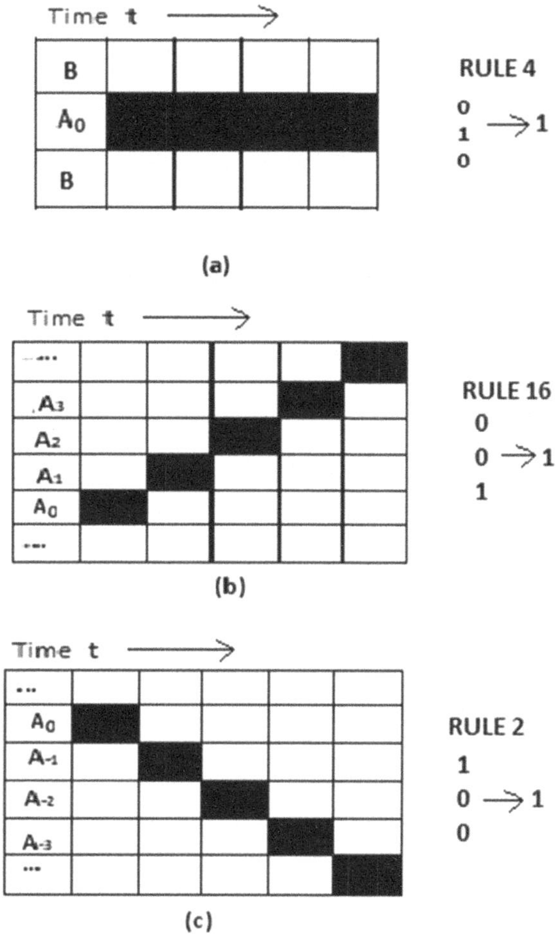

Fig. 1 Crisp CA models For $\lambda > 0, y_0 > 0$

4.2 First Order FFDE and FCA Models

On fuzzifying the FDE (3) given by, two cases arise.

- Case-I: $\tilde{y}_0$ is a fuzzy triangular number and $\lambda > 0$ is a crisp constant. Here, the solution of FFDE (4) will be (5). And, for $\alpha \in (0, 1]$ we get the α-cut solutions of the form (11).
- Case-II: $\tilde{\lambda}$ is fuzzy triangular number and $y_0 > 0$ is a crisp initial value. Here, the solution of FFDE (13) will be (14). And, for $\alpha \in (0, 1]$ we get the α-cut solutions similar to the form (19).

If $\tilde{y}_0$ is real then all possible fuzzy phase points $\tilde{y}_t$ are real.

Let the fuzzy phase points be arranged in the increasing order of their values and be denoted in terms of variable $\tilde{x}$ as follows: For any fuzzy triangular number

$\tilde{y}_t$, $\exists i \in \mathbb{Z}$, such that
$\tilde{y}_t = \tilde{x}_i$,
$\tilde{y}_{t+1} = \begin{cases} \tilde{x}_{i+1} & if\ \ \tilde{y}_t < \tilde{y}_{t+1} \\ \tilde{x}_{i-1} & if\ \ \tilde{y}_{t+1} < \tilde{y}_t \end{cases}$
where each $\tilde{x}_i$ is a fuzzy triangular number.

The values of the fuzzy phase points are such that

$$\ldots < \tilde{x}_{i-1} < \tilde{x}_i < \tilde{x}_{i+1} < \ldots$$

Let $\tilde{x}_i = (c_{i1}/c_{i2}/c_{i3})$ where $c_{i1} < c_{i2} < c_{i3}$.
For some $\alpha \in (0, 1]$, α-cut operation on $\tilde{x}_i$ gives

$$\tilde{x}_i[\alpha] = [c_{i1} + (c_{i2} - c_{i1})\alpha, c_{i3} - (c_{i3} - c_{i2})\alpha]$$

Fuzzy CA (FCA) model for an FFDE are as follows: The ith cell of the FCA representing the α-cut $\tilde{x}_i[\alpha]$, is denoted by $\tilde{A}_i$ and the state of the cell $\tilde{A}_i$ at a particular time t is denoted by $\tilde{A}_i(t)$.

$\tilde{A}_i(t)$ is said to be in the ON stage provided at time t the system is within $\tilde{x}_i[\alpha]$ for $\alpha \geq 0.25$, otherwise it is in the OFF stage.

- Case 1: $\lambda = 1$
  The only fuzzy phase point is $\tilde{x}_0$ corresponding to $\tilde{y}_0$ and it is represented by $\tilde{A}_0$. If $\tilde{\lambda} \approx 1$ then also the variations in the values of the fuzzy phase points are negligible.
  Hence for both cases the FCA has transition function $min(1 - c_{i-1}, c_i, 1 - c_{i+1})_{(010)}$ from DNF-fuzzification of Wolfram's **RULE 4** (Fig. 2b).
- Case 2: $\lambda > 1$, $\tilde{y}_0 > 0$ or $\tilde{\lambda} > 1$, $y_0 > 0$
  Here for $\lambda > 1$, $\tilde{y}_0 > 0$ we get,

$$\tilde{y}_0 < \tilde{y}_1 < \tilde{y}_2 < \cdots < +\infty$$

  The corresponding fuzzy phase points are considered to be $\tilde{x}_0, \tilde{x}_1, \tilde{x}_2, \ldots$ and the FCA will have cells $\tilde{A}_0, \tilde{A}_1, \tilde{A}_2, \ldots$.
  Hence this FCA has transition function $min(c_{i-1}, 1 - c_i, 1 - c_{i+1})_{(100)}$ from DNF-fuzzification of Wolfram's **RULE 16**(Fig. 3b).
  For $\tilde{\lambda} > 1$, $y_0 > 0$, we get a fuzzy system from $\tilde{y}_1$ onwards such that,

$$\tilde{y}_1 < \tilde{y}_2 < \cdots < +\infty$$

  The corresponding fuzzy phase points are considered to be $\tilde{x}_1, \tilde{x}_2, \ldots$ and the FCA will be similar to (Fig. 3b).
- Case 3: $0 < \lambda < 1$, $\tilde{y}_0 > 0$ or $0 < \tilde{\lambda} < 1$, $y_0 > 0$
  Here for $0 < \lambda < 1$, $\tilde{y}_0 > 0$ we get,

$$\tilde{y}_0 > \tilde{y}_1 > \tilde{y}_2 > \cdots > 0$$

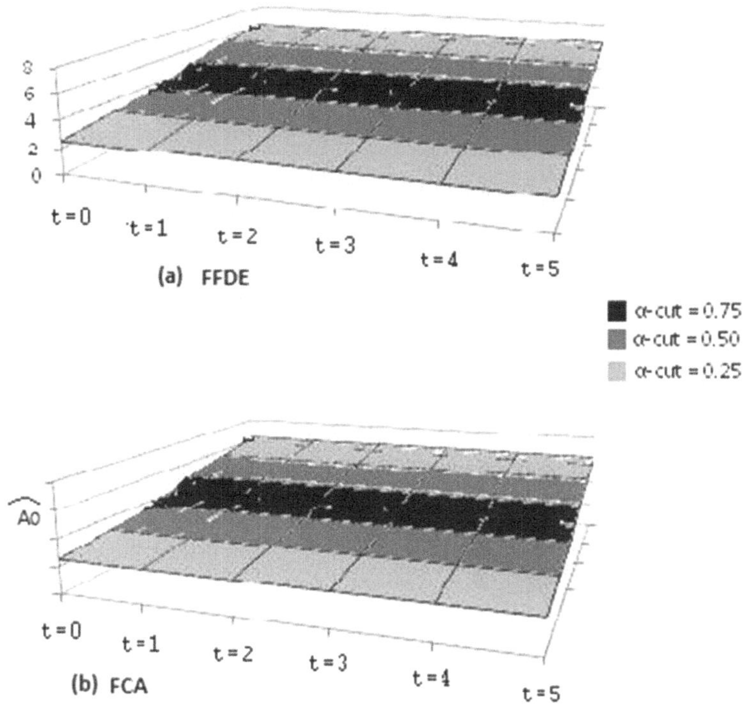

Fig. 2 **a** FFDE, **b** FCA For ($\lambda = 1, \tilde{y_0} > 0$)

The corresponding fuzzy phase points are considered to be $\tilde{x}_0, \tilde{x}_{-1}, \tilde{x}_{-2}, \ldots$ and the FCA will have cells $\tilde{A}_0, \tilde{A}_{-1}, \tilde{A}_{-2}, \ldots$.
Hence this FCA has transition function $min(1 - c_{i-1}, 1 - c_i, c_{i+1})_{(001)}$ from DNF-fuzzification of Wolfram's **RULE 2**(Fig. 4b).
For $0 < \tilde{\lambda} < 1$, $y_0 > 0$, we get a fuzzy system from $\tilde{y}_1$ onwards such that,

$$\tilde{y}_1 > \tilde{y}_2 > \cdots > 0$$

The corresponding fuzzy phase points are considered to be $\tilde{x}_{-1}, \tilde{x}_{-2}, \tilde{x}_{-3}, \ldots$ and the FCA will be similar to (Fig. 4b).

5 Output and Results

We have made an estimation of the suspected number of virus-infected people having different infection levels, on the basis of the calculated infection rate of the virus.

It is known that the spread of any virus depends on the basic reproduction number (R_0) of the virus which indicates how contagious the virus is. In general, the health condition of a virus-infected person is categorized as critical or mild. For COVID-19

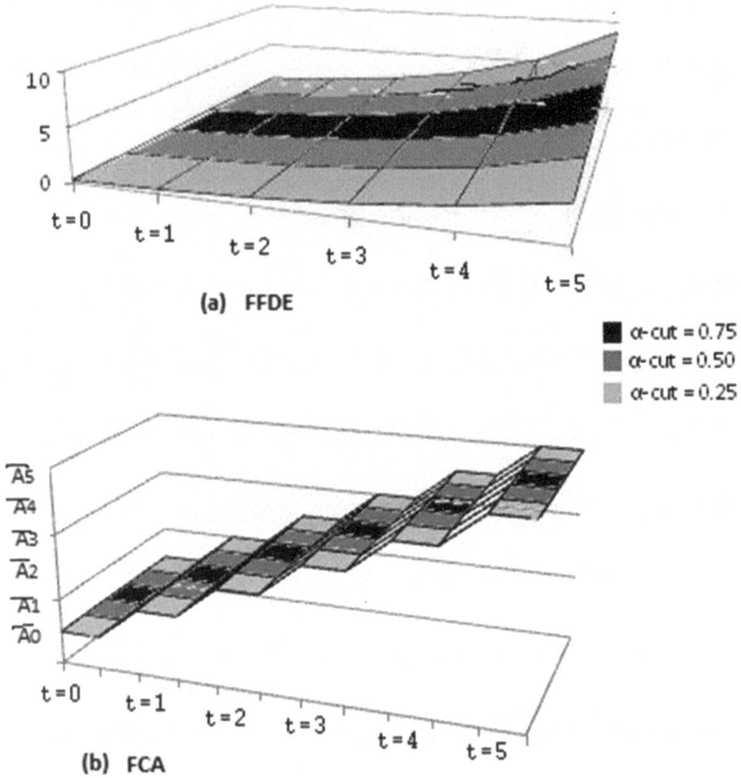

Fig. 3 **a** FFDE, **b** FCA For $(\lambda > 1, \tilde{y_0} > 0)$ Or $(\tilde{\lambda} > 1, y_0 > 0)$

virus, usually around 2% of the active cases have critical conditions while the rest 98% are mild [24]. Among the cases having mild conditions, there can be different levels of infection manifested by different grades of symptoms.

FCA model (which are temporally hybrid) representing the spread of MERS and COVID-19 virus, indicating a gradation of infection, have been designed here.

5.1 Fuzzy Model Representing Growth-Trend of the Number of Virus-Infected People Within a Short Span of Time

The R_0 value of any virus, can vary between different intervals of time which constitute a considerably larger period of time (reported in Sect. 5.2). However, within any short time interval the rise or fall in the number of the virus-infected individuals may apparently seem to occur at a constant rate, say ρ. The virus-infected population

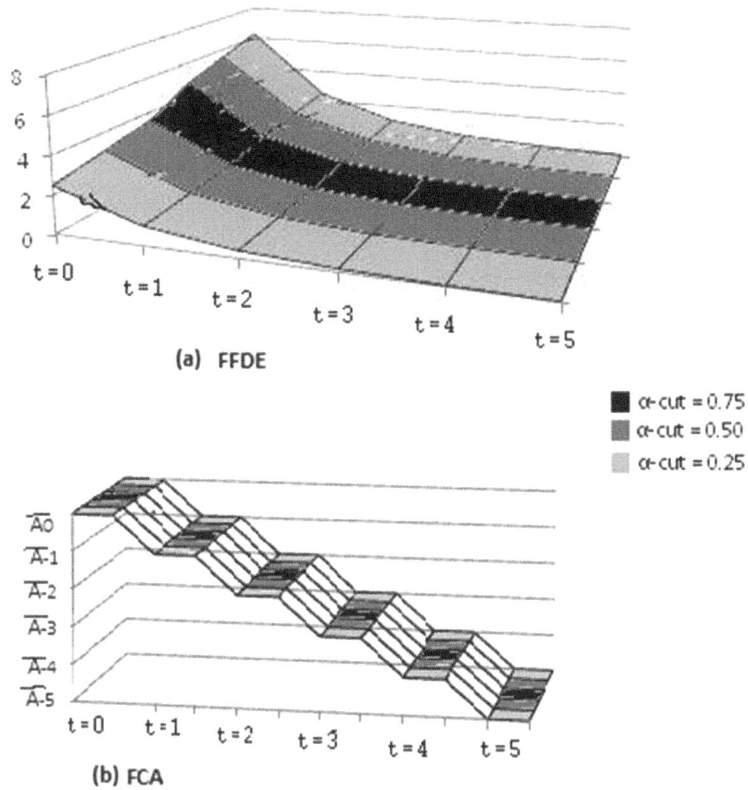

Fig. 4 **a** FFDE, **b** FCA For $(0 < \lambda < 1, \tilde{y}_0 > 0)$ Or $(0 < \tilde{\lambda} < 1, y_0 > 0)$

grows or decays according as $\rho > 1$ or $\rho < 1$, and it almost remains at the same level if ρ is nearly 1.

An FFDE for the growth-trend of number of infected people within a short time, has been obtained by fuzzifying an FDE (of the form 3), given as:

$$y_{t+1} = \rho y_t, \quad \rho > 0, \ t = 0, 1, 2, \ldots \tag{25}$$

where, 'y_t' is the reported number of people being actively infected by the virus at time t. If the initial number of people reported to be actively infected be $y_0 > 0$, then the solution of (25) at time t, will be

$$y_t = \rho^t y_0 \tag{26}$$

- Case-I: $\tilde{y}_0 > 0$ is fuzzy and ρ is crisp.
  The solution of the corresponding FFDE $\forall t \geq 0$ will be $\tilde{y}_t = \rho^t \tilde{y}_0$. For some $\alpha \in (0, 1]$,

$$\tilde{y}_t[\alpha] = \rho^t \tilde{y}_0[\alpha] \tag{27}$$

- Case-II: $y_0 > 0$ is crisp and $\tilde{\rho}$ is fuzzy.
  Then $\tilde{y}_1 = \tilde{\rho} y_0$ and the solution of the corresponding FFDE $\forall t \geq 1$ will be $\tilde{y}_t = \tilde{\rho}^t y_0$. For some $\alpha \in (0, 1]$,

$$\tilde{y}_t[\alpha] = (\tilde{\rho}[\alpha])^t . y_0 \tag{28}$$

Let us suppose $\tilde{y}_t[\alpha]$ represents the suspected number of actively infected people provided $\alpha \geq 0.25$. We further assume that $\tilde{y}_t[\alpha]$ represents

- highly infected population if $\alpha \geq 0.75$
- moderately infected population if $0.50 \leq \alpha < 0.75$
- slightly infected population if $0.25 \leq \alpha < 0.50$.

Among the highly infected people, the cases which become critical can be indicated by $\alpha \geq 0.98$ (in case of COVID-19).

And at $\alpha = 1.0$, the α-cut operation on $\tilde{y}_t$, denoted by $\tilde{y}_t[1]$ coincides with the crisp value y_t (which indicates the reported active cases).

Let R_0 be the basic reproduction rate of a virus from any time interval (T) to the next time interval $(T + 1)$ where each interval has an n-day span. If ρ be the constant growth rate of the number of infected individuals (Y) at time T, for a period of n days, then

$$R_0 Y \approx (\rho)^n Y \Leftrightarrow R_0^{(1/n)} \approx \rho \tag{29}$$

5.1.1 FCA Model Representing COVID-19 Spread for a Short Period

The 2019 Novel Coronavirus (2019-nCoV or COVID-19) also known as Severe Acute Respiratory Syndrome Coronavirus 2 (SARS-CoV-2) was first reported towards the end of 2019 Wuhan city in the Hubei province of China. Around March 2020, COVID-19 emerged to be a world-wide pandemic. Then by the second week of April 2020, the curve for the number active cases in China almost flattened. At that time, in some countries like Germany, the number of active COVID-19 cases started falling since the growth-rate fell below 1. However in countries like India, USA, Singapore, the growth-rate being above 1, the number of active cases was still on the rise.

Here the trend of growth of number of COVID-19 patients for a short period from 11/04/2020 to 15/04/2020 for India, Germany and China has been depicted. The number of active cases y_t, at time t, has been recorded from [24]. The value of ρ has been calculated from (26) for $t = 4$.

(1) **India** having $\rho > 1$ from 11/04/20–15/04/20

The number of active cases on 11/04/2020 was 7189 and on 15/04/2010 was 10,440. Considering the scale of 1000:1, $y_0 = 7.189$ and $y_4 = 10.440$ gives $\rho =$

Table 3 $\tilde{y}_0 = (6.789/7.189/7.589)$; $\rho = 1.098$

Time t	$\tilde{y}_t[0.25]$	$\tilde{y}_t[0.50]$	$\tilde{y}_t[0.75]$
0(11/4)	[6.889,7.489]	[6.989,7.389]	[7.089,7.289]
1(12/4)	[7.564,8.223]	[7.674,8.113]	[7.784,8.003]
2(13/4)	[8.305,9.029]	[8.426,8.908]	[8.547,8.788]
3(14/4)	[9.119,9.914]	[9.252,9.781]	[9.384,9.649]
4(15/4)	[10.013,10.885]	[10.158,10.740]	[10.304,10.594]

1.098. Let $\tilde{y}_0 = (y_0 - 0.4/y_0/y_0 + 0.4)$ and $\tilde{\rho} = (\rho - 0.02/\rho/\rho + 0.02)$ be triangular fuzzy numbers.

Case-I: Let $\tilde{y}_0 = (6.789/7.189/7.589)$ be fuzzy and $\rho = 1.098$ be a crisp constant. Thus $\tilde{y}_0[\alpha] = [6.789 + 0.4\alpha, 7.589 - 0.4\alpha]$ and $\forall t \geq 1$, $\tilde{y}_t[\alpha]$ has been calculated from (27). The pattern of values of slightly, moderately and highly infected active cases during the stipulated time period has been given in Table 3. Here, $\tilde{y}_0 < \tilde{y}_1 < \tilde{y}_2 < \tilde{y}_3 < \tilde{y}_4$.

Thus the fuzzy phase points are $\tilde{x}_0, \tilde{x}_1, \ldots, \tilde{x}_4$. The corresponding FCA will have cells $\tilde{A}_0, \ldots, \tilde{A}_4$ and the ON states of these cells will be $\tilde{A}_0(0)$, $\tilde{A}_1(1)$, $\tilde{A}_2(2)$, $\tilde{A}_3(3)$, $\tilde{A}_4(4)$. This FCA will be as shown in (Fig. 5a).

Case-II: Let $y_0 = 7.189$ be crisp and $\tilde{\rho} = (1.078/1.098/1.118)$ be fuzzy. Thus $\tilde{\rho}[\alpha] = [1.078 + 0.02\alpha, 1.118 - 0.02\alpha]$ and $\forall t \geq 1$, $\tilde{y}_t[\alpha]$ has been calculated from (28). The pattern of values of slightly, moderately and highly infected active cases during the stipulated time period has been given in Table 4. Here $\tilde{y}_1 < \tilde{y}_2 < \tilde{y}_3 < \tilde{y}_4$.

The corresponding FCA will be similar to as shown in (Fig. 5a).

(2) **Germany** having $\rho < 1$ from 11/04/20–15/04/20

The number of active cases on 11/04/2020 was 65181 and on 15/04/2020 was 58349. Considering the scale of 1000:1, $y_0 = 65.181$ and $y_4 = 58.349$ gives $\rho = 0.973$. Let $\tilde{y}_0 = (y_0 - 0.4/y_0/y_0 + 0.4)$ and $\tilde{\rho} = (\rho - 0.01/\rho/\rho + 0.01)$ be triangular fuzzy numbers.

Case-I: Let $\tilde{y}_0 = (64.781/65.181/65.581)$ and $\rho = 0.973$ be a crisp constant. Thus $\tilde{y}_0[\alpha] = [64.781 + 0.4\alpha, 65.581 - 0.4\alpha]$ and $\forall t \geq 1$, $\tilde{y}_t[\alpha]$ has been calculated from *(27)*. The pattern of values of slightly, moderately and highly infected active cases during the stipulated time period has been given in *Table* 5. Here, $\tilde{y}_0 > \tilde{y}_1 > \tilde{y}_2 > \tilde{y}_3 > \tilde{y}_4$

Thus the fuzzy phase points are $\tilde{x}_0, \tilde{x}_{-1}, \ldots, \tilde{x}_{-4}$. The corresponding FCA will have cells $\tilde{A}_0, \ldots, \tilde{A}_{-4}$ and the ON states of these cells will be $\tilde{A}_0(0)$, $\tilde{A}_{-1}(1)$, $\tilde{A}_{-2}(2)$, $\tilde{A}_{-3}(3)$, $\tilde{A}_{-4}(4)$. This FCA will be as shown in (Fig. 5b).

Case-II: Let $y_0 = 65.181$ be crisp and $\tilde{\rho} = (0.963/0.973/0.983)$ be fuzzy.

Thus $\tilde{\rho}[\alpha] = [0.963 + 0.01\alpha, 0.983 - 0.01\alpha]$ and $\forall t \geq 1$, $\tilde{y}_t[\alpha]$ has been calculated from (28). The pattern of values of slightly, moderately and highly infected active cases during the stipulated time period has been given in Table 6. Here, $\tilde{y}_1 > \tilde{y}_2 > \tilde{y}_3 > \tilde{y}_4$.

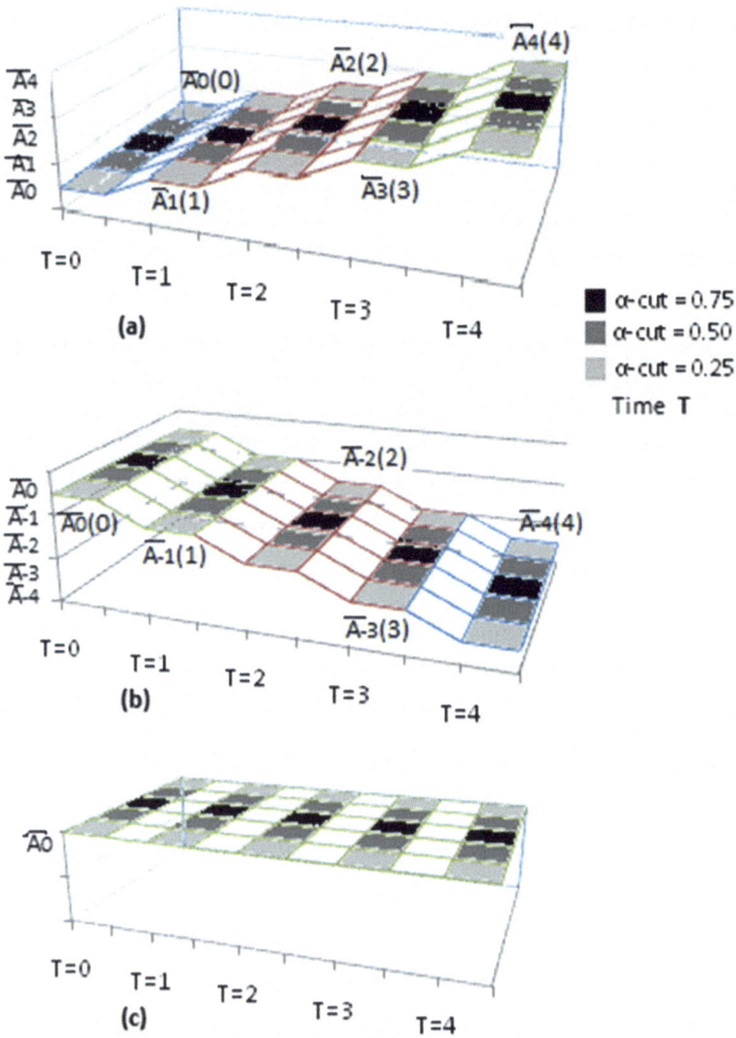

Fig. 5 FCA for short period COVID-19 growth-trend from 11/04/2020 To 15/04/2020 in **a** India With $\rho > 1$, **b** Germany With $\rho < 1$, **c** China With $\rho \approx 1$

The corresponding FCA will be similar to as shown in (Fig. 5b).

(3) **China** having $\rho \approx 1$ from 11/04/20–15/04/20

The number of active cases on 11/04/2020 was 1138 and on 15/04/2020 was 1107. Considering the scale of 1000:1, $y_0 = 1.138$ and $y_4 = 1.107$ gives $\rho \approx 1$. Let $\tilde{y}_0$ and $\tilde{\rho} = (\rho - 0.03/\rho/\rho + 0.03)$ be triangular fuzzy numbers.

Case-I: If $\tilde{y}_0$ be fuzzy and $\rho = 1.0$ be a crisp constant, then $\forall t,\ \tilde{y}_t = \tilde{y}_0$.

The only fuzzy point corresponding to $\tilde{y}_0$ is $\tilde{x}_0$.

Table 4 $y_0 = 7.189$; $\tilde{\rho} = (1.078/1.098/1.118)$

	$\tilde{\rho}[0.25]$= [1.083,1.113]	$\tilde{\rho}[0.50]$= [1.088,1.108]	$\tilde{\rho}[0.75]$= [1.093,1.103]
Time t	$\tilde{y}_t[0.25]$	$\tilde{y}_t[0.50]$	$\tilde{y}_t[0.75]$
1(12/4)	[7.786,8.001]	[7.822,7.965]	[7.858,7.929]
2(13/4)	[8.432,8.906]	[8.510,8.826]	[8.588,8.746]
3(14/4)	[9.132,9.912]	[9.259,9.779]	[9.387,9.647]
4(15/4)	[9.890,11.032]	[10.074,10.835]	[10.260,10.641]

Table 5 $\tilde{y}_0 = (64.781/65.181/65.581)$; $\rho = 0.973$

Time t	$\tilde{y}_t[0.25]$	$\tilde{y}_t[0.50]$	$\tilde{y}_t[0.75]$
0(11/4)	[64.881,65.481]	[64.981,65.381]	[65.081,65.281]
1(12/4)	[63.129,63.713]	[63.227,63.616]	[63.324,63.518]
2(13/4)	[61.425,61.993]	[61.519,61.898]	[61.614,61.803]
3(14/4)	[59.766,60.319]	[59.858,41.657]	[59.950,60.135]
4(15/4)	[58.153,58.690]	[58.242,40.533]	[58.332,58.511]

Table 6 $y_0 = 65.181$; $\tilde{\rho} = (0.963/0.973/0.983)$

	$\tilde{\rho}[0.25]$ = [0.965,0.980]	$\tilde{\rho}[0.50]$ = [0.968,0.978]	$\tilde{\rho}[0.75]$ = [0.970,0.975]
Time t	$\tilde{y}_t[0.25]$	$\tilde{y}_t[0.50]$	$\tilde{y}_t[0.75]$
1(12/4)	[62.90,63.877]	[63.095,63.747]	[63.226,63.551]
2(13/4)	[60.698,62.60]	[61.076,62.345]	[61.329,61.963]
3(14/4)	[58.574,61.348]	[59.122,60.973]	[59.489,60.414]
4(15/4)	[56.524,60.121]	[57.230,59.632]	[57.704,58.903]

Case-II: Let $y_0 = 1.138$ be crisp and $\tilde{\rho} = (0.97/1.0/1.03)$ be fuzzy. Thus $\tilde{\rho}[\alpha] = [0.97 + 0.03\alpha, 1.03 - 0.03\alpha]$ and $\forall t \geq 1$, $\tilde{y}_t[\alpha]$ has been calculated from (28). The pattern of values of slightly, moderately and highly infected active cases during the stipulated time period has been given in Table 7. Here the variations in the values of $\tilde{y}_t$ in the stipulated period are negligible. The corresponding FCA for both cases will have only one cell $\tilde{A}_0$ as shown in (Fig. 5c).

5.2 *Fuzzy Model Representing Spread of Virus over a Considerably Large Period of Time*

It is known that the number of people infected by the virus grows or falls according as $R_0 > 1$ or $R_0 < 1$.

Table 7 $y_0 = 1.138$; $\tilde{\rho} = (0.97/1.0/1.03)$

	$\tilde{\rho}[0.25] =$ [0.977,1.022]	$\tilde{\rho}[0.50] =$ [0.985,1.015]	$\tilde{\rho}[0.75] =$ [0.992,1.007]
Time t	$\tilde{y}_t[0.25]$	$\tilde{y}_t[0.50]$	$\tilde{y}_t[0.75]$
1(12/4)	[1.112,1.163]	[1.121,1.155]	[1.129,1.146]
2(13/4)	[1.086,1.187]	[1.104,1.172]	[1.120,1.154]
3(14/4)	[1.061,1.215]	[1.088,1.190]	[1.111,1.162]
4(15/4)	[1.037,1.241]	[1.071,1.208]	[1.102,1.170]

An FFDE representing spread of virus population over a period of time, has been obtained by fuzzifying the FDE (of the form 20) given as:

$$y_{t+1} = R_{0(t)} y_t, \quad R_{0(t)} > 0, \ t = 0, 1, 2, \ldots \tag{30}$$

where, 'y_t' is the reported number of people being actively infected by the virus at time t, and '$R_{0(t)}$' is the basic reproduction number of the virus at time t. If the initial number of people tested to be actively infected be $y_0 > 0$, the following two cases are considered:

- Case-I: $\tilde{y}_0 > 0$ is fuzzy and $\forall t \geq 0, \ R_{0(t)}$ is crisp.
  The FFDE $\forall t \geq 0$ will be $\tilde{y}_{t+1} = R_{0(t)} \tilde{y}_t$ and for some $\alpha \in (0, 1]$,

$$\tilde{y}_{t+1}[\alpha] = R_{0(t)} \tilde{y}_t[\alpha] \tag{31}$$

- Case-II: $y_0 > 0$ is crisp and $\forall t \geq 0, \ \tilde{R}_{0(t)}$ is fuzzy.
  Then $\tilde{y}_1 = \tilde{R}_{0(0)} y_0$ and the FFDE $\forall t \geq 1$ will be $\tilde{y}_{t+1} = \tilde{R}_{0(t)} \tilde{y}_t$.
  For some $\alpha \in (0, 1]$,

$$\tilde{y}_1[\alpha] = (\tilde{R}_{0(t)}[\alpha]) y_0 \ ; \ \ \forall t \geq 1, \tilde{y}_{t+1}[\alpha] = \tilde{R}_{0(t)}[\alpha].\tilde{y}_t[\alpha] \tag{32}$$

$\tilde{R}_{0(t)}[\alpha].\tilde{y}_t[\alpha]$ has been computed using Definition (2.11).

Here $\tilde{y}_t[\alpha]$ represents the suspected number of actively infected people provided $\alpha \geq 0.25$ such that they are assumed to be as given in Sect. (5.1).

Through these FFDE we depict the spread of MERS virus and COVID-19 virus and hence design their corresponding FCA which are temporally hybrid.

5.2.1 FCA Model Representing Spread of MERS Virus

Middle East Respiratory Syndrome Coronavirus(MERS-CoV or MERS) was first reported in 2012 in Saudi Arabia. A significant outbreak of MERS have been observed in Saudi Arabia and South Korea in and around 2015. Though, at the onset of these

Table 8 $\tilde{y}_0 = (0.3/1/1.7)$; $R_{0(t)} = \frac{y_{t+1}}{y_t}$ be crisp with $R_{0(0)} = 5.7$

Time t	y_t	$R_{0(t)}$	$\tilde{y}_t[0.25]$	$\tilde{y}_t[0.50]$	$\tilde{y}_t[0.75]$
0	1	5.7	[0.47, 1.52]	[0.65, 1.35]	[0.82, 1.17]
1	5.7	3.5	[2.71, 8.69]	[3.70, 7.69]	[4.70, 6.70]
2	20	1.5	[9.47, 30.42]	[12.97, 26.93]	[16.46, 23.44]
3	30	2.5	[14.21, 45.63]	[19.45, 40.40]	[24.68, 35.16]
4	75	0.5	[35.53, 114.08]	[48.64, 100.99]	[61.71, 87.89]
5	37	0.3	[17.76, 57.04]	[24.32, 50.50]	[30.86, 43.95]
6	11	0.55	[5.33, 17.11]	[7.29, 15.15]	[9.26, 13.18]
Day 50	6	–	[2.93, 9.41]	[4.01, 8.33]	[5.09, 7.25]

outbreaks, the reproduction number ranged from 1.0 to 5.7, it dropped below 1 within 2–6 weeks [4, 23]. Out of 2449 total reported cases of MERS there has been 845 deaths [23] which is around 34% of the total cases.

Here the dynamics of the MERS virus for South Korea and Riyadh (Saudi Arabia) for a period of 50 days in 2015 have been analysed where a 1-week period is considered as a unit time step [4].

The number of cases y_t at time t, has been recorded from [4]. If the initial cases be y_0, then let the fuzzy initial value be $\tilde{y}_0 = (0.3y_0/y_0/1.7y_0)$.

Initially, $R_0(0)$ has been used as given in (see [4]) and its given value range corresponds to the limits of the considered fuzzy $\tilde{R}_{0(0)}$. For any $t \geq 1$, the crisp $R_{0(t)}$ values have been calculated from (30).

(1) **South Korea** from May 11, 2015–July 22, 2015

Let the initial number of cases be $y_0 = 1$. Also, $\tilde{R}_{0(0)} = (3.0/5.7/9.0)$ and $\forall t \geq 1$, $\tilde{R}_{0(t)} = (0.52R_{0(t)}/R_{0(t)}/1.6R_{0(t)})$ has been considered.
Case-I: Let $\tilde{y}_0 = (0.3/1/1.7)$ and $R_{0(t)}$ be crisp with $R_{0(0)} = 5.7$
Thus $\tilde{y}_0[\alpha] = [0.3 + 0.7\alpha, 1.7 - 0.7\alpha]$ and $\forall t \geq 1$, $\tilde{y}_t[\alpha]$ has been calculated from (31). The pattern of values of slightly, moderately and highly infected active cases during the stipulated time period has been given in Table 8.

Here,

$$\tilde{y}_0 < \tilde{y}_1 < \tilde{y}_7 < \tilde{y}_6 < \tilde{y}_2 < \tilde{y}_3 < \tilde{y}_5 < \tilde{y}_4.$$

Thus the fuzzy phase points are $\tilde{x}_0, \tilde{x}_1, \ldots, \tilde{x}_7$. The corresponding FCA will have cells $\tilde{A}_0, \tilde{A}_1, \ldots, \tilde{A}_7$ and the ON states of these cells will be $\tilde{A}_0(0)$, $\tilde{A}_1(1)$, $\tilde{A}_2(7)$, $\tilde{A}_3(6)$, $\tilde{A}_4(2)$, $\tilde{A}_5(3)$, $\tilde{A}_6(5)$, $\tilde{A}_7(4)$ as shown in (Fig. 6a).

Case-II: Let $y_0 = 1$ be crisp and $\tilde{R}_{0(t)} = (0.52R_{(t)}/R_{0(t)}/1.6R_{0(t)})$ be triangular fuzzy numbers with $\tilde{R}_{0(0)} = (3.0/5.7/9.0)$. Thus $\forall t \geq 1$, $\tilde{y}_t[\alpha]$ has been calculated from (32). The pattern of values of slightly, moderately and highly infected active cases during the stipulated time period has been given in Table 9. Since the pattern

Table 9 $y_0 = 1$; $\tilde{R}_{0(t)} = (0.52R_{0(t)}/R_{0(t)}/1.6R_{0(t)})$

Time t	$\tilde{R}_{0(t)}$	$\tilde{R}_{0(t)}[0.25].\tilde{y}_t[0.25]$	$\tilde{R}_{0(t)}[0.50].\tilde{y}_t[0.50]$	$\tilde{R}_{0(t)}[0.75].\tilde{y}_t[0.75]$
0	(3.0/5.7/9.0)	[3.675, 8.175] × 1	[4.35, 7.35]× 1	[5.025, 6.525]× 1
1	(1.8/3.5/5.6)	[2.225, 5.075] [3.7, 8.2]	[2.65, 4.55] [4.3, 7.3]	[3.075, 4.025] [5.0, 6.5]
2	(0.8/1.5/2.4)	[0.975, 2.175] [8.2, 41.6]	[1.15, 1.95] [11.4, 33.2]	[1.325, 1.725] [15.4, 26.2]
3	(1.3/2.5/4.0)	[1.6,3.625] [8.0, 90.5]	[1.9, 3.25] [13.1, 64.7]	[2.2, 2.875] [20.4, 45.2]
4	(0.3/0.5/0.8)	[0.35, 0.725] [12.8, 328.1]	[0.4, 0.65] [24.9, 210.3]	[0.45, 0.575] [44.9, 130.0]
5	(0.2/0.3/0.5)	[0.225, 0.45] [4.5, 237.8]	[0.25, 0.4] [10.0, 136.7]	[0.275, 0.35] [20.2, 74.7]
6	(0.3/0.55/0.9)	[0.362, 0.812] [1.0, 107.0]	[0.425, 0.725] [2.5, 54.7]	[0.487, 0.637] [5.6, 26.1]
Day 50	–	$\tilde{y}_7[0.25] =$ [0.4, 86.9]	$\tilde{y}_7[0.50] =$ [1.1, 39.7]	$\tilde{y}_7[0.75] =$ [2.7, 16.6]

of the α-cut values of the fuzzy phase points from Tables 8 and 9 are similar, the corresponding FCA will be similar to as shown in (Fig. 6a).

(2) **Riyadh** from July 13, 2015–August 31, 2015

Let the initial number of cases be $y_0 = 2$. Also, $\tilde{R}_{0(0)} = (2.0/2.9/5.0)$ and $\forall t \geq 1$, $\tilde{R}_{0(t)} = (0.7R_{0(t)}/R_{0(t)}/1.7R_{0(t)})$ has been considered.
Case-I: Let $\tilde{y}_0 = (0.6/2/3.4)$ and $R_{0(t)}$ be crisp with $R_{0(0)} = 2.9$
Thus $\tilde{y}_0[\alpha] = [0.6 + 1.4\alpha, 3.4 - 1.4\alpha]$ and $\forall t \geq 1$, $\tilde{y}_t[\alpha]$ has been calculated from (31). The pattern of values of slightly, moderately and highly infected active cases during the stipulated time period has been given in Table 10.

Here,

$$\tilde{y}_0 < \tilde{y}_7 < \tilde{y}_1 < \tilde{y}_2 < \tilde{y}_6 < \tilde{y}_3 < \tilde{y}_4 \approx \tilde{y}_5$$

Thus the fuzzy phase points are $\tilde{x}_0, \tilde{x}_1, \ldots, \tilde{x}_6$. The corresponding FCA will have cells $\tilde{A}_0, \tilde{A}_1, \ldots, \tilde{A}_6$ and the ON states of these cells will be $\tilde{A}_0(0)$, $\tilde{A}_1(7)$, $\tilde{A}_2(1)$, $\tilde{A}_3(2)$, $\tilde{A}_4(6)$, $\tilde{A}_5(3)$, $\tilde{A}_6(4)$, $\tilde{A}_6(5)$ as shown in (Fig. 6b).
Case-II: Let $y_0 = 2$ be crisp and $\tilde{R}_{0(t)} = (0.7R_{0(t)}/R_{0(t)}/1.7R_{0(t)})$ be triangular fuzzy numbers with $\tilde{R}_{0(0)} = (2.0/2.9/5.0)$. Thus $\forall t \geq 1$, $\tilde{y}_t[\alpha]$ has been calculated from (32). The pattern of values of asymslightly, moderately and highly infected active cases during the stipulated time period has been given in Table 11. Since the pattern of the α-cut values of the fuzzy phase points from Tables 10 and 11 are similar, the corresponding FCA will be similar to as shown in (Fig. 6b).

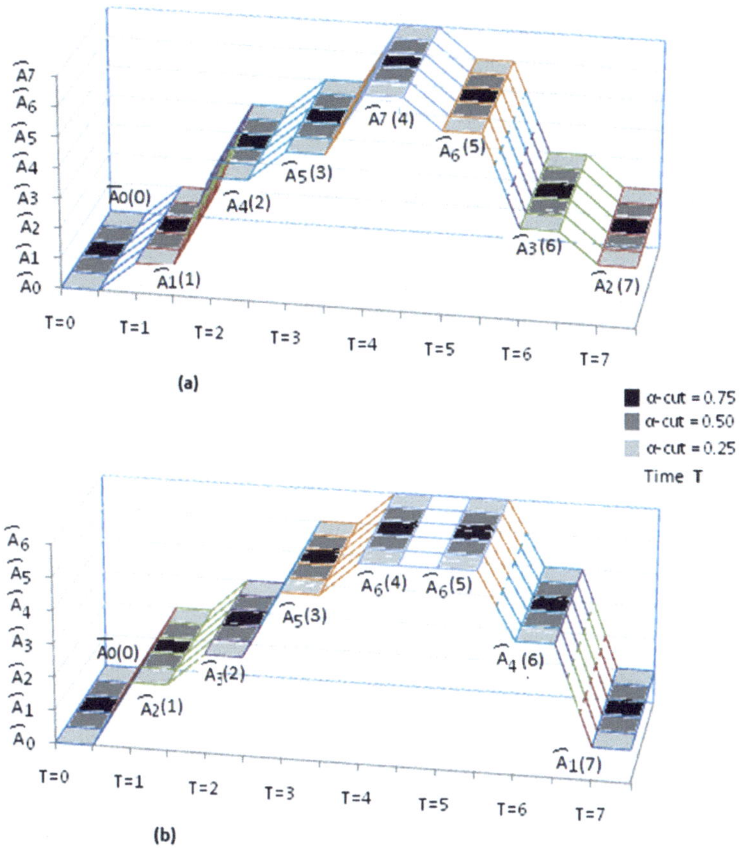

Fig. 6 FCA for spread of MERS during 2015 in **a** South Korea, **b** Riyadh (Saudi Arabia)

Table 10 $\tilde{y}_0 = (0.6/2/3.4)$; $R_{0(t)} = \frac{y_{t+1}}{y_t}$ be crisp with $R_{0(0)} = 2.9$

Time t	y_t	$R_{0(t)}$	$\tilde{y}_t[0.25]$	$\tilde{y}_t[0.50]$	$\tilde{y}_t[0.75]$
0	2	2.9	[0.95, 3.05]	[1.3, 2.7]	[1.65, 2.35]
1	5.8	1.4	[2.78, 8.84]	[3.77, 7.83]	[4.78, 6.81]
2	8	2.5	[3.89, 12.38]	[5.29, 10.96]	[6.69, 9.53]
3	20	1.4	[9.72, 30.95]	[13.22, 27.4]	[16.72, 23.82]
4	28	1.0	[13.61, 43.33]	[18.51, 38.36]	[23.41, 33.35]
5	28	0.54	[13.61, 43.33]	[18.51, 38.36]	[23.41, 33.35]
6	15	0.2	[7.35, 23.40]	[10.0, 20.71]	[12.64, 18.01]
Day 50	3	–	[1.47, 4.68]	[2.0, 4.14]	[2.53, 3.6]

Table 11 $y_0 = 2$; $\tilde{R}_{0(t)} = (0.7R_{0(t)}/R_{0(t)}/1.7R_{0(t)})$

Time t	$\tilde{R}_{0(t)}$	$\tilde{R}_{0(t)}[0.25].\tilde{y}_t[0.25]$	$\tilde{R}_{0(t)}[0.50].\tilde{y}_t[0.50]$	$\tilde{R}_{0(t)}[0.75].\tilde{y}_t[0.75]$
0	(2.0/2.9/5.0)	[2.225, 4.475] × 2	[2.43, 3.95]× 2	[2.675, 3.425]× 2
1	(1.0/1.4/2.4)	[1.1, 2.15] [4.4, 8.9]	[1.2, 1.9] [4.9, 7.9]	[1.3, 1.65] [5.3, 6.8]
2	(1.8/2.5/4.3)	[1.975, 3.85] [4.8, 19.1]	[2.15, 3.4] [5.9, 15.0]	[2.325, 2.95] [6.9, 11.2]
3	(1.0/1.4/2.4)	[1.1, 2.15] [9.4, 73.5]	[1.2, 1.9] [12.7, 51.0]	[1.3, 1.65] [16.0, 33.0]
4	(0.7/1.0/1.7)	[0.775, 1.525] [10.3, 158.0]	[0.85, 1.35] [15.2, 96.9]	[0.925, 1.175] [20.8, 54.4]
5	(0.4/0.54/0.9)	[0.435, 0.81] [8.0, 241.0]	[0.47, 0.72] [12.9, 130.8]	[0.505, 0.63] [19.2, 63.9]
6	(0.1/0.2/0.3)	[0.125, 0.275] [3.4, 195.2]	[0.15, 0.25] [6.1, 94.2]	[0.175, 0.225] [9.7, 40.3]
Day 50	–	$\tilde{y}_7[0.25] =$ [0.4, 53.7]	$\tilde{y}_7[0.50] =$ [0.9, 23.5]	$\tilde{y}_7[0.75] =$ [1.7, 9.1]

5.2.2 FCA Model Representing Spread of COVID-19 Virus

COVID-19 which emerged at China's Wuhan towards the end of 2019, became a pandemic around March 2020. Though more that 5.6 million people have been affected till recently, the global reproduction number which was around 1.66 in March has dropped below 1.1 by the beginning of May.

Here the dynamics (according to [24]) of the active cases of COVID-19 virus for India, USA and Germany for an entire period of 49 days(referred to as large period) from March 22, 2020 to May 09, 2020, has been analysed where a 4-day gap(referred to as short period) is considered as a unit time step. The number of active cases y_t at time t has been recorded from [24] and the $R_{0(t)}$ value at each time step t has been calculated from (30).

Again, from (29), we get, $R_{0(t)} \approx \rho^4$.

(1) India on 22/03/2020, had 365 active cases and 31 closed cases out of total reported 396 cases. On 09/05/2020 there were 41,406 active and 21,402 closed out of 62,808 cases[24]. The average percentage of closed cases during this period is found to be nearly 20%. Considering the scale of 1000:1, the initial cases are $y_0 \approx 0.36$. Here, $\tilde{y}_0 = (0.2y_0/y_0/1.8y_0)$ and $\tilde{R}_{0(t)} = (R_{0(t)} - 0.02/R_{0(t)}/R_{0(t)} + 0.02)$ have been considered.

Case-I: Let $\tilde{y}_0 = (0.07/0.36/0.65)$ be fuzzy and $R_{0(t)}$ be crisp with $R_{0(0)} = 1.83$. Thus $\tilde{y}_0[\alpha] = [0.07 + 0.29\alpha, 0.65 - 0.29\alpha]$ and $\forall t \geq 1$, $\tilde{y}_t[\alpha]$ has been calculated from (31). The pattern of values of slightly, moderately and highly infected active cases during the stipulated time period has been given in Table 12. Here,

Table 12 $\tilde{y}_0 = (0.07/0.36/0.65)$; $R_{0(t)} \frac{y_{t+1}}{y_t}$ is crisp with $R_{0(0)} = 1.83$

Time t	y_t	$R_{0(t)}$	$\tilde{y}_t[0.25]$	$\tilde{y}_t[0.50]$	$\tilde{y}_t[0.75]$
0(22/03)	0.36	1.83	[0.142, 0.577]	[0.215, 0.505]	[0.287, 0.432]
1(26/03)	0.66	1.69	[0.260, 1.056]	[0.393, 0.924]	[0.525, 0.791]
2(30/03)	1.12	2.48	[0.439, 1.785]	[0.664, 1.562]	[0.887, 1.337]
3(03/04)	2.78	1.70	[1.089, 4.427]	[1.647, 3.874]	[2.20, 3.316]
4(07/04)	4.72	1.52	[1.851, 7.526]	[2.80, 6.586]	[3.74, 5.637]
5(11/04)	7.19	1.45	[2.814, 11.44]	[4.256, 10.011]	[5.685, 8.568]
6(15/04)	10.44	1.36	[4.08, 16.588]	[6.171, 14.516]	[8.243, 12.424]
7(19/04)	14.20	1.22	[5.549, 22.56]	[8.393, 19.742]	[11.210, 16.897]
8(23/04)	17.31	1.23	[6.77, 27.523]	[10.239, 24.085]	[13.676, 20.614]
9(27/04)	21.37	1.22	[8.327, 33.853]	[12.594, 29.625]	[16.821, 25.355]
10(01/05)	26.03	1.29	[10.159, 41.301]	[15.365, 36.142]	[20.522, 30.933]
11(05/05)	33.57	1.23	[13.105, 53.278]	[19.821, 46.623]	[26.473, 39.904]
12(09/05)	41.41	–	[16.120, 65.532]	[24.38, 57.346]	[32.562, 49.082]

$$\tilde{y}_0 < \tilde{y}_1 < \cdots < \tilde{y}_{12}$$

Thus the fuzzy phase points are $\tilde{x}_0, \tilde{x}_1, \ldots, \tilde{x}_{12}$. The corresponding FCA will have cells $\tilde{A}_0, \tilde{A}_1, \ldots, \tilde{A}_{12}$ and the ON states of these cells will be $\tilde{A}_0(0), \tilde{A}_1(1), \ldots, \tilde{A}_{12}(12)$ as shown in (Fig. 7a).

Case-II: Let $y_0 = 0.36$ be crisp and $\tilde{R}_{0(t)} = (R_{0(t)} - 0.02/R_{0(t)}/R_{0(t)} + 0.02)$ be fuzzy triangular numbers with $\tilde{R}_{0(0)} = (1.81/1.83/1.85)$. Thus $\forall t \geq 1$, $\tilde{y}_t[\alpha]$ has been calculated from (32). The pattern of values of slightly, moderately and highly infected active cases during the stipulated time period has been given in Table 13. Since the pattern of the α-cut values of the fuzzy phase points from Tables 12 and 13 are similar, the corresponding FCA will be similar to as shown in (Fig. 7a).

(2) USA on 22/03/2020, had 33,150 active cases and 690 closed cases out of total reported 33,840 cases. On 09/05/2020 there were 1,015,164 active and 332,145 closed out of 1,347,309 cases [24]. The average percentage of closed cases during this period is found to be nearly 13%. Considering the scale of 1000:1, the initial cases are $y_0 \approx 33.15$. Here, $\tilde{y}_0 = (0.13y_0/y_0/0.87y_0)$ and $\tilde{R}_{0(t)} = (R_{0(t)} - 0.04/R_{0(t)}/R_{0(t)} + 0.04)$ have been considered.

Table 13 $y_0 = 0.36$; $\tilde{R}_{0(t)} = (R_{0(t)} - 0.02/R_{0(t)}/R_{0(t)} + 0.02)$

Time t	$\tilde{R}_{0(t)}$	$\tilde{R}_{0(t)}[0.25].\tilde{y}_t[0.25]$	$\tilde{R}_{0(t)}[0.50].\tilde{y}_t[0.50]$	$\tilde{R}_{0(t)}[0.75].\tilde{y}_t[0.75]$
0(22/03)	(1.81/1.83/1.85)	[1.815, 1.845]× 0.36	[1.82, 1.84]× 0.36	[1.825, 1.835]×0.36
1(26/03)	(1.67/1.69/1.71)	[1.675, 1.705] [0.653, 0.664]	[1.68, 1.70] [0.655, 0.662]	[1.685, 1.695] [0.657, 0.661]
2(30/03)	(2.46/2.48/2.50)	[2.465, 2.495] [1.094, 1.132]	[2.47, 2.49] [1.10, 1.125]	[2.475, 2.485] [1.107, 1.120]
3(03/04)	(1.68/1.70/1.72)	[1.685, 1.715] [2.698, 2.826]	[1.690, 1.710] [2.717, 2.801]	[1.695, 1.705] [2.740, 2.783]
4(07/04)	(1.50/1.52/1.54)	[1.505, 1.535] [4.546, 4.846]	[1.510, 1.530] [4.592, 4.79]	[1.515, 1.525] [4.644, 4.745]
5(11/04)	(1.43/1.45/1.47)	[1.435, 1.465] [6.841, 7.438]	[1.44, 1.460] [6.934, 7.329]	[1.445, 1.455] [7.036, 7.236]
6(15/04)	(1.34/1.36/1.38)	[1.345, 1.375] [9.817, 10.897]	[1.350, 1.37] [9.985, 10.70]	[1.355, 1.365] [10.167, 10.528]
7(19/04)	(1.20/1.22/1.24)	[1.205, 1.235] [13.204, 14.984]	[1.210, 1.230] [13.480, 14.659]	[1.215, 1.225] [13.776, 14.371]
8(23/04)	(1.21/1.23/1.25)	[1.215, 1.245] [15.911, 18.505]	[1.22, 1.24] [16.311, 18.031]	[1.225, 1 .235] [16.738, 17.604]
9(27/04)	(1.20/1.22/1.24)	[1.205, 1.235] [19.332, 23.039]	[1.210, 1.23] [19.899, 22.358]	[1.215, 1.225] [20.504, 21.741]
10(01/05)	(1.27/1.29/1.31)	[1.275, 1.305] [23.295, 28.453]	[1.28, 1.30] [24.078, 27.50]	[1.285, 1.295] [24.912, 26.633]
11(05/05)	(1.21/1.23/1.25)	[1.215, 1.245] [29.701, 37.131]	[1.22, 1.24] [30.820, 35.750]	[1.225, 1.235] [32.012, 34.490]
12(09/05)	–	$\tilde{y}_{12}[0.25]$ = [36.087,46.228]	$\tilde{y}_{12}[0.50]$ = [37.60,44.33]	$\tilde{y}_{12}[0.75]$ = [39.215,42.595]

Case-I: Let $\tilde{y}_0 = (4.3/33.15/62.0)$ be fuzzy and $R_{0(t)}$ be crisp with $R_{0(0)} = 2.5$. Thus $\tilde{y}_0[\alpha] = [4.3 + 28.85\alpha, 62.0 - 28.85\alpha]$ and $\forall t \geq 1$, $\tilde{y}_t[\alpha]$ has been calculated from (31). The pattern of values of slightly, moderately and highly infected active cases during the stipulated time period has been given in Table 14. Here,

$$\tilde{y}_0 < \tilde{y}_1 < \cdots < \tilde{y}_{12}$$

Thus the fuzzy phase points are $\tilde{x}_0, \tilde{x}_1, \ldots, \tilde{x}_{12}$. The corresponding FCA will have cells $\tilde{A}_0, \tilde{A}_1, \ldots, \tilde{A}_{12}$ and the ON states of these cells will be $\tilde{A}_0(0)$, $\tilde{A}_1(1)$,…,$\tilde{A}_{12}(12)$ as shown in (Fig. 7a).

Case-II: Let $y_0 = 33.15$ be crisp and $\tilde{R}_{0(t)} = (R_{0(t)} - 0.04/R_{0(t)}/R_{0(t)} + 0.04)$ be triangular fuzzy numbers with $\tilde{R}_{0(0)} = (2.46/2.5/2.54)$. Thus $\forall t \geq 1$, $\tilde{y}_t[\alpha]$ has been calculated from *(*32*)*. The pattern of values of slightly, moderately and highly infected active cases during the stipulated time period has been given in Table 15. Since the pattern of the α-cut values of the fuzzy phase points of Tables 14 and 15 are similar,

Table 14 $\tilde{y}_0 = (4.3/33.15/62.0)$; $R_{0(t)} = \frac{y_{t+1}}{y_t}$ is crisp with $R_{0(0)} = 2.5$

Time t	y_t	$R_{0(t)}$	$\tilde{y}_t[0.25]$	$\tilde{y}_t[0.50]$	$\tilde{y}_t[0.75]$
0(22/03)	33.15	2.5	[11.512, 54.787]	[18.725, 47.575]	[25.937, 40.362]
1(26/03)	82.87	1.91	[28.78,136.967]	[46.812, 118.937]	[64.842, 100.905]
2(30/03)	158.56	1.65	[54.97, 261.607]	[89.411, 227.170]	[123.848, 192.729]
3(03/04)	262.26	1.42	[90.7, 431.652]	[147.528, 374.830]	[204.349, 318.003]
4(07/04)	371.82	1.31	[128.794, 612.946]	[209.49, 532.259]	[290.176, 451.564]
5(11/04)	485.43	1.18	[168.720, 802.959]	[274.432, 697.259]	[380.131, 591.549]
6(15/04)	571.06	1.15	[199.09, 947.492]	[323.83, 822.766]	[448.555, 698.028]
7(19/04)	656.75	1.13	[228.953, 1089.616]	[372.404, 946.181]	[515.838, 802.732]
8(23/04)	745.15	1.09	[258.717, 1231.266]	[420.817, 1069.185]	[582.897, 907.087]
9(27/04)	808.52	1.11	[282.0, 1342.08]	[458.691, 1165.412]	[635.358, 988.725]
10(01/05)	895.11	1.07	[313.02, 1489.709]	[509.147, 1293.607]	[705.247, 1097.485]
11(05/05)	953.56	1.06	[334.931, 1593.989]	[544.787, 1384.159]	[754.614, 1174.309]
12(09/05)	1015.16	–	[355.027, 1689.628]	[577.474, 1467.209]	[799.891, 1244.768]

the corresponding FCA will be similar to as shown in (Fig. 7a).

(3) Germany on 22/03/2020, had 24,513 active cases and 360 closed cases out of total reported 24,873 cases. On 09/05/2020 there were 20,475 active and 150,849 closed out of 171,324 cases [24]. The average percentage of closed cases during this period is found to be nearly 44%. Considering the scale of 1000:1, the initial cases $y_0 \approx 24.51$. Here, $\tilde{y}_0 = (0.44y_0/y_0/1.56y_0)$ and $\tilde{R}_{0(t)} = (R_{0(t)} - 0.02/R_{0(t)}/R_{0(t)} + 0.02)$ have been considered.

Case-I: Let $\tilde{y}_0 = (10.8/24.51/38.2)$ be fuzzy and $R_{0(t)}$ be crisp with $R_{0(0)} = 1.55$. Thus $\tilde{y}_0[\alpha] = [10.8 + 13.71\alpha, 38.2 - 13.69\alpha]$ and $\forall t \geq 1, \tilde{y}_t[\alpha]$ has been calculated from (31). The pattern of values of slightly, moderately and highly infected active cases during the stipulated time period has been given in Table 16. Here, $\tilde{y}_0 < \cdots < \tilde{y}_4$ and $\tilde{y}_5 > \cdots > \tilde{y}_{12}$ giving

$$\tilde{y}_{12} < \tilde{y}_0 \approx \tilde{y}_{11} < \tilde{y}_{10} < \tilde{y}_1 \approx \tilde{y}_9 < \tilde{y}_8 < \tilde{y}_2 \approx \tilde{y}_7 < \tilde{y}_6 < \tilde{y}_3 \approx \tilde{y}_5 < \tilde{y}_4$$

Table 15 $y_0 = 33.15$; $\tilde{R}_{0(t)} = (R_{0(t)} - 0.04/R_{0(t)}/R_{0(t)} + 0.04)$

Time t	$\tilde{R}_{0(t)}$	$\tilde{R}_{0(t)}[0.25].\tilde{y}_t[0.25]$	$\tilde{R}_{0(t)}[0.50].\tilde{y}_t[0.50]$	$\tilde{R}_{0(t)}[0.75].\tilde{y}_t[0.75]$
0(22/03)	(2.46/2.5/2.54)	[2.47, 2.53] × 33.15	[2.48, 2.52] × 33.15	[2.49, 2.51]× 33.15
1(26/03)	(1.87/1.91/1.95)	[1.88, 1.94] [81.880, 83.869]	[1.89, 1.93] [82.212, 83.538]	[1.90, 1.92] [82.543, 83.206]
2(30/03)	(1.61/1.65/1.69)	[1.62, 1.68] [153.934, 162.706]	[1.63, 1.67] [155.381, 161.228]	[1.64, 1.66] [156.832, 159.756]
3(03/04)	(1.38/1.42/1.46)	[1.39, 1.45] [249.373, 273.346]	[1.40, 1.44] [253.271, 269.251]	[1.41, 1.43] [257.204, 265.195]
4(07/04)	(1.27/1.31/1.35)	[1.28, 1.34] [346.628, 396.352]	[1.29, 1.33] [354.579, 387.721]	[1.30, 1.32] [362.658, 379.229]
5(11/04)	(1.14/1.18/1.22)	[1.15, 1.21] [443.684, 531.112]	[1.16, 1.2] [457.407, 515.669]	[1.17, 1.19] [471.455, 500.582]
6(15/04)	(1.11/1.15/1.19)	[1.12, 1.18] [510.237, 642.646]	[1.13, 1.17] [530.592, 618.803]	[1.14, 1.16] [551.602, 595.693]
7(19/04)	(1.09/1.13/1.17)	[1.10, 1.16] [571.465, 758.322]	[1.11, 1.15] [599.569, 724.0]	[1.12, 1.14] [628.826, 691.004]
8(23/04)	(1.05/1.09/1.13)	[1.06, 1.12] [628.612, 879.654]	[1.07, 1.11] [666.522, 832.6]	[1.08, 1.10] [704.285, 787.745]
9(27/04)	(1.07/1.11/1.15)	[1.08, 1.14] [666.329, 985.212]	[1.09, 1.13] [712.109, 924.186]	[1.10, 1.12] [760.628, 866.52]
10(01/05)	(1.03/1.07/1.11)	[1.04, 1.10] [719.635, 1123.142]	[1.05, 1.09] [776.199, 1044.33]	[1.06, 1.08] [836.691, 970.502]
11(05/05)	(1.02/1.06/1.10)	[1.03, 1.09] [748.420, 1235.456]	[1.04, 1.08] [815.009, 1138.320]	[1.05, 1.07] [886.892, 1048.142]
12(09/05)	–	$\tilde{y}_{12}[0.25] =$ [770.823, 1346.647]	$\tilde{y}_{12}[0.50] =$ [847.609, 1229.386]	$\tilde{y}_{12}[0.75] =$ [931.237, 1121.512]

Thus the different fuzzy phase points are $\tilde{x}_{-1}$, $\tilde{x}_0$, $\tilde{x}_1$, …,$\tilde{x}_7$. The corresponding FCA will have cells $\tilde{A}_{-1}$, $\tilde{A}_0$, $\tilde{A}_1$, …, $\tilde{A}_7$ and the ON states of these cells will be $\tilde{A}_{-1}(12)$, $\tilde{A}_0(0)$, $\tilde{A}_0(11)$, $\tilde{A}_1(10)$, $\tilde{A}_2(1)$, $\tilde{A}_2(9)$, $\tilde{A}_3(8)$, $\tilde{A}_4(2)$, $\tilde{A}_4(7)$, $\tilde{A}_5(6)$, $\tilde{A}_6(3)$, $\tilde{A}_6(5)$, $\tilde{A}_7(4)$ as shown in (Fig. 7b).

Case-II: Let $y_0 = 24.51$ be crisp and $\tilde{R}_{0(t)} = (R_{0(t)} - 0.02/R_{0(t)}/R_{0(t)} + 0.02)$ be triangular fuzzy numbers with $\tilde{R}_{0(0)} = (1.53/1.55/1.57)$. Thus $\forall t \geq 1$, $\tilde{y}_t[\alpha]$ has been calculated from (32). The pattern of values of slightly, moderately and highly

Table 16 $\tilde{y}_0 = (10.8/24.51/38.2)$; $R_{0(t)} = \frac{y_{t+1}}{y_t}$ be crisp with $R_{0(0)} = 1.55$

Time t	y_t	$R_{0(t)}$	$\tilde{y}_t[0.25]$	$\tilde{y}_t[0.50]$	$\tilde{y}_t[0.75]$
0(22/03)	24.51	1.55	[14.227, 34.777]	[17.655, 31.355]	[21.082, 27.932]
1(26/03)	38.0	1.39	[22.052, 53.904]	[27.365, 48.60]	[32.677, 43.295]
2(30/03)	52.74	1.24	[30.652, 74.927]	[38.037, 67.554]	[45.421, 60.180]
3(03/04)	65.31	1.06	[38.008, 92.909]	[47.166, 83.767]	[56.322, 74.623]
4(07/04)	69.57	0.94	[40.288, 98.484]	[49.996, 88.793]	[59.701, 79.100]
5(11/04)	65.18	0.90	[37.871, 92.575]	[46.996, 83.465]	[56.119, 74.354]
6(15/04)	58.35	0.91	[34.084, 83.317]	[42.296, 75.118]	[50.507, 66.919]
7(19/04)	53.10	0.83	[31.016, 75.818]	[38.489, 68.357]	[45.961, 60.896]
8(23/04)	44.25	0.86	[25.743, 62.929]	[31.946, 56.736]	[38.148, 50.544]
9(27/04)	38.13	0.80	[22.139, 54.119]	[27.474, 48.793]	[32.807, 43.468]
10(01/05)	30.44	0.82	[17.711, 43.295]	[21.979, 39.034]	[26.246, 34.774]
11(05/05)	24.91	0.82	[14.523, 35.502]	[18.023, 32.008]	[21.522, 28.515]
12(09/05)	20.47	–	[11.901, 29.112]	[14.779, 26.246]	[17.648, 23.382]

infected active cases during the stipulated time period has been given in Table 17. Since the pattern of the α-cut values of the fuzzy phase points of Tables 16 and 17 are similar, hence the corresponding FCA will be similar to as shown in (Fig. 7b).

6 Conclusion

The basic reproduction number associated with any virus outbreak changes after a short period of time. We have designed an FCA which turned out to be temporally hybrid, representing the growth of the number of infected population from MERS virus outbreak in 2015, and for Covid-19 virus. However, a moderately large time period may be divided into short equal time intervals. In each of these equal time intervals there will be growth of the number of infected population which may be designed by an FCA. So alternate use of FCA and temporally hybrid FCA will

Table 17 $y_0 = 24.51$; $\tilde{R}_{0(t)} = (R_{0(t)} - 0.02/R_{0(t)}/R_{0(t)} + 0.02)$

Time t	$\tilde{R}_{0(t)}$	$\tilde{R}_{0(t)}[0.25].\tilde{y}_t[0.25]$	$\tilde{R}_{0(t)}[0.50].\tilde{y}_t[0.50]$	$\tilde{R}_{0(t)}[0.75].\tilde{y}_t[0.75]$
0(22/03)	(1.53/1.55/1.57)	[1.535, 1.565] × 24.51	[1.54, 1.56] × 24.51	[1.545, 1.555] × 24.51
1(26/03)	(1.37/1.39/1.41)	[1.375, 1.405] [37.623, 38.358]	[1.38, 1.40] [37.745, 38.236]	[1.385, 1.395] [37.868, 38.113]
2(30/03)	(1.22/1.24/1.26)	[1.225, 1.255] [51.732, 53.893]	[1.23, 1.25] [52.088, 53.530]	[1.235, 1.245] [52.447, 53.168]
3(03/04)	(1.04/1.06/1.08)	[1.045, 1.075] [63.372, 67.636]	[1.05, 1.07] [64.068, 66.912]	[1.055, 1.065] [64.772, 66.194]
4(07/04)	(0.92/0.94/0.96)	[0.925, 0.955] [66.224, 72.709]	[0.93, 0.95] [67.271, 71.596]	[0.935, 0.945] [68.334, 70.497]
5(11/04)	(0.88/0.90/0.92)	[0.885, 0.915] [61.257, 69.437]	[0.89, 0.91] [62.562, 68.016]	[0.895, 0.905] [63.892, 66.620]
6(15/04)	(0.89/0.91/0.93)	[0.895, 0.925] [54.212, 63.535]	[0.90, 0.92] [55.680, 61.895]	[0.905, 0.915] [57.183, 60.291]
7(19/04)	(0.81/0.83/0.85)	[0.815, 0.845] [48.520, 58.77]	[0.82, 0.84] [50.112, 56.943]	[0.825, 0.835] [51.751, 55.166]
8(23/04)	(0.84/0.86/0.88)	[0.845, 0.875] [39.544, 49.661]	[0.85, 0.87] [41.092, 47.832]	[0.855, 0.865] [42.695, 46.064]
9(27/04)	(0.78/0.80/0.82)	[0.785, 0.815] [33.415, 43.453]	[0.79, 0.81] [34.928, 41.614]	[0.795, 0.805] [36.504, 39.845]
10(01/05)	(0.80/0.82/0.84)	[0.805, 0.835] [26.231, 35.414]	[0.81, 0.83] [27.593, 33.707]	[0.815, 0.825] [29.021, 32.075]
11(05/05)	(0.80/0.82/0.84)	[0.805, 0.835] [21.116, 29.571]	[0.81, 0.83] [22.350, 27.977]	[0.815, 0.825] [23.652, 26.462]
12(09/05)	–	$\tilde{y}_{12}[0.25]$ = [16.998, 24.692]	$\tilde{y}_{12}[0.50]$ = [18.104, 23.221]	$\tilde{y}_{12}[0.75]$ = [19.276, 21.831]

completely explain the model. Use of the concept of α-cut enabled us to introduce a gradation of the number of infected people. Changing the values of α will give a different gradation.

Study of the models obtained by replacing basic reproduction number with effective reproduction number may be an interesting exercise.

Acknowledgements We are very thankful to Prof. Sitabhra Sinha of IMSc. Chennai, India, for providing the relevant data regarding the R_0 values of COVID-19.

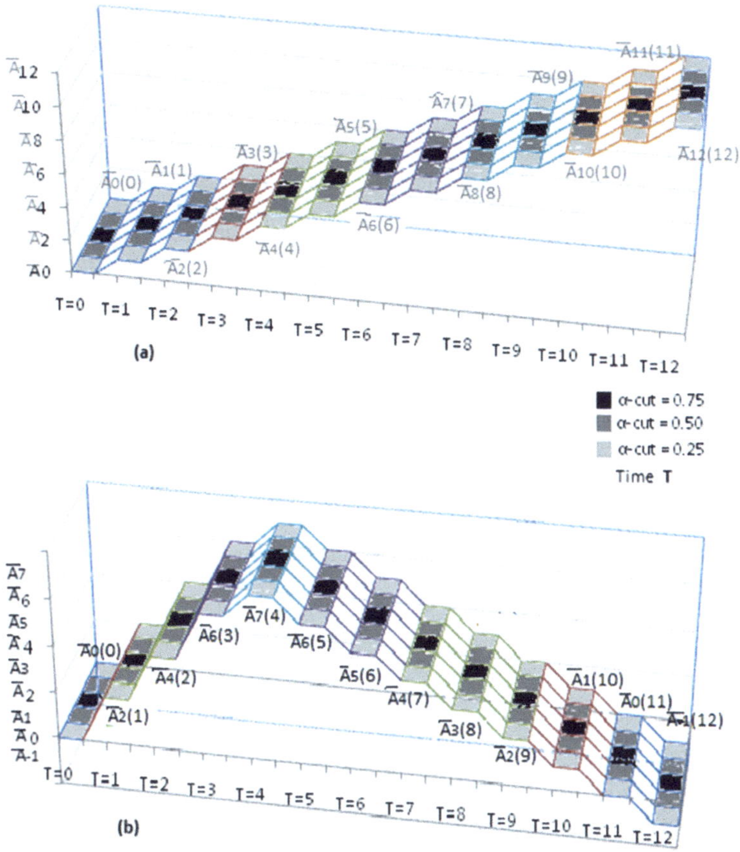

Fig. 7 FCA for spread Of COVID-19 from 22/03/2020 to 09/05/2020 in **a** India/USA, **b** Germany

References

1. Barros, et al.: Fuzzy Modelling in Population Dynamics. Ecol. Modelling **128**, 27–33 (2000)
2. Barros, Bassanezi: Tonelli : Attractors and Asymptotic Stability for Fuzzy Dynamical Systems. Fuzzy Sets and Systems **113**, 473–483 (2000)
3. Basu S etal : Different Types of Linear Fuzzy Cellular Automaton and their Applications, Fundamenta Informaticae, 87(2008), 185–205
4. Bernard-Stoecklin S. et al : Comparative Analysis of Eleven Healthcare-Associated Outbreaks of Middle East Respiratory Syndrome Coronavirus (Mers-Cov) from 2015 to 2017, Scientific Reports (2019), 9:7385, url : https://doi.org/10.1038/s41598-019-43586-9
5. Betel, Flocchini : On the Relationship between Boolean and Fuzzy Cellular Automata, 15th International Workshop On Cellular Automata and. Discrete Complex Systems (2009) ; Electronic notes in TCS, Vol 252,(Oct 2009), 5–21
6. Buckley, J., Qu, Y.: On Using α-cuts to Evaluate Fuzzy Equations. Fuzzy Sets and Systems **38**, 309–312 (1990)
7. Buckley et al : Fuzzy Difference Equations : The Initial Value Problem, J. of Advanced Computational intelligence, Vol.5, No.6, 2001

8. Buckley etal : Fuzzy MathematicsCA in Economics and Engineering, Studies in Fuzziness and Soft Computing,Vol 91,(2002), ISBN: 978-3-7908-2505-3
9. Buckley J : Fuzzy Probability and Statistics, Springer-Verlag Berlin Heidelberg (2006), ISBN: 13 978-3-540-30841-6
10. Catteneo etal : Cellular automata in fuzzy backgrounds, Physica D 105 (1997) 105–120
11. Dutta P. et al : Fuzzy Arithmetic with and without using α-cut method: A Comparative Study , International Journal of Latest Trends in Computing (E-ISSN: 2045-5364) 99, Vol 2, Issue 1, March 2011
12. Ghosh, S., Basu, S.: Evolution Patterns of Some Boolean Cellular Automata Having Atmost One Active Cell To Model Simple Dynamical Systems. Bull. Cal. Math Soc. **108**(6), 449–464 (2016)
13. Ghosh S, Basu S: Evolution Patterns of Finite Celled Synchronous Cellular Automata Having Atmost One Active Cell, Proceedings of The 10th International Conference MSAST 2016, pp 154–164 (Dec. 2016)
14. Ghosh S, Basu S: Some Algebraic Properties of Linear Synchronous Cellular Automata, arXiv:1708.09751v1 [nlin CG] (30 AUG. 2017)
15. Kari, J.: Theory of cellular automata: A Survey. Theo. Comp. Sci. **334**, 3–33 (2005)
16. von Neumann, J., : The General and Logical Theory of Automata, Hixon Symposium, : Published in, vol. V. Theory of Automata and Numerical Analysis, Pergamon Press, Design of Computers (1948)
17. von Neumann J.: Theory of Self-Reproducing Automata, University of Illinois Press, Illinois (1966) Edited and completed by A.W.Burks
18. Ulam S.M. : On some mathematical problems connected with patterns of growth of figures; Proc. Symp. Appl Math., Amer. Math. Soc. 14, 215–224 (1962)
19. Wolfram Stephen : Cellular Automata as models of complexity, Nature,(1984) vol. 311, no. 4 pp. 419–424
20. Stephen, Wolfram: Theory and Applications of Cellular Automata. World Scientific, Singapore (1986)
21. Wolfram S: A New Kind of Science,Wolfram Media (2002)
22. Zadeh, L.: A : Fuzzy Sets. Information and Control **8**, 338–353 (1965)
23. Middle East respiratory syndrome coronavirus (MERS-CoV), WHO MERS Global Summary and Assessment of Risk , (July 2019), WHO/MERS/RA/19.1
24. Worldometer For COVID-19, url : https://www.worldometers.info (2020)

Author Index

© The Editor(s) (if applicable) and The Author(s), under exclusive license
to Springer Nature Singapore Pte Ltd. 2020

C. Chakraborty et al. (eds.), *Internet of Medical Things for Smart Healthcare*,
Studies in Big Data 80, https://doi.org/10.1007/978-981-15-8097-0

The manufacturer's authorised representative in the EU is Springer Nature Customer Service Centre GmbH, Europaplatz 3, 69115 Heidelberg, Germany. If you have any concerns regarding our products, please contact ProductSafety@springernature.com

Printed and bound by CPI Group (UK) Ltd, Croydon, CR0 4YY
30/09/2026
02225506-0004